EMERGENCY MANAGEMENT OF SKIN AND SOFT TISSUE WOUNDS

EMERGENCY MANAGEMENT OF SKIN AND SOFT TISSUE WOUNDS

AN ILLUSTRATED GUIDE

Ernest N. Kaplan, M.D.
Clinical Associate Professor of Surgery
Division of Plastic and Reconstructive Surgery
Stanford University School of Medicine
Stanford, California

Vincent R. Hentz, M.D.
Associate Professor of Surgery
Division of Plastic and Reconstructive Surgery
Stanford University School of Medicine
Stanford, California

Little, Brown and Company
Boston / Toronto

Copyright © 1984 by Ernest N. Kaplan and Vincent R. Hentz
First Edition

All rights reserved. No part of this book may be reproduced in any form or by any electronic or mechanical means, including information storage and retrieval systems, without permission in writing from the publisher, except by a reviewer who may quote brief passages in a review.

Library of Congress Catalog Card No. 84-81668
ISBN 0-316-48278-1
Printed in the United States of America
MUR

CONTENTS

Preface vii

1. Fundamentals of Wound Management 1
2. Preoperative Preparation 21
3. Simple Lacerations 53
4. Complex Lacerations 93
5. Amputations and Skin Loss 123
6. Penetrating Injuries and Deep Transections 185
7. Closed and Blunt Injuries 249
8. Postoperative Care and Dressings 293

Index 339

PREFACE

In most communities in the United States, the hospital emergency department, in addition to its traditional role in treating major trauma, has become the central focus for the initial management of almost *all* acute injuries, especially open injuries such as lacerations, avulsions, and amputations. In the past, the task of managing "minor" acute injuries fell to the general practitioner, junior house staff, or medical student. Today there is an increased awareness that the physician who first sees, diagnoses, and treats the acute injury must bear the greatest responsibility for the ultimate outcome of the injury. Furthermore, an increasingly sophisticated public is demanding quality care from experienced physicians and nurses for even minor injuries. In some areas, and perhaps for the wrong reasons, many patients with even minor lacerations expect that a "plastic surgeon" will be called to treat their wounds. There has been a change in the patient's attitude about the role of the emergency department in managing his or her injury. This change in attitude has already spawned a new specialty, emergency medicine, with its own board examination.

In recognizing these changes in both the management of minor trauma and the patient's attitude, the authors, both practicing plastic surgeons, have attempted to provide emergency department physicians, nurses, hospital house officers, and medical students with a rational, step-by-step approach to the proper management of most injuries to the soft tissues and their related structures. Because most injuries seen in the emergency department occur to the head, face, and extremities (the exposed areas of the body), the diagnosis and management of injuries to these areas are stressed. The beginning chapters deal with general principles of wound management. Subsequent chapters detail the sequence of diagnosis and treatment of specific types of wounds. Basic biology related to wound healing, local anesthetics, and sepsis are included in the appropriate chapters. For example, Chapter 4, Complex Lacerations, considers debridement and antibiotics. Chapter 6, Penetrating Injuries and Deep Transections, describes the healing of transected tendons, nerves, and ligaments, and Chapter 7, Closed and Blunt Injuries, includes aspects of bone healing.

The text is not designed to serve as an encyclopedic compendium to the management of all minor afflictions. For example, the management of burns, soft tissue infections, and snake and insect bites is not discussed. Similarly, this text is not designed to serve merely as a "cookbook." We have endeavored to provide practical advice so that the initial management can be carried out in an orderly and successful fashion, stressing the principles of good wound management upon which the plastic surgeon's true reputation rests.

Many members of the Division of Plastic and Reconstructive Surgery at Stanford University School of Medicine have given freely of their time and effort in the preparation of this manuscript. We would like to express our gratitude to Nancy Berndt, Terry Flaviano, Paula Louie, Mary McKenna, and Mary McGee for their assistance. A special acknowledgment is given to Joan Wieder for her steadfastness in organizing and editing the manuscript. We particularly acknowledge the excellent work and cooperation of our illustrator John Volkert, and Halcyon Winters.

In addition, we thank Dr. Russel Pardoe for his efforts in conceptualizing and helping to write the initial manuscript.

E. N. K.
V. R. H.

EMERGENCY MANAGEMENT OF SKIN AND SOFT TISSUE WOUNDS

NOTICE

The indications and dosages of all drugs in this book have been recommended in the medical literature and conform to the practices of the general medical community. The medications described do not necessarily have specific approval by the Food and Drug Administration for use in the diseases and dosages for which they are recommended. The package insert for each drug should be consulted for use and dosage as approved by the FDA. Because standards for usage change, it is advisable to keep abreast of revised recommendations, particularly those concerning new drugs.

1. FUNDAMENTALS OF WOUND MANAGEMENT

Successful management of traumatic wounds requires an understanding of many basic principles, which leads to conceptualization of a management plan and performance of the surgical technique.

This chapter provides the basis of management of the patient with a soft tissue injury, including general principles, goals, priorities, and definitions.

PRIORITIES OF PATIENT MANAGEMENT

Never overlook a potentially life-threatening injury by concentrating on a more dramatic but less important soft tissue injury. Every patient requires thorough examination before treatment.

Priorities of care have been established for multiple system injuries according to the threat to life each injury represents. The priorities in sequence are

Stabilization of the patient against life-threatening conditions
General history and physical examination
Assessment of the tissue injury
Definition of goals and chronology (i.e., treatment plan)
Institution of wound care
Follow-up and reassessment

Patient Stabilization (Lifesaving Priorities)

The lifesaving priorities often are referred to as the ABCs of emergency care (*a*irway, *b*reathing, and *c*irculation); however, the priorities should also include a more extensive but still relatively cursory examination. The following list summarizes the sequence of steps:

1. Establish and maintain a patent airway by clearing obstructions to breathing and positioning tongue and mandible.
2. Ensure effective ventilation by using an artificial respiration bag or mouth-to-mouth breathing, identifying and treating tension pneumothorax, and dressing open chest wounds.
3. Establish adequate circulation by stopping mass bleeding, establishing normal cardiac function, and restoring blood volume.
4. Evaluate for intracranial and spinal injury.
5. Examine for intraabdominal injury.
6. Examine for extremity injuries; stabilize fractures and ensure adequate limb perfusion.

Finally, the wound itself can be examined carefully and a plan of action established. If other life-threatening conditions exist, the wound should be covered with sterile gauze and the greater priorities attended to.

Table 1-1. Examination and treatment of wound emergencies

Rapid general assessment for emergencies
    Head-neck examination and stabilization for spinal injury
    Airway evaluation and treatment
    Bleeding and shock assessment
Initial screening assessment for urgent problems
    Circulatory sufficiency
        Compartment syndromes
        Obstruction of major vessels
        Compressive hematomas
    Prevention of infection
        Antibiotics
        Wound sepsis and dressings
Consultants and tests
    Complex problems requiring operating room management or surgical specialists
    Radiologic exams for fractures
    Laboratory tests
    Circulatory assessment
        Doppler
        Arteriograms
Intraoperative wound assessment and care
    Reassessment of circulation and treatment
        Clinical assessment
        Fluorescein test
    Skin cover
    Bone and joint stabilization
    Muscle and tendon repair
    Nerve repair

PRINCIPLES OF EXAMINATION AND TREATMENT—ESTABLISHING PRIORITIES

All open injuries, particularly severe blunt injuries, should undergo complete examination and systematic, sequential treatment. The recommended sequence is shown in Table 1-1.

Head and Neck Injury—Emergency Measures

When the patient arrives in the emergency department with facial injuries, it is often difficult to determine the extent and site of injury. There may be massive edema and hematoma as well as multiple lacerations, abrasions, and contusions. Therefore, follow a systematic approach that eliminates the problems of life-threatening injuries, and progress to the less severe injuries. The initial screening examination must determine if there is any life-threatening situation that requires immediate care before other diagnostic evaluations take place. The two emergency situations that commonly occur as a direct result of a trauma are airway obstruction and massive bleeding. Also, *always be aware that a cervical spine injury (if present) may be aggravated by examination or manipulation of the airway.*

CERVICAL SPINE EXAMINATION AND STABILIZATION

Examine the neck quickly before manipulating the patient. If there are signs of local injury with deformity, pain, or spasm, or if there are peripheral motor or sensory deficits, *the neck should be immobilized.* Cervical x-rays should be obtained after stabilization and management of airway obstruction and bleeding.

AIRWAY OBSTRUCTION

The brain can tolerate only a few minutes of anoxia before cell death and irreversible brain damage occur. Therefore, a rapid assessment and correction of airway obstruction is mandatory. Moreover, hypoxia can cause cardiac arrhythmias and must be corrected before cardiac therapy begins. The emergency care for cardiopulmonary resuscitation (CPR) should be instituted (basic and advanced life support) for these patients. CPR is not discussed here, although the patient with maxillofacial injuries and a compromised airway without manifest cardiac dysfunction is considered in Table 1-2. The following steps should be taken:

1. Check whether the upper airway is obstructed by foreign material.
    a. Open the patient's mouth and examine for obstruction from tongue, dentures, blood clots, vomitus, or other foreign materials in the oral cavity. Remove any obstructions.
    b. *Place the conscious patient in a prone position with the head turned to the side.* The tongue will drop forward with the mandible. This maneuver may quickly relieve airway obstruction caused by the tongue; also, oral hemorrhage does not pool and clot in the upper airway but flows out of the mouth.
    c. Place either a nasopharyngeal or oropharyngeal airway to maintain the position of the tongue.
2. Check for lower airway obstruction.
    a. If the patient cannot be ventilated by mouth-to-mouth methods or with mask and bag, there is airway obstruction in the hypopharynx or trachea. It is probable that there has been aspiration of a foreign body (against the glottis or into the trachea) or that there is laryngotracheal injury. Impact or pressure injury against the neck can cause laryngotracheal injury and immediate airway obstruction.
        (1) To diagnose, look for
            (a) Subcutaneous emphysema
            (b) Hoarseness or aphonia
            (c) Edema and ecchymosis with loss of palpable thyroid cartilage landmark
            (d) Hemoptysis
            (e) Associated cervical fracture
            (f) Dysphagia and drooling caused by associated esophageal injury
        (2) To treat
            (a) Take soft tissue lateral neck x-ray, if time allows.
            (b) Minimize manipulation to avoid complete airway obstruction.
            (c) Use endotracheal intubation.
            (d) Perform tracheostomy.
    b. In the absence of laryngotracheal injury, a sharp blow to the back should be followed by the Heimlich maneuver. Turning the patient upside down also might dislodge the obstruction.

Table 1-2. Causes and treatment of airway obstructions

Possible cause of airway obstruction	Physical finding	Emergency measures (in order of priority)
Mandibular fracture with posterior displacement	Mandibular deformity with dental malocclusion	1. Prone positioning 2. Pull tongue forward with instrument 3. Nasotracheal tube 4. Tracheostomy
Nasomaxillary fracture	Massive bleeding from nose or mouth Facial ecchymosis and deformity	1. Compression of maxilla 2. Nasal packing 3. Blood replacement
Aspiration of foreign body	Inspiratory stridor Wheezing Paradoxical chest movement Pain	*If complete obstruction:* 1. Put head down or turn patient upside down 2. Firm blow to back 3. Grasp object with instrument 4. Cricothyrotomy *If patient not in immediate danger:* 1. Maintain position. Second and third measures listed above may cause complete obstruction; do not attempt to manipulate unless prepared for immediate cricothyrotomy or tracheostomy
Laryngotracheal crush	Hoarseness Aphonia Hemoptysis Dysphagia Cervical and chest ecchymosis Subcutaneous emphysema Pain	1. Endotracheal tube 2. Cricothyrotomy or tracheostomy

    c. Laryngoscopy and intubation with an endotracheal tube should be attempted.
    d. As a final measure, an emergency cricothyrotomy or tracheostomy may be required.

MASSIVE BLEEDING AND SHOCK

Massive bleeding may accompany injury to several head and neck sites. The nature of the wound or the anatomic site may preclude use of the usual conservative hemostatic measures, such as direct pressure or immobilization.

Bleeding from oral or facial injury can be quite profuse and cause hypotensive shock and airway obstruction from clots around the trachea, or blood can be swallowed with subsequent vomiting and aspiration into the lungs. The most massive bleeding occurs with nasomaxillary fractures and tongue lacerations.

General measures include

1. Placing the patient face down to prevent aspiration of blood clots into the trachea and to prevent swallowing of blood with subsequent hematemesis
2. Performing a careful physical examination to determine the bleeding site, including a check of the nasal cavity
3. Typing and cross-matching blood and starting an intravenous line

Assessment of Injury

After the patient has been stabilized, a general assessment and careful local examination of the injury should be undertaken. Moreover, a systematic examination must be recorded in a legible form. A simple sketch of the injured part should be part of the record.

The general history and physical examination should identify systemic factors that may affect the outcome of wound repair or healing.

HISTORY OF INJURY

An accurate history of the injury is the first step in the evaluation; answers to the principal questions of how, where, when, and what heavily influence the subsequent physical examination and treatment. Necessary information includes

Mechanism of injury
When it occurred
Where it occurred
Occupation
Avocation
Past medical history that influences healing (e.g., allergies; disease processes, such as diabetes; use of steroids or other medications; bleeding disorders)

INITIAL EXAMINATION (PREANESTHESIA)

An initial thorough examination identifies injured structures whose functions cannot be evaluated when the patient is anesthetized. Nerve damage and tendon transection must be evaluated before anesthesia.

As much information as possible is gained without subjecting the patient to severe discomfort. The wound should not be probed or manipulated, especially in a child. Grossly contaminated wounds require early institution of antibiotics, and badly displaced fractures or dislocations require splinting or stabilization to decrease the likelihood of additional damage.

FINAL EVALUATION FOLLOWING ANESTHESIA

Once the patient or injured part is anesthetized, a final evaluation verifies and enlarges on the initial assessment.

Ducts can be probed for evidence of disruption, and nerves and tendons may be identified by direct inspection. Ligament stability can be tested completely only following anesthesia.

DIAGNOSIS OF INJURIES TO SPECIFIC TISSUES

A tissue-oriented systematic examination should be used to evaluate any injured part. To assess accurately the severity of the trauma, it is necessary to test for integrity and function of the integral components—circulation, skin cover, bone and joint, nerve and tendon, ducts, and other specific structures such as the globe. To be complete, consider every structure deep to any skin wound to be divided or injured until ruled out by specific tests!

1. Circulation. Perfusion of the injured tissues may be compromised by diffuse contusion to small vessels or injury to a major artery from direct damage.
   a. Signs of vascular injury
      (1) *Minimal ooze or large hematoma.* A minimal ooze or a large hematoma may be the only visible sign of a vascular transection. Massive pulsatile bleeding is not usually seen in the emergency room. This is because such severe injury often results in death from exsanguination, and the less severe injuries often abate spontaneously because of vasospasm, intravascular clot, or periarterial hematoma. Moreover, emergency first aid measures such as tourniquets and pressure bandages may temporarily control bleeding.
      (2) *Distal vascular skin insufficiency.* The site or extremity distal to the injury may be pale or cyanotic and cold.
      (3) *Absent distal pulse.* Absence of distal pulse may be caused by transection or vasospasm. Moreover, presence of a pulse does not exclude vascular injury because collateral or retrograde flow can occur.
      (4) *Neurologic injury.* Adjacent major nerves may be damaged, suggesting that the associated vessel may also be injured. Paresis can also occur from compression by a hematoma.
   b. Diagnostic testing
      (1) *Doppler flowmeter.* Using a Doppler flowmeter is a relatively simple noninvasive method of assessing flow in vessels larger than 1 mm near the skin surface. Nonetheless, the apparent sign of flow across the injury site does not preclude a major injury.
      (2) *Arteriograms.* These radiologic studies may be of value for deep injuries involving the neck, peritoneal, retroperitoneal, or chest areas. They can be helpful in determining these sites of injury. However, a normal arteriogram does not negate the presence of severe vascular injury.
      (3) *"Stabograms."* The tract of a penetrating injury can be injected with a water-soluble radiopaque dye to delineate the direction and depth of the tract. This helps to determine if the stab wound is near a major vessel.
      (4) *CAT scan.* Computerized axial tomography may be indicated for certain soft tissue injuries.

2. Skin cover. The assessment of injury to the skin should determine the answer to the following questions:
   a. Is there actual skin loss or have the edges retracted?
   b. Will the skin still present survive? The chapters on amputation, skin defects, and wounds discuss the assessment and treatment of such wounds.
3. Bony skeleton and joints. The diagnosis and assessment of injury to the underlying skeleton differ somewhat according to the area of the body injured. The presence of one or several of the following signs or symptoms is early evidence of fracture or dislocation. These signs and symptoms include:
   a. Instability—abnormal motion indicates the presence of a fracture or dislocation
   b. Deformity—the normal contours may be absent
   c. Pain—with stress on the underlying skeleton
   d. Hematoma—about the site of a fracture

   The diagnosis of specific bony injuries is discussed in Chapter 7, Blunt Trauma.
4. Diagnosis of nerve injury. Nerve injuries are diagnosed by correlation of the anatomy about the site of injury with motor and sensory testing. These tests determine whether or not there is an injury and at what level the injury has occurred. They do not, however, indicate whether there is a complete nerve transection (neurotmesis) or whether there is a partial disruption (axonotmesis) or a temporary functional loss (neuropraxia). This distinction of type of injury is made on the basis of historical information and, more importantly, operative exploration.

   The history of previous trauma or injury may indicate that any physical findings of peripheral nerve damage are related to previous events and not to the immediate injury.
   a. *Sensory.* A sensory examination of the injured region is usually performed using the modalities of pain (pinprick) and light touch (cotton-tip application). To perform these tests adequately, the physician must have a detailed knowledge of the distribution of cutaneous sensory nerves or charts or maps of sensory nerve distributions.

      Testing should begin in the areas of suspected anesthesia and progress from anesthetic areas to normal areas, drawing out the areas of demarcation with a marking pen. Testing should be repeated at intervals before a decision is made to perform surgery, to determine if there is a neuropraxic-type injury with a gradual return of sensibility.
   b. *Motor.* The individual muscle groups within and distal to the area of injury should be tested independently. If there is a functional muscular deficit, the testing may not distinguish between a nerve injury and a direct injury to the muscle or tendon. This distinction can be made only with the cumulative evidence of sensory and other testing, and finally by intraoperative exploration.
   c. *Sudomotor.* Sweating usually disappears within 5 minutes after a complete disruption of a nerve. A careful examination of the skin for droplets of sweat, and palpation for moisture or dry friction usually are sufficient. Visual inspection can be aided with the use of the magnifying lens or operating magnifying glasses. The Ninhydrin

and starch iodine tests are color tests that provide similar information but are not generally used.
5. Ducts, tendons, and ligaments. The assessment of injuries to these specific tissues is discussed at length in Chapter 6, Penetrating Injuries.

Tissue Priorities

The sequence of wound care is designed to produce the optimal cosmetic and functional results. The prime goal is to achieve rapid and complete skin healing to minimize deposition of scar and development of infection. After achieving wound cover by direct closure, skin flap, or skin graft, the series of priorities are

1. Skin cover
2. Skeletal stabilization
3. Musculotendinous repairs
4. Nerve and duct repair

These priorities should be achieved during the context of the surgery; however, the actual sequence of repair may be quite different. Skin closure is clearly the last maneuver of a multiple tissue injury.

If direct skin closure cannot be accomplished and a skin graft or temporary dressing is required, nerve and tendon repair may have to be delayed until skin cover is achieved.

WOUND CLASSIFICATION

The succeeding chapters discuss the diagnosis and management of soft tissue wounds. The organization of this discussion is based on a system of wound classification that provides a format for subsequent treatment.

An *open wound* is an injury in which the protective epithelial surface has been broken and must be reconstituted.

Closed wounds are caused by blunt trauma or thermal insults and have an intact epithelial surface. Subcutaneous hemorrhages, tissue disruption, and fractures are typical injuries.

A wound caused by a piece of broken glass could be described as a superficial, tidy, simple, clean, sharp laceration; a lawn mower injury could be described as an untidy, contaminated, complex, compound, blunt amputation; a bullet wound could be described as an untidy, clean, complex, compound, high-energy penetration.

These descriptions improve communication among physicians and have implications regarding wound preparation and treatment strategy. A more detailed description of these terms of classification follows.

Clinical Type of Wound

These categories are for convenient reference and not absolute identification. A specific injury may be a combination of these types. The clinical distinctions are primarily a function of the direction of trauma. *Lacerations* are caused by an object moving across the skin, *penetrations* are from objects moving into the skin, and *amputations* are from objects moving parallel to the skin. Other factors, such as the energy and size of the object causing injury, determine if a laceration, penetration, or amputation occurs.

LACERATIONS

A laceration is defined as a linear physical disruption of the skin surface with a separation of the wound edges but no loss of tissue. Although the injury may penetrate into the deeper tissue, the direction of tissue damage tends to be greatest in line with the surface. Lacerations are most commonly caused by sharp, thin objects such as glass or metals, which slice through the tissue with minimal energy. The condition of this type of wound is quite variable. Although it is usually tidy, it may be clean or contaminated, simple or complex in configuration, and either superficial, deep, or compound.

Lacerations also can be caused by blunt trauma, such as a fall against the edge of a table or other object. These blunt lacerations are caused by higher impact energy and thus are more likely to be untidy, complex, and contaminated. They are often superficial but can frequently have associated fractures and other deep compound injuries.

PENETRATING INJURIES

These wounds are characterized by a minimal surface disruption and considerable underlying compound injuries from penetration perpendicular to the skin. The penetration can be caused by a rigid, slender, sharp, low energy source, such as slivers, knives, or nails, or a high energy source, such as bullets, missiles, and pressurized paint or grease injectors. Determination of the extent and type of a deep compound injury is essential. Treatment is directed at reestablishing continuity of transected deep structures. Surface wound care is a lesser problem, although untidy wounds may require debridement.

AMPUTATION—TISSUE LOSS

These wounds are caused by injury parallel to the surface (skin loss) or transversely across a prominence or appendage (amputation). All variations of high or low energy objects can cause amputation. Treatment is directed at replacing missing skin and soft tissue or reattaching the amputated part.

Mechanism of Wound

The mechanism has numerous direct and indirect implications regarding the extent and treatment of the injury.

SHARP VERSUS BLUNT

The condition of the wound is greatly influenced by the mechanism. Untidy, contaminated, complex, compound wounds are most commonly from blunt, high energy sources, such as bullets or falls, whereas tidy, clean, simple, superficial wounds are most commonly from sharp, low energy sources. However, almost any wound condition can occur from each mechanism.

HIGH ENERGY VERSUS LOW ENERGY

Unique problems are associated with the high energy injuries. The extent and severity of damage is often greater than would be suspected by track of bullet or missile. Vascular thrombosis, fractures, and other injuries are common. Additional details of the various high energy sources are discussed in Chapter 7.

Condition of Wound

TIDY VERSUS UNTIDY

Tidy wounds are created by sharp objects and do not contain devitalized tissue or debris. The wound can be a laceration, amputation, or penetration. If the wound is tidy and of recent origin, it can be cleaned and closed with the expectation of rapid primary healing.

An untidy wound usually results from more forceful impact, crush, tearing, or avulsion. As a result, there is usually devitalized tissue, loss of tissue, and, more frequently, injury to deeper structures. Debridement and irrigation must be pursued aggressively, and delayed closure is often required.

Complete debridement converts an untidy wound into a tidy wound. The underlying damaged structures can be repaired and the skin closed, with full expectation of primary healing.

Some injuries cannot be debrided adequately because of the difficulty of recognizing the limits of devitalized tissue. This occurs in injuries with high levels of energy, such as high-velocity missile injuries, thermal injuries, and explosives. In these injuries adequate initial debridement and wound drainage take precedence over immediate skin coverage. In this type of injury, repeated inspection is required to complete the debridement of tissues that subsequently become devitalized.

In principle, whenever the efficacy of debridement is uncertain, a sterile dressing is applied and the wound inspected 24, 48, and 72 hours later. The need for any additional debridement will be evident, and the wound can be closed at that time (delayed primary closure) or at a later time (secondarily).

CLEAN VERSUS CONTAMINATED

This classification represents a general assessment of the numbers of bacteria in the wound and, therefore, the likelihood of a subsequent infection. A clean wound has "few" bacteria, whereas a contaminated wound has many. The degree of bacterial presence (and thus classification into one of these categories) can be assessed according to the mechanism of injury, time since injury, or wound culture or microscopic examination of a smear taken from the wound.

NONCOMPLEX VERSUS COMPLEX

This classification is related to the anatomic location and geometric configuration of the wound and provides a measure of the technical difficulty of the repair. A *noncomplex wound* is (1) located at a favorable site, such as a flat surface, and away from critical facial, limb, or hand anatomy; (2) linear or with a minimal curve or angle; and (3) perpendicular to the skin surface, without undercut.

Closure of noncomplex wounds does not require technical manipulation, extensive debridement, or additional incisions, and a good result usually can be expected.

A *complex wound* is (1) located in an adverse site, such as in a convexity or concavity, in a flexion crease, across a boundary between structures, or at an angle to normal skin wrinkles and lines of tension; (2) nonlinear, with skin flaps, edge irregularities, or multiple adjacent lacerations; and (3) oblique to the skin surface, with one side having an undercut and the other an oblique scything.

Complex wounds result in a bad scar or deformity unless specific additional surgical maneuvers are performed.

SIMPLE VERSUS COMPOUND

This classification is a description of the depth of the wound and an indication of whether structures other than dermis and fat have been lacerated. In simple wounds only skin and fat are injured, and in compound wounds other anatomic structures are damaged, such as major vessels, nerves, ducts or glands, muscle, tendon, or body cavities.

The management of simple, noncomplex wounds of the skin may be delegated to physicians or paramedical personnel who possess the basic knowledge and skills of wound closure. A compound injury signifies greater potential danger or likelihood of secondary complications, and its optimal care frequently must await the availability of a specialist.

In subsequent chapters we make use of many of these descriptive classes of wounds, especially tidy-untidy and simple-compound. Any system of wound classification that is used consistently can serve the primary purpose of communication.

WOUND HEALING

The primary goal of wound care is to aid the natural processes. We cannot accelerate the healing of a cleanly incised, carefully repaired wound. However, the emergency physician may influence positively or negatively, the course of many wounds. The successful outcome of wound management depends on a clear understanding of the basic processes of wound healing and the proper application of the general principles of wound care.* These are set forth in this and succeeding chapters. Failure to understand these basic processes or heed these general principles may result in delayed wound healing and secondary complications, which are distressing consequences to physician, patient, and family.

Regeneration and Repair

Wound healing occurs by either repair or regeneration of damaged tissues. Regeneration is replication of the original cell type, and repair is replacement with collagen scar interposed between the tissues.

Regeneration occurs in nerves, epithelium, bone, and liver; the mesothelial surfaces of joints, bursae, pleura, and peritoneum; and the endothelium of blood vessels.

Repair occurs in the dermis and fat, tendons, fascia, cartilage, and all other internal organs. To some degree each of these tissues may remodel the collagen so that it closely resembles the healing tissue.

---

*For a more detailed analysis of the biology of wound healing, refer to E. E. Peacock and W. Van Winkle, Jr., *Surgery and Biology of Wound Repair* (Philadelphia: Saunders, 1972).

Surgical Terminology

FIRST INTENT (PRIMARY CLOSURE)
Healing by first intent is more commonly referred to as primary healing or primary closure. A cleanly incised and surgically reapproximated (primarily closed) wound heals by epithelialization and scar repair.

SECOND INTENT
If a wound is not surgically closed, it heals by granulation, wound contraction, and epithelialization. This usually occurs in infected wounds or tissue avulsions.

THIRD INTENT (SECONDARY OR DELAYED CLOSURE)
Healing by third intent is more commonly referred to as delayed closure. This involves a purposeful or inadvertent initial delay in surgical closure. During this delay period, the wound begins to granulate and contract. Later, the wound is surgically closed to hasten wound healing. Delayed or secondary wound closure is useful when potential wound contamination, as opposed to wound infection, is a factor.

Normal Wound Healing

Normal wound healing is the result of an interrelated sequence of physical and biochemical events that produces the structural mechanism of repair, the protein moiety, collagen. Each sequential step in the process is in part an inductor for succeeding steps; thus delay, interruption, or absence of an event may slow or halt wound healing. The earliest events include natural hemostasis and the development of an inflammatory process that sets the stage for wound repair by the processes of collagen production, wound contraction, and epithelialization described later in this chapter.

Because most investigations into wound healing have used as their model the cutaneous wound, the basic processes of healing are here described for this wound.

HEMOSTASIS
A knife has sliced the skin, and blood pours from the wound. Within minutes the bleeding begins to subside, and by the time the patient has reached the emergency department, there is little or no bleeding. A series of natural events (hemostasis) has occurred that prevents exsanguination. This process of hemostasis has three components: vascular spasm, platelet clumping, and coagulation.

1. Vascular spasm. Almost immediately after transection of a blood vessel, the circular smooth muscle contracts, thus narrowing the vascular lumen and reducing the flow of blood. Vascular spasm is effective only if there is complete transection of a vessel. Partially transected vessels may bleed more profusely and for a longer time than a completely transected vessel.
2. Platelet clumping. The normal platelet count in human blood varies from 150,000 to 300,000 cells per cubic millimeter. An injury to the intimal layer of a blood vessel exposes the collagen fibrils, which then protrude into the vascular lumen. It is thought that an electrical charge

on the collagen molecule causes platelets to adhere to collagen. This platelet adherence results in release of adenosine diphosphate (ADP). ADP causes continuing aggregation and adherence of platelets.

These events may be ineffective in producing hemostasis if, for example, the bleeding from a partially transected vessel cannot be slowed by spasm, or if there are insufficient platelets or a depressed concentration of clotting factor. (See section on coagulation factors later in this chapter.)

INFLAMMATORY RESPONSE

Leukocytes enter the wound at the time of injury and concurrent with the process of hemostasis. The blood clot that initially fills the wound contains blood-borne leukocytes in concentrations equivalent to the normal ratio of these cells in whole blood. Neutrophils, lymphocytes, and macrophages defend against pathogenic bacteria and foreign material. This is done by macrophagic phagocytosis and release of enzymes and antibodies. The macrophage also may play an essential role in inducing fibroblastic and capillary migration. The role of the prostaglandin system is just beginning to be understood.

Within 10 to 20 minutes nearby vessels begin to dilate and become more permeable to leukocyte migration and in response to histamines released by local mast cells and platelets. Circulating leukocytes then actively migrate between endothelial cells into the wound. Additional tissue leukocytes, usually macrophages, enter the wound and engulf foreign material.

COLLAGEN FORMATION

1. Fibroblastic migration. Shortly after injury, undifferentiated mesenchymal cells located primarily in the adventitia of blood vessels become identifiable as fibroblasts. These local fibroblasts migrate into the wounds using the fibrin strands of the original clot as a scaffold. The fibroblasts are accompanied by capillary ingrowth. This combination of fibroblasts and capillaries is called granulation tissue.

    After the third postinjury day, the first evidence of fibroblastic activity or the products of fibroblastic synthesis can be identified. The fibroblast is believed to be involved in various aspects of wound healing, including
    a. Collagen production
    b. Collagen breakdown by collagenase
    c. Wound contraction by myofibroblasts
    d. Ground substance production by mucopolysaccharides and glycoproteins
    e. Elastin production
    f. Elastin breakdown by elastase

    It is not clear whether these independent fibroblastic processes can be performed simultaneously or in sequence by any individual fibroblast, or whether populations of cells become specialized to perform only one of these functions.

    Of the six fibroblastic functions listed above, only the first three are discussed, because most is known about these, and there are means of modifying these activities to the benefit or detriment of the healing wound.

2. Collagen production. The intracellular synthesis of collagen begins within the fibroblasts shortly after injury and proceeds for 5 days. There is continuing collagen production in the fibroblast.

By the fifth day postinjury, fine monomeric collagen molecules are present in the extracellular tissues, and there is a rapid increase in the collagen content of the wound. In most wounds the total collagen content reaches a stable level by 3 weeks. The continued absence of an epithelialized cover causes continued collagen production with increased scar formation (hypertrophic scars or keloids).

Collagen production never entirely ceases. Rather, a balance is reached between collagen production and collagen breakdown. Additional strength achieved after 2 to 4 weeks is related to cross-linking of collagen into structurally strong units. Additional strength does not occur from added collagen. Abnormal accumulation occurs with keloids and hypertrophic scars. With these, collagen content of the wound increases for many months or years after injury.

WOUND CONTRACTION

Contraction is caused by fibroblasts pulling the skin margins centrally. Wound contraction is not the same as wound contracture. Contracture refers to the deformity caused by wound contraction or shortening of muscles or ligaments.

Wound contraction involves the movement of the entire skin thickness, not just epithelial cells. Epithelialization and contraction are independent processes. The movement of the skin thickness does not occur at the same rate along all margins. A circular defect may contract to form a long thin ellipse, and a square defect may contract in a stellate form or to form a long thin rectangle. The form of contraction is dependent on the tension of the surrounding skin. The contraction process must occur on healthy granulation tissue and probably occurs most actively along the edges of the wound.

It was once speculated that the collagen molecule itself was capable of shortening and accounted for the contraction process. It is known that a specialized fibroblast—the myofibroblast—which possesses several of the properties of smooth muscle cells, causes contraction.

EPITHELIALIZATION

Epithelium maintains fluid and electrolyte balance by preventing evaporation and acts as a barrier against physical, chemical, or biologic agents. Epithelialization is a true regenerative process, in which there is replication of normal cells, in contrast to scar formation, which is a reparative process.

Epithelium is regenerated across an open wound from the germinal cells at the basement membrane and from the skin appendages (sweat glands, hair follicles, sebaceous glands).

The mechanism leading to reepithelialization can be considered to be four independent but overlapping events: mobilization, mitosis, migration, and maturation.

1. Mobilization. Mobilization occurs along the margins of the laceration or open wound. Germinal cells enlarge and detach themselves from the basement membrane and from skin appendages.

2. Mitosis. Mitosis of epidermal cells occurs along the margins of the wound and rarely in those that are actively migrating.
3. Migration. Migration, which occurs by an active ameboid process, is limited by contact inhibition. Epidermal cells continue to migrate until they contact another epidermal cell. When a cell is surrounded by other epidermal cells, migration and mitosis cease and maturation begins.

    The plane across which the epidermal cells migrate is determined by the local wound condition. In the *cleanly incised and primarily closed wound*, a fibrin clot (scab) fills the space between the skin margins. Using fibrin as a scaffold, the epithelial cells migrate across the wound within 24 to 36 hours.

    In wound healing by second intent, the rate of migration varies with wound condition:

    a. In the nonoccluded, open wound there is desiccation of the superficial dermis, and the epidermal cells must burrow through an intact deep layer of dermis. This burrowing process is facilitated by collagenase and other proteolytic enzymes released by epithelium.
    b. In the moist or occluded wound, the dermis does not desiccate, and the epidermal cells are capable of migrating on the surface fibrin scab at the interface of the dermis and scab. This process does not require the presence of collagenase. The rate of epithelialization in moist occluded wounds may be 2 to 3 mm per day, which is twice the rate of that in nonoccluded dry wounds.

    Therefore, the rate of wound healing and the quality of the healed epidermis can be modified by the type of wound care and dressings. The application of this principle is described in conjunction with specific types of injuries.

    It is also important to recognize that each skin suture represents a puncture-type wound that allows epidermal proliferation along the suture tract. Thus, the type of suture and length of time the sutures are in the skin have considerable importance in the formation of stitch marks. This application of the epidermal regeneration principle is discussed in the section on sutures (see p. 39).
4. Maturation. Maturation begins to occur in epithelial cells that are not undergoing mitosis or migration. Thus, the initial peripheral region of the epidermis undergoes maturation with a tendency toward thickening of the epidermal layer and normal stratification and maturation, whereas the more central areas maintain their monolayer arrangement. The regenerated epithelium, although stratified, does not develop projections into the dermis (rete ridges) and is therefore more susceptible to shearing.

Factors Affecting Wound Healing

Generally, wound healing cannot be accelerated in the normal person, although the rate differs from one part of the body to another. Several anatomic and physiologic factors seem to play a role.

AGE
All wounds gain tensile strength more rapidly in the young child than in the adult.

SEX

There may be a greater incidence of hypertrophic scars in women than in men. For example, during a hormonally active period (e.g., girls aged 11–13), scarring seems to be more pronounced.

RACE

The more darkly pigmented races have a distinctly higher incidence of abnormal states of wound healing, particularly collagen overproduction or reduced collagenolysis, including hypertrophic scarring and keloid formation. There appears to be no racial difference, however, in the rate of gain of tensile strength in various wounds.

ANATOMIC LOCATION

Several aspects of wound location influence the rate of healing.

1. Vascularity. Wounds about the head and neck heal faster than wounds of the feet. This allows safe removal of sutures in facial lacerations at a time at which removal of sutures in a foot wound would result in wound dehiscence. This is related to the difference in vascularity from region to region—the head and neck region is more richly vascularized than the lower extremity.
2. Proximity to contamination. Wounds about the perineal region, particularly the rectum, heal more slowly—they seem to epithelialize at a slower rate. Granulation tissue proliferation is marked. Contraction may affect wound closure, resulting in stricture.
3. Numbers of epithelial appendages. Abrasions and, possibly, second degree burns may reepithelialize more rapidly in areas possessing greater numbers of skin appendages. Certainly the facial skin in the bearded region and in the hair-bearing areas of the scalp reepithelialize a deeper, partial-thickness burn more rapidly than does the neck or chest skin.
4. Laxity of surrounding skin. Wound contraction occurs more readily in areas in which tissues are loosely adherent to underlying structures, such as over the abdomen. Where there are strong attachments to rigid underlying structures, as in the scalp or over the anterior tibial crest, contraction is limited. The presence of a flexion crease enhances the ability of the tissues in the area to contract.

Abnormal Wound Healing

A delay in healing of a traumatic wound can result in complications of varying magnitude. The effect of debridement of the wound, antisepsis, and use of prophylactic antibiotics are mentioned. Factors more intrinsic to the wound are discussed in terms of local and systemic factors.

LOCAL FACTORS CAUSING AVASCULARITY

Tissue avascularity delays wound healing. Avascularity may be the result of such factors as tension at wound closure, irradiation, and fibrosis.

1. Tension on the sutured wound. Excessive tension on closed wounds is clinically detectable. The wound edges are blanched or there is blanch-

ing about each suture. The blanched areas are relatively avascular, and their rate of healing is seriously impaired or healing is prevented. Extreme tension results in actual necrosis of previously uninjured skin edge and may lead to dehiscence of the wound when the skin sutures are removed.

2. The irradiated wound. The effects of ionizing radiation on normal tissues have been extensively studied. Two temporal tissue responses occur. During the initial weeks a short period of intense inflammation occurs. Injury occurring at this time is highly susceptible to delay or failure of healing. During the weeks to months following exposure to sufficient levels of ionizing radiation, an obliterative vasculitis occurs. The severity of the ischemia corresponds to the dosage and method of irradiation. The result is an ischemic tissue in which wound healing is delayed. If vasculitis is very severe, the wound may never heal.

3. Wound infection. Bacterial contamination occurs in almost all open injuries. Whether the bacterial contamination is controlled by the normal inflammatory process and resolves or progresses to clinical infection is determined by three factors: bacterial concentration and virulence, host defense mechanisms, and the condition of the wound. A clean minimal injury in a healthy person usually produces a transient inflammatory reaction. Extensive trauma with tissue necrosis and vascular ischemia in the presence of pathogenic bacteria results in an environment-favoring infection. In this situation, the physician has the opportunity to influence wound healing positively by establishing better wound conditions through antiseptic preparation of the wound, debridement of devitalized tissue, removal of foreign material, and bolstering of the host's defense mechanisms.

   Gross clinical infection with abscess formation certainly prohibits wound healing. A severe infection, particularly with *Streptococcus* or *Staphylococcus*, results in many adverse changes. Bacterial toxins, cellular toxins, and products of bacterial and cellular metabolism cause hypoxia, tissue lysis, and vascular thrombosis. These occurrences also delay healing. Lesser degrees of infection are more frequent but also reduce the rate of gain of wound tensile strength.

SYSTEMIC FACTORS

Some of the local factors mentioned above can be altered at the time of wound repair. Unfortunately, most systemic factors cannot be altered at the time of injury. Their deleterious effects on wound healing must be recognized because their presence may require considerable alteration in the management of the wound.

Table 1-3 lists several systemic disease processes that affect wound healing. Table 1-4 lists a number of drugs known to have a considerable influence on wound healing. The list grows every year. Review of the patient's medical history at the time of initial examination is necessary to avoid mistreating the patient who is taking such agents.

1. Keloids and hypertrophic scars. Previously discussed abnormal healing has been characterized by insufficient or delayed production of collagen. Excessive collagen is characteristic of keloids and hypertrophic scars. These are disorders of the balance of collagen production and

Table 1-3. Systemic diseases that affect wound healing

Disease	Mechanism
Systemic infection	Inflammatory response
Malignancy	Nutritional deficiencies
Diabetes	Peripheral vascular compromises
Anemia (hypoperfusion)	Impaired oxygen
Uremia, hyperbilirubinemia	Toxic metabolites
Distant trauma	Probable secondary effect, including impaired perfusion
Nutritional deficiency	
Protein	Essential amino acid deficiency
Vitamin C	Abnormal collagen production
Zinc	Coenzyme deficiency

Table 1-4. Effects of certain drugs on wound healing

Drug	Effect
Steroids (cortisone)	Suppresses inflammation, protein synthesis, contraction, and epithelialization
Aspirin	Suppresses inflammation
Colchicine	Arrests cell replication, suppresses collagen transport
Chemotherapeutic agents	Arrest cell replication, suppress inflammation, suppress protein synthesis

collagen breakdown. Table 1-5 compares the characteristics of keloids and hypertrophic scars.

Hypertrophic scars are caused by particular wound conditions and locations. Wound care and surgical manipulations sometimes can prevent hypertrophic scars, whereas little or nothing can be done to prevent keloids. The surgeon's responsibility is to recognize that darkly pigmented people are susceptible, and specific history must be sought. If a patient is known to have formed keloids, no unnecessary wound manipulations and additional incisions should be made. The patient who exhibits a tendency toward hypertrophic scar or keloid formation should be forewarned.

2. Coagulation factors. Uneventful wound healing may be compromised if a coagulation abnormality is overlooked. If a history of specific bleeding disorders is obtained, if the bleeding persists for greater than 15 minutes after all the appropriate measures have been completed, or if observation of the bleeding indicates that clot is not being formed, it is likely that a specific coagulation defect is the cause of bleeding.
3. Diagnosis of bleeding disorders
   a. History. Some patients relate a history of previous bleeding and a specific disorder. In those patients it is reasonable to start treatment based on that information, but to draw blood tests for confirmation. The use of aspirin in the 2 weeks before injury is perhaps the most common cause of minimal bleeding.

   Other patients describe episodes of bleeding that may or may not be related to the emergency situation. Specific questions regarding

Table 1-5. Characteristics of keloids and hypertrophic scars

	Keloid	Hypertrophic scar
Genetic predisposition	Dark-skinned races	
Causes	Any laceration	Tension parallel with scar
		Delayed healing
		Contamination and foreign body
Site	Chest, shoulder, and ear are common but occurs anywhere	Across concavities
		Perpendicular to flexion crease
Growth pattern	Overgrows boundaries of original scar	Stays within boundaries
Symptoms	Pain, paresthesia, pruritus	Minimal pruritus
Natural history	Progressive for decades	Often resolves spontaneously
Pathology	Thick, short, disorganized whorls of collagen	Parallel long bundles of collagen
	Hyalin-ground substance	
	Atypical giant fibroblasts	Normal fibroblasts
Treatment	Pressure ± Steroid injections (triamcinolone [Kenalog, Aristocort])	Time (1–2 years)
	Excision occasionally required	Excision and Z-plasty
	Radiation: 600–900 rads (3 doses of 200–300 rads) after surgery and during first week	

bites, drug ingestions, and family history are of particular importance.

b. *Diagnostic tests.* A battery of six tests usually provides the information required to make a specific diagnosis that allows appropriate emergency treatment. The first four identify the existence of almost all bleeding disorders. The exact cause may not be determined by these six tests, but a treatment plan that can control the hemorrhage can be established. Additional tests may be required to establish the diagnosis and cause. These tests include the following:

  (1) *PTT (partial thromboplastin time)* is a test of the intrinsic clotting system. Normal values vary with individual laboratories from 25 to 80 seconds. A prolongation of the PTT usually indicates an abnormality of one of the factors in the intrinsic system. The PTT is prolonged in such potentially troublesome disorders as hemophilia, factor VIII deficiency, and von Willebrand's disease.

  (2) The *Quick test (protime)* measures the extrinsic system, primarily factor VII. The most common bleeding disorders associated with a prolonged protime are those related to hepatic disease.

  (3) A *platelet count and smear*—a carefully prepared Wright's stain performed as part of a complete blood count—allows an estimate of platelet numbers but does not determine the cause of platelet deficiency, which usually requires a detailed history, physical examination, and other diagnostic testing.

(4) *Bleeding time* is a very general test that measures the total in vivo mechanism. It is very nonspecific and may be normal in many of the coagulation disorders. The most common abnormalities of bleeding time occur with von Willebrand's disease and thrombocytopenias.
(5) *Fibrin split products* is a test for fibrinolysis.
(6) *Urinalysis for hemoglobin and myoglobin* is a test for hemolysis with the indirect implication of concurrent toxic or hypersensitivity reaction against platelets.

The two most common types of bleeding disorders are factor deficiency states and platelet abnormalities. Only a few of these conditions are common enough to warrant discussion. Diagnosis of even the common conditions usually requires confirmation by a specialist before definitive treatment starts. However, some knowledge of the most commonly presenting conditions, such as factor VIII deficiency (classic hemophilias), decreased platelet adhesiveness (von Willebrand's disease), or factor VII or V deficiency (chronic liver disease), allows proper selection of diagnostic tests and the initiation of a satisfactory treatment regimen. This information is available in standard hematology textbooks, for example, *Clinical Hematology* (7th ed.), by M. M. Wintrobe (Philadelphia: Lea & Febiger, 1974).

2. PREOPERATIVE PREPARATION

Most injuries seen in the emergency room are relatively straightforward in their presentation. Assessment of the extent of injury is readily made, and treatment is initiated within a reasonable period of time. Just as the sequence of steps of the initial assessment should be consistent regardless of the nature of the wound, certain consistencies in subsequent wound assessment and management must be maintained. For many injuries, the final assessment and treatment can be performed only following local wound preparation and under anesthesia.

The proper steps in the preoperative preparation of both the patient and the wound, and the principles that dictate choice of agents and instruments for prevention of infection, patient and wound preparation, and wound closure are discussed in this chapter.

PREOPERATIVE EVALUATION

Basic Goals

The principles governing the preoperative evaluation of patients and wounds are discussed in Chapter 1. In short, the history and initial evaluation must be detailed enough to allow (1) classification of the wound, such as clean and tidy versus untidy and contaminated, and identification of special circumstances of the wound (for example, a wound caused by a human bite) or special patient considerations (for example, a patient undergoing cancer chemotherapy) that may influence adversely the outcome of standard care. Such factors raise the index of suspicion that here is a wound or patient whose treatment requires more than "the ordinary."

The examination must provide the data base that enables us to make sequential systematic therapeutic decisions regarding management of the wound. Such decisions involve answers to questions about practical considerations, such as the following:

1. Will special tests be required to complete the diagnosis?
2. Is hemostasis adequate for final assessment and/or treatment?
3. Are additional treatments other than wound care and/or closure necessary to permit successful wound healing?

A decision to undertake any of these measures frequently depends on identification of the problems in hemostasis and wound infection discussed in Chapter 1. The principles of hemostasis are discussed in Chapter 1 and in subsequent sections concerning specific types of wounds. A far more frequent cause of concern is whether to add prophylactic antibiotics to prevent infection in addition to carrying out the traditional mechanical regimens of wound care, irrigation, and debridement.

Prevention of Infection

PREDICTING PROBLEMS

All wounds, whether caused by trauma or surgically created, are contaminated with bacteria, but few become infected. The factors influencing the establishment of an infected wound are discussed in Chapter 1; they include the virulence and degree of bacterial contamination, the nature of the wound, and factors of general host resistance. As is stressed in this and in subsequent chapters, the physician can prevent the development of infection in a traumatic wound by examining each of these three factors and modifying treatment accordingly. Two factors—the nature of the wound and the degree of bacterial contamination—are more easily and immediately modified than factors of general host resistance.

The tenets of proper mechanical wound management are discussed later in this and following chapters. However, as part of patient preparation, some determination of the need for prophylactic antibiotics must be made. Decisions regarding the use of prophylactic antibiotics are predicated on the relative influence of each of these above-mentioned factors in the specific patient. Because we do not know the exact nature or virulence of the contaminating organisms in most acute wounds, and because we cannot easily influence factors of general host resistance, the major factor that influences the need for prophylactic antibiotics is the nature of the wound. Thus, classifying the wound helps determine the need for prophylactic antibiotics.

GUIDELINES FOR ADMINISTRATION OF ANTIBIOTICS

There are no hard and fast rules governing either the decision to use prophylactic antibiotics or the type of antibiotic chosen. Prophylactic antibiotics are strongly indicated for

1. Traumatic wounds with heavy contamination, especially those contaminated by soil or those associated with crushed tissues of marginal viability
2. Untidy wounds in which adequate debridement cannot be completed or must be delayed
3. Wounds entering joint spaces or compound fractures, including intraoral compound fractures
4. Wounds in which treatment has been considerably delayed (beyond 6–12 hours)
5. Most animal and all human bite wounds

Additional relative indications can be determined by analyzing patient factors, including:

1. The compromised host (for example, the patient with a severely suppressed immunologic system, such as patients taking chemotherapeutic agents for cancer)
2. Patients for whom an infection might be disastrous (for example, someone with rheumatoid valvular disease)

Selectivity is advised in the use of prophylactic antibiotics. General rules are:

1. Use a bactericidal drug if possible.
2. Give in therapeutic doses for 3 to 5 days.
3. Choose the drug most likely to be effective against the organisms that most commonly contaminate the wounds. Gram-positive cocci predominate as the major cause of wound infections in the most common types of traumatic wounds.

CHOICE OF ANTIBIOTIC AGENT

Because the penicillinase-producing organism *Staphylococcus aureus* so predominates within traumatic wounds, penicillin G is no longer the drug of choice. The orally administered drugs of choice for most wounds are dicloxacillin or, for patients allergic to penicillin, one of the cephalosporins. The exceptions to this general rule include:

1. Human bites. See Chapter 6 regarding penetrating injuries.
2. Farm machinery injuries. Recent work indicates that because the contaminating flora is so varied, aggressive surgical debridement, frequent observation, and antibiotics prescribed on the basis of culture results comprise the treatment of choice.
3. Major burn wounds. Penicillins remain the drugs of choice for prophylaxis against *Streptococcus*.

For those allergic to both penicillins and cephalosporins, erythromycin or lincomycin is the drug of choice. It must be emphasized that there is no such thing as a "prophylactic dosage." The usual therapeutic schedule should be followed. Table 2-1 lists the commonly used antibiotics, their mode of action, the usual dose and schedule of administration, and potential side effects. Table 2-2 lists the drugs usually chosen for common types of infection.

It should be stressed over and over again that in the management of traumatic wounds, antibiotics are only adjuvants. They cannot replace good wound care.

IMMUNIZATION FOR TETANUS

When obtaining the history for any patient with a traumatic wound, questions regarding the adequacy of tetanus prophylaxis must be included. The recommendations of the World Health Organization, the American College of Surgeons, or other agencies are usually posted in emergency departments and are summarized here.

1. Previously immunized patients
   a. Patients with minimal wounds who have been immunized or who have received boosters within the previous 5 years probably require no additional immunization; those with severe wounds with obvious risk of tetanus should receive 0.5 ml of tetanus toxoid.
   b. Patients who have been immunized or who have received boosters within the last 10 years. Give 0.5 ml of tetanus toxoid.
   c. Patients immunized more than 10 years before the present wound. In

Table 2-1. Commonly used antibiotics

Antibiotic	Usual adult dosage	Mode of action	Complications of use and side effects
Penicillins			
Penicillin G	2–30 million units per day, parenterally, in 4–6 divided doses	Bactericidal; inhibits cell wall synthesis	Allergic reactions frequent
Penicillin V	400,000 units, 4–6 hr, orally	Same as above	Allergic reactions frequent
Dicloxacillin	1–4 gm/day, in 4–6 divided doses (oral only)	Same as above; best absorption from the GI tract of all the synthetic penicillins	Allergic reactions frequent
Ampicillin	2–12 gm/day, in 4–6 divided doses	Effective against some gram-negative organisms	Allergic reactions frequent; diarrhea
Cephalosporins			
Cephalothin	2–6 gm/day, parenterally in 4–6 divided doses	Bactericidal; resistant to penicillinase	Allergic reactions resembling those of penicillin
Cephalexin	1–4 gm/day, orally	Same as above	Same as above
Tetracyclines			
Tetracycline	1–2 gm/day, in 4–6 divided doses, orally	Bacteriostatic	GI disturbances; stains teeth in children; hepatotoxicity in excess dosage
Erythromycins			
Erythromycin	1–4 gm/day, in 4 divided doses	Bacteriostatic	GI and hepatic disturbances
Aminoglycosides			
Gentamicin	1.5–3 mg/kg/day, intramuscularly, in 4 divided doses	Bactericidal	Vestibular auditory nerve damage; may be nephrotoxic
Kanamycin	1–1.5 mg/kg/day, intramuscularly, in 2–3 divided doses	Bactericidal	Same as above

most instances, give 0.5 ml of tetanus toxoid; if the wound is severe, with severe contamination and a high risk of tetanus, give 250 units of human tetanus–immune globulin in addition to 0.5 ml of tetanus toxoid.

2. Unimmunized or partly immunized patients
   a. Wounds in which the risk of tetanus is very small. Give tetanus toxoid, 0.5 ml. The patient must have subsequent doses of toxoid to complete immunization, and this should be scheduled.
   b. Severe wounds in which the risk of tetanus is great. Give 0.5 ml of tetanus toxoid, and schedule the patient for completion of immunization. Also give 250 units of tetanus–immune globulin, and antibiotics to restrict the growth of organisms that promote the formation and growth of tetanus spores, particularly organisms that create anaerobic conditions.

VACCINATION FOR RABIES

The next most common concern involves recommendations for the use of rabies vaccines. Indications vary from region to region, so the local, county, or state department of health should be contacted for advice. Advice can be obtained directly from the Centers for Disease Control of the United States Public Health Department in Atlanta, Georgia. The tele-

Table 2-2. Antibiotics used for common infections

Appearance or source of infection	Usual organism	Results of Gram stain	Drugs used	
			First choice	Second choice
Erysipelas	*Streptococcus*	Gm$^+$ cocci	Penicillin G or V; dicloxacillin	Erythromycin or cephalosporin
Cellulitis	*Streptococcus* or *Staphylococcus*	Gm$^+$ cocci	Penicillin G or V; dicloxacillin	Cephalosporin
Subcutaneous abscess, not hospital-acquired organism	*Staphylococcus* penicillinase or nonpenicillin product	Gm$^+$ cocci	Oral dicloxacillin	Cephalosporin or lincomycin
Infected human bite	Polymicrobial and spirochetal	Mixed flora	Dicloxacillin and gentamicin	Cephalosporin; clindamycin
Crepitant myositis	Clostridia	Gm$^+$ bacilli	Penicillin G or V	Erythromycin; tetracycline; cephalosporin
Lymphangitis	*Streptococcus*; *Staphylococcus*	GM$^+$ cocci; Gm$^+$ cocci	Dicloxacillin	Cephalosporin
Infected animal bite, cat bite	Polymicrobial with *Pasteurella multocida*, often associated with cat bites	Mixed flora GM$^-$ bacilli	Dicloxacillin	Cephalosporin Tetracycline
Infection 2° to retained foreign body	Polymicrobial—predominantly *Staphylococcus*	Mixed flora	Dicloxacillin	Cephalosporin; lincomycin; clindamycin
Acute necrotizing fasciitis	Polymicrobial	Mixed flora	Cephalosporin; gentamicin	Lincomycin; clindamycin

phone numbers for the CDC are 404-633-3311 (weekdays) and 404-633-2176 (during off-hours).

Record Keeping

The maintenance of good records is crucial to the continuing care of a patient with a traumatic wound. This is particularly important if the patient is ultimately to be transferred to the care of a specialist. Recording of the history and physical examination data never should be relegated to the end of the day or even the end of the initial treatment. Just as it is important to develop a systematic method of evaluating and treating wounds, a systematic method of recording the examination should be developed. For most wounds, a sketch is one of the best methods of recording information.

PATIENT PREPARATION

Patient Consent and Education

It is often said that an ugly facial scar, a distorted eye or lip, or loss of hand function offers a mute testimony to malpractice. Is this so? Of course not! What, then, can physicians in the emergency department do to protect themselves against such unjustified claims of malpractice or negligence, or statements such as, "Why didn't you call in a plastic surgeon?"

The answers to these questions are quite simple yet frequently overlooked because of oversight, the hurry of getting back to a warm bed in the middle of the night, or the absolute necessity of attending to a more critically injured area or other patient.

Establishing rapport with the patient (and family) is the essence not only of avoiding legal action, but more importantly, of achieving the most successful treatment of the injury.

1. *Explain carefully and in simple lay terminology the nature of the injury*, possible outcomes, and possible complications.
2. *Explain alternative means of treatment* or the availability (or nonavailability) of other specialists. This allows the patient to participate in therapeutic decisions.
3. *Treat only those injuries for which you are confident of the appropriate treatment* (unless it is an absolute emergency). Be honest to yourself and the patient about your training and capabilities in handling specific problems.
4. *Make no promises about the outcome!* Statements such as, "Everything will be as good as new," or "You'll never be able to see the scar" are an invitation to misunderstanding.
5. After completion of the above discussions, the *patient or guardian should sign an advised consent form.*
6. To protect yourself additionally and provide for satisfactory follow-up, make sure that critical *diagnostic and therapeutic information has been documented adequately* in the emergency department records.

Patient Comfort

Most patients have considerable anxiety or specific fears regarding their injuries, deformities, loss of function, or fear of pain, or nonspecific anxieties regarding this new experience. Several measures can be taken to make the experience as comfortable as possible.

COMMUNICATION

Communication with the patient and establishing confidence in your abilities are usually of great benefit. A thorough step-by-step explanation in layperson terms and reassurance before any assessment or treatment takes place are essential.

During surgery or administration of anesthesia, continuous verbal communication has a hypnotic and distracting effect. Discussion about school, jobs, family, current events, or other pleasant subjects distracts the patient from surgical activities. When caring for an injured child, additional efforts at reassurance pay large dividends. The positive influence of a calm parent is equally beneficial. However, each event must be individualized; an agitated parent present during examination and treatment certainly magnifies an injured child's anxiety.

POSITION

A well-padded table with appropriate pillow support for the head and neck and the legs provides the patient with initial physical comfort. Furthermore, the patient gains confidence that you are concerned about his or her general well-being and not simply interested in the wound and technique of treatment.

Tying a child down on a "mummy board" with leather restraints (or a dozen adult hands immobilizing the child's hands, feet, and head) is rarely, if ever, indicated. Talk to the child and give a simple but truthful explanation. A verbal prelude to avoid surprise about pain, and care not to cover the child's eyes may be all that is required to do the surgical work successfully, without the need for immobilization. If this is not possible, sedation or general anesthesia should be considered.

ANALGESIC MEDICATION

Some patients require sedation for relief of anxiety or analgesics for relief of pain.

Before administering any medication, *be sure that there are no associated injuries that might be masked or worsened by medication.* Respiratory depression, hypotension, abdominal pain, state of consciousness, or other neurologic signs can be altered or caused by narcotic analgesics (e.g., morphine, meperidine [Demerol]) and most sedatives (e.g., barbiturates, phenothiazines). If, in your opinion, medications are required, however, the following dose schedules can be recommended for anxious adults and uncooperative children:

Meperidine (Demerol): 1.5 to 2 mg per kilogram IM, *or*
Morphine: 0.15 to 2 mg per kilogram IM, *combined with*
Diazepam (Valium): 0.03 to 0.15 mg per kilogram IM, *or*
Hydroxyzine (Vistaril): 0.75 to 1 mg per kilogram IM

For the uncooperative child, an effective combination of drugs is:

Meperidine (Demerol): 2 mg per kilogram IM
Promethazine (Phenergan): 1 mg per kilogram IM
Chlorpromazine (Thorazine): 1 mg per kilogram IM

It is important to wait at least 30 minutes following IM injection before proceeding with care.

Monitoring

Before attention is focused on actual wound repair, it is most important that the surgeon be aware of the patient's general condition and be prepared for other therapies if that deteriorates. This awareness must continue throughout the therapy.

CLINICAL ASSESSMENT

In most instances, the patient's clinical condition can be followed accurately by observing the vital signs and other physical characteristics. The color of the blood and pulsations of bleeding wounds or soft tissues give an indication of the patient's state of oxygenation, pulse rate, and blood pressure.

By continuously talking with the patient and observing facial expressions and skin and lip color, the patient's state of consciousness and vascular status can be evaluated.

These clinical assessments can be carried out by the physician, assistant, nurse, or other trained person. Furthermore, these should be done even if special mechanical monitoring is also being performed.

MECHANICAL MONITORS

Blood pressure cuffs, pulse monitors, and ECG monitors are useful when available and may be necessary for severely injured patients.

INTRAVENOUS INFUSIONS

A continuous IV is not needed for most simple emergency department problems. However, an IV should be used if the physician anticipates problems for medication use or circulatory insufficiency, or if medications are to be administered.

Tourniquets

The bloodless field afforded by a tourniquet enhances visualization of injured and uninjured structures in both upper and lower limbs. This allows more accurate wound assessment and facilitates treatment. There are dangers of tissue ischemia from the use of a tourniquet, however, which increase according to the time the tourniquet is inflated. Therefore, all aspects of care that can be accomplished without the tourniquets should be done before inflation. A tourniquet should not be used with ischemic injuries.

ARM OR LEG TOURNIQUET

Without anesthesia at the tourniquet site, the cooperative adult can tolerate 30 minutes of tourniquet inflation. If treatment requires use of a tourniquet for longer than 30 minutes, an axillary block or general anesthesia is necessary. The longer the procedure, the greater the possibility of ischemic damage to muscle vessels and nerves from the tourniquet. However, 2 hours of tourniquet inflation can be tolerated safely. Once tourniquet pain occurs, the tourniquet may be deflated for 5 to 10 minutes and then reinflated. It is extremely dangerous to give additional doses of analgesics, especially narcotics, in an effort to alleviate tourniquet pain. Analgesics in this situation are usually ineffective, and when the tourniquet is released and the painful stimulant gone, you may discover that the patient has a narcotic overdose. If the procedure is nearly completed, several layers of elastic bandage can be wrapped tightly around the forearm, and then the upper tourniquet can be deflated. This bandage should be left in place only briefly (5–10 minutes).

An outline of the equipment and procedure for use of arm or leg tourniquets follows.

1. Equipment. Although a blood pressure cuff elevated 50 to 100 mm Hg above systolic pressure will suffice in an emergency, more reliable tourniquets are commercially available. The double cuff is particularly useful for IV regional blocks.

PREOPERATIVE PREPARATION

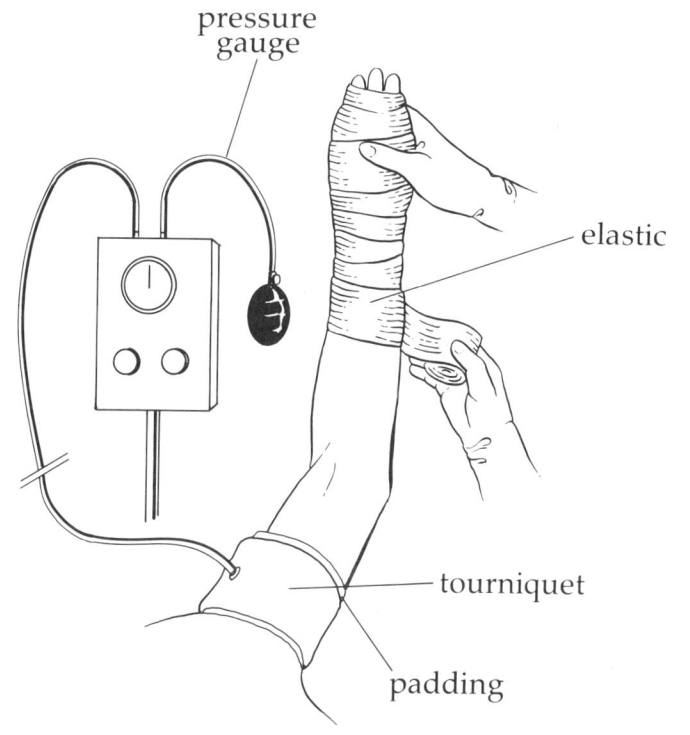

Figure 2-1. The six sequential steps for use of a tourniquet include: (1) Pretest of accuracy of pressure gauge, (2) pretest for air leaks, (3) smooth layer of padding, (4) snug application of tourniquet, (5) exsanguination, (6) inflation to a level 50–100 mm Hg above systolic blood pressure.

2. Procedure. Fig. 2-1 shows the proper application of a tourniquet on an arm. The six steps of its application are as follows:
   a. Check the tourniquet pressure gauge for reliability, preferably against a mercury rather than an aneroid manometer. The pressure source should be checked to ensure that it will last throughout the procedure.
   b. Pretest the entire system for air leaks.
   c. Protect the arm with cast padding or bias-cut stockinette. The padding is smoothly wrapped around the upper arm as close to the shoulder as possible. Avoid wrinkling the padding.
   d. After the padding is in place, wrap the tourniquet snugly over it.
   e. Elevate the arm for 30 seconds and/or wrap with an elastic bandage so that venous blood may be exsanguinated. A sterile Ace bandage or Esmarch bandage can be used, beginning at the fingers and wrapping proximally toward the tourniquet.
   f. Inflate the tourniquet to a pressure sufficient to permit a bloodless field. As a rule of thumb, the arm tourniquet can be inflated 50 to 100 mm Hg above systolic pressure. The same principles apply to lower extremity tourniquets, but inflation pressures should be 50 to 100 mm higher than those recommended for the upper limb.

DIGITS

A finger tourniquet of a soft rubber drain secured with a heavy clamp can be maintained safely for 15 to 30 minutes (Fig. 2-2). However, the rubber drain must be at least ½-inch wide and should not be knotted or twisted. *It should be applied just tightly enough to occlude arterial inflow.* A narrow rubber band should not be used! These tend to disappear into the skin and have

Figure 2-2. A soft 1 cm-wide rubber drain, used as a finger tourniquet for distal injuries or for the incision and drainage of infections. The drain should not be twisted or knotted and should be applied just tightly enough to occlude arterial inflow.

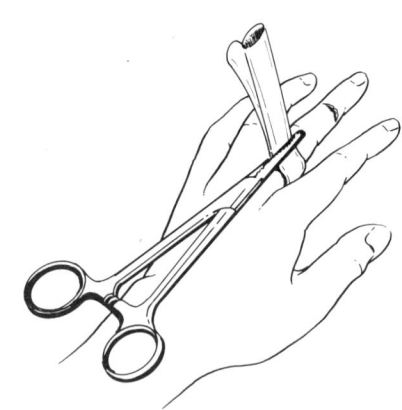

Figure 2-3. Hair around a wound should be trimmed closely with a pair of scissors, not shaved.

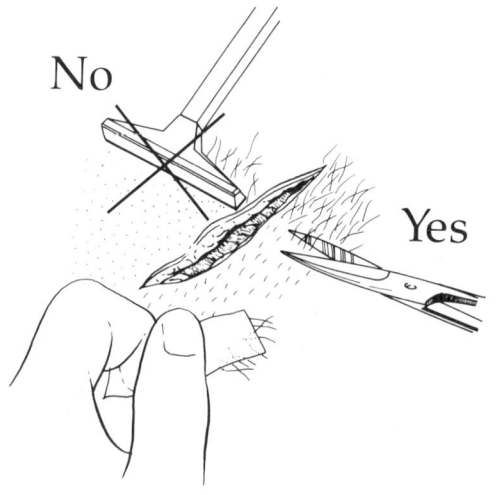

been included in the dressing following wound closure with, quite naturally, disastrous consequences. For more proximal wounds, the arm tourniquet is used. Finger tourniquets are *rarely* necessary for most soft tissue injuries and should be used only when visualization of a nerve or other important structure is necessary.

OPERATIVE FIELD PREPARATION

Hair Trimming

The hair around a wound should be trimmed, not shaved (Fig. 2-3). A scissor trim of long scalp hair or body hair within 1 to 2 cm of the wound prevents entanglement with suture material and prevents incorporation into the wound. Long hair not in the immediate vicinity of the wound can be plastered with ointment, braided, or taped out of the way.

Shaving predisposes to increased wound infection caused by destruction of the natural epidermal barrier and inadvertent cuts in the skin. The

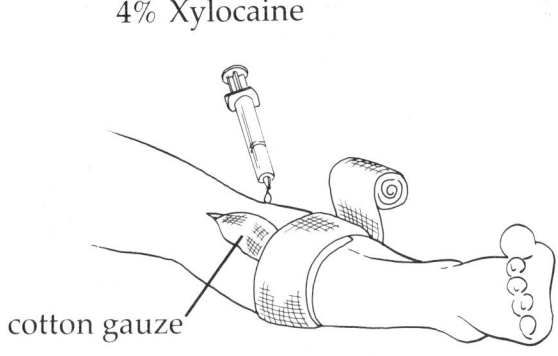

Figure 2-4. Open wounds packed with sterile cotton gauze to prevent contamination during skin preparation and draping. Covering the wound may also relieve patient anxiety. Gauze packs assist in hemostasis and, if presoaked with a topical anesthetic such as 4% Xylocaine, provide some wound anesthesia.

longer the interval between shaving and wound closure, the higher the infection rate. A 10-fold increase in infection rate can occur if a wound is shaved 12 or more hours before a routine elective surgical procedure. The risk is minimized in wounds shaved immediately before their closure.

Furthermore, natural landmarks such as the junction of the scalp and forehead, or, most importantly, of the eyebrows, are destroyed. This could lead to malalignment or a step deformity at the junction of hair-bearing or non-hair-bearing skin.

Packing

Insert sterile gauze and pack into the open wound while preparing for the surgical procedure (Fig. 2-4). The gauze serves four purposes. It prevents contamination from airborne hospital bacteria; it may be soaked with an anesthetic agent to provide topical anesthesia; it helps provide pressure for hemostasis; and it reduces patient anxiety.

A 2 × 2 gauze pad is placed into the wound gently and soaked with 4% lidocaine (Xylocaine). The initial use of topical anesthesia simplifies the task of injection of local anesthesia. If hemostasis is necessary, a pressure wrap with an elastic bandage is applied.

Skin Preparation—Wound Antisepsis

The skin of the entire operative field should be prepped with an antiseptic solution. To avoid confusing terminology, several definitions are discussed, followed by a discussion of the classes of antiseptics and some guidelines for their proper usage.

DEFINITIONS

Antisepsis refers to any process that is directed at inactivating or destroying living organisms for the purpose of preventing infection. Antisepsis can be achieved with antiseptics, disinfectants, immunizations, antibiotics, sterilization, or surgical debridement.

Antiseptics are chemical agents that are topically applied to skin or wounds to prevent growth and multiplication of microorganisms in or on living tissues. The term does not usually differentiate between agents that are bactericidal and those that are bacteriostatic. Most antiseptics are inorganic chemicals, but some are organic compounds. Antiseptics have a spectrum of biologic activity against many bacteria, fungi, and viruses.

Before 1837, when Pasteur discovered that microorganisms cause infection, it was believed that "effluvia" (noxious vapors) was the cause of infection. The term *disinfectant* was introduced in the seventeenth century to refer to a substance used to destroy or mask the vile odors thought to cause infection.

A *disinfectant* or *germicide* is a chemical agent that destroys or inactivates organisms on the surface of inanimate objects, unlike an antiseptic, which is used on living tissue. The same agent can be both a disinfectant and an antiseptic.

Sterilization is the process of total destruction of all forms of living organisms. Sterilization can be achieved with chemical agents, such as formaldehyde, or physical agents, such as extreme heat and ionizing radiation.

Agents used for sterilization or disinfection of inanimate objects require the application of the highest concentration possible for a rapid kill, as long as it does not cause physical damage to the object treated or toxicity to persons handling the material. In contrast, the use of agents in living tissue involves the lowest concentration that is effective and not toxic.

CLASSES OF ANTISEPTICS
1. Heavy metals
    a. *Mercurials*. Inorganic and organic mercurial compounds have been used as disinfectants and antiseptics since Roman times. Inorganic mercuric chloride (corrosive sublimate) is the active chemical. Mercuric compounds were used for the treatment of syphilis.

    The organic mercurials merbromin (Mercurochrome) and thimerosal (Merthiolate) were used for surgical skin preparation before hexachlorophene and the iodophors and are now used occasionally for treatment of skin graft donor sites.

    The organic mercurials are weakly bactericidal, with poor activity as systemic antimicrobials. They are inactivated by organic materials.
    b. *Silver ion*. In ancient times, silver containers were used on an empiric basis to store water for purification—a dilute solution of silver ion is slowly bactericidal. In the late nineteenth century, 1% silver nitrate drops were used to prevent and treat gonococcal ophthalmia neonatorum.
    c. *Silver nitrate*. In 1965 an important advance in the topical therapy of burn wounds occurred with the introduction of 0.5% silver nitrate. Saturated dressings of 0.5% silver nitrate solution were applied to the burn wounds. Complications included dehydration, which raised the concentrations of silver nitrate to caustic levels; silver staining; chloride depletion by precipitation; and methemoglobinemia from microbial reduction of nitrates to nitrites. A silver nitrate caustic stick is used for cauterization and removal of hypertrophic granulation tissue.
    d. *Silver sulfadiazine*. This is a unique combination of an antiseptic (silver) and an antibiotic (sulfadiazine). Nonionized low-solubility silver salt is used in a 1% cream for topical antibacterial treatment of burns, especially for *Pseudomonas aeruginosa* and other gram-negative organisms. It is effective against gram-positive and gram-negative bacteria

and fungi. It is not painful on application and does not stain skin dressings or bedding.

   e. *Zinc, aluminum, bismuth, and antimony* are used as astringent agents because they coagulate surface skin proteins.

2. Halogens

   a. *Chlorine.* Sodium and calcium hypochlorite solutions have been used for nearly 2 centuries. In the early nineteenth century, the French used chlorinated lime to clean hospital wards and bathrooms. Semmelweiss in Vienna reduced puerperal fever by handwashes with hydrochlorite solution. During World War I, Carrel and Dakin used a 0.5% solution for the irrigation of wounds. Chlorination is the most widely used method of water sanitation.

   Hypochlorous acid dissociates into hydrogen and hypochlorite ion. Hypochlorous acid has a rapid bactericidal action, and hypochlorite is also bactericidal. Dilute hypochlorite solutions (0.1–0.5%) are used in hydrotherapy tanks in the treatment of burn patients and packing of necrotic wounds.

   Hypochlorite solutions have little role in the emergency department or in home care because of the rapid inactivation of the active agent by organic molecules. Their hospital use has been largely supplanted by newer agents, such as the iodophors described below.

   b. *Iodine* is bactericidal against the broad spectrum of pathogens, including most bacteria, fungi, and viruses. It is also active against bacterial and fungal spores. It has a rapid action, but causes stains, skin irritation, and corrosion of metals. Free iodine (I_2) is the effective germicidal agent. Like chlorine, iodine is inactivated by organic material. Iodine is minimally soluble in water. It is soluble in alcohol as a 2% solution, which is more bactericidal than similar concentrations of chlorine or bromine. A 0.5% to 1% iodine solution in 70% ethyl or isopropyl alcohol is the most effective preoperative skin preparation but should be used only on the intact skin surrounding the wound. Both alcohols and free iodines are extremely toxic to living tissues and never should be allowed to contact an open wound or used around the eye. The higher concentrations of iodine (2%) even injure intact skin. The proper techniques of application include painting the solution or tincture on the intact skin surrounding the wound, allowing this to dry, and removing residual iodine with a final wipe of alcohol, wiping the skin until most of the brown pigment is removed. Great care must be taken to avoid pooling of iodine-containing solutions or tincture in body creases, such as about the neck, axillae, or groin. If left in contact with tissues in these areas for sufficient time, severe chemical injury occurs.

   c. *Iodophors* are iodines with an organic carrier. Iodophors slowly release free iodine when diluted with water and have the same broad spectrum of activity as iodine. They are nonirritating to mucosa and conjunctiva except in sensitive people. They cause temporary staining. Common preparations of povidone-iodine are Betadine, Ioprep, and Septadyne. These organic iodines are now the most commonly used antiseptics in emergency rooms. Both a detergent form for preparation of surrounding intact skin, and a nondetergent antiseptic "paint" are available. The antiseptic paint, usually diluted half and half with normal saline, can be used directly in the wound—even in large wounds—as a soaking or irrigating solution. They are minimally tissue-toxic, and if residual iodophor is rinsed from the wound with normal saline, almost no cellular damage occurs. They can be used around the eye but should not be used, undiluted, directly in the eye. One pitfall in their use is that the brown color imparted to the skin may make the assessment of tissue viability more difficult, especially if these solutions are allowed to dry on the skin. Therefore, when the viability of skin flaps or wound margins are in doubt, the solution should be rinsed or wiped off with a saline-soaked gauze before it dries on the skin.

Iodophors are now commonly used as topical antiseptics on wounds left open and allowed to heal by secondary intent or those to be closed by delayed primary closure. Because loss of the brown color indicates inactivation of the active agent, the solution should be renewed at frequent intervals (or a new dressing soaked with the solution applied) when used for these purposes.

  d. *Iodoform (triiodomethane).* A 5% or 10% iodoform gauze strip is used most commonly as a pack or wick following incision and drainage of subcutaneous abscesses. Contact with body fluids liberates the active free iodine.

  Absorption of iodine through large-surface-area open wounds, such as burns, can cause acidosis.

3. Phenolic compounds
  a. *Phenol* (carbolic acid) has limited antiseptic use because of its systemic toxicity. It is rapidly absorbed through intact and damaged skin and mucosa. It is used in chemical face peeling for the aged face. A 2% solution is an excellent disinfectant for fecal contamination of inanimate objects because it is not inactivated by organic material.
  b. *Hexachlorophene* is a bis-phenol in a 1% solution with bacteriostatic activity against gram-positive organisms. Considerable activity is lost in the presence of organic materials such as pus and serum. It is, therefore, not useful in open wounds. Moreover, hexachlorophene has extreme CNS toxicity and is contraindicated on open wounds. Hexachlorophene can be absorbed through damaged skin, especially large burn areas, and through the intact skin of premature infants. Therefore, it is also contraindicated in these situations.

  It accumulates on the skin for 3 to 4 days, after which the level remains relatively constant. It reduces the bacterial flora of the skin and is useful in staphylococcal skin infections, especially in newborn nurseries. It is also used as a surgical hand scrub in a detergent base. It is only effective if used repeatedly.

  The action of hexachlorophene is antagonized by quaternary ammonium salts and soaps.

4. *Alcohols* are bactericidal against vegetative forms, but they are not sporicidal. Therefore, they are not adequate for the sterilization of surgical instruments. They also are not effective against the hepatitis viruses. Alcohol is toxic to phagocytic macrophages and therefore should not be used as an antiseptic in open wounds.

  Isopropyl alcohol has slightly greater bactericidal activity than ethyl alcohol. It is also more toxic. Unlike ethyl alcohol, the bactericidal action of isopropyl alcohol increases with concentrations greater than 70%.

Alcohol is useful as a skin preparation before hypodermic injections or venipuncture. Because it is volatile, it dries rapidly.

5. *Biguanides*—chlorhexidine (Hibitane). Gram-positive organisms are more susceptible to chlorhexidine than gram-negative organisms, and resistance does not develop. At low bactericidal levels, chlorhexidine affects cell membranes. Recommended concentrations are 0.2% to 0.4%.

6. *Quaternary ammonium compounds* are cationic surface active agents. Benzalkonium chloride (Zephirin) is frequently used as an antiseptic and as the tincture for skin preparation. It is virucidal for rabies virus and is recommended for the irrigation of bites from rabid animals.

At low concentrations, the quaternary ammonium salts are bacteriostatic and fungistatic. At medium concentrations they are bactericidal, fungicidal, and virucidal against lipophilic viruses. They are not sporicidal nor are they effective against tubercle bacillus. They are inactivated by soaps.

At bactericidal levels, they are more effective against gram-positive organisms. The recommended concentration is 0.1% to 1%.

7. *Oxidizing agents (hydrogen peroxide).* A 3% solution is an effective disinfectant for inanimate objects such as contact lenses. Hydrogen peroxide is not effective against living organisms, which contain inactivating catalases and peroxidases. Catalase is present in all tissues including red and white blood cells. The mechanical detergent action associated with the release of oxygen gas bubbles is probably of greater value than any antiseptic action in living tissue.

A useful rule of thumb to guide antiseptic technique, is: "Do not put anything in a wound that you would not first put in your eye." Therefore, for most cleanly incised, tidy, uncontaminated wounds, such as sharp lacerations and slicing injuries, only the skin surrounding the wound needs preparation with an antiseptic solution. The wound itself should be cleaned by irrigation with normal saline.

Our recommendations for specific use of these agents are as follows:
a. Skin prep (patient's wound, surgeon's hand)
   (1) Chlorhexidine (Hibiclens)
   (2) Iodophor—povidone-iodine (Betadine, Isoprep, Septadyne)
   (3) Hexachlorophene
b. Wound packing
   (1) Iodophor (most wounds)
   (2) Silver sulfadiazine (dry wounds)
c. Abrasions and burns
   (1) Silver sulfadiazine
   (2) Hypochlorite solution

Drapes

A sterile cloth should surround the operative field. The purposes of a drape are prevention of contamination from the surrounding areas and provision of a sterile surface for placement of sutures and instruments.

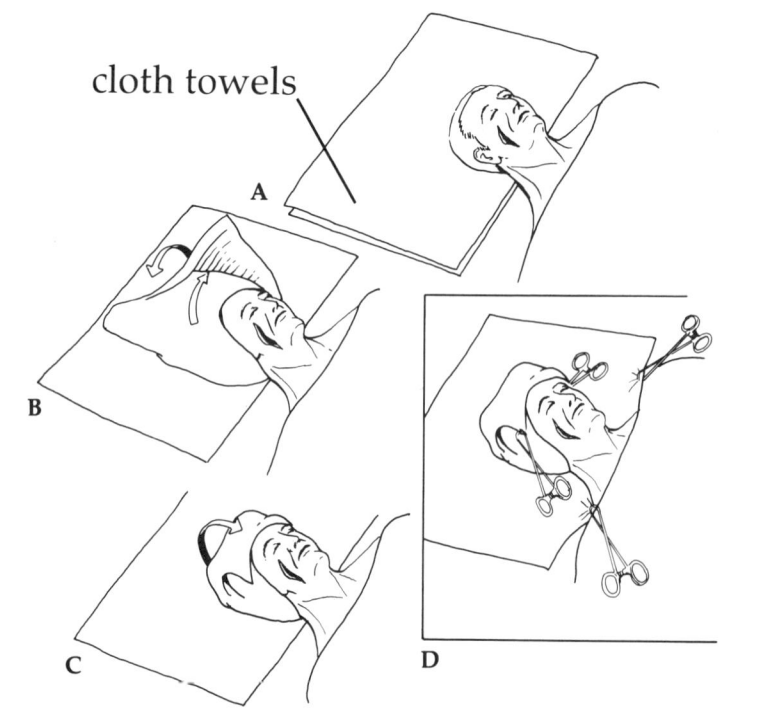

Figure 2-5. Method for application of a head drape.
A. Place two sterile towels under the head.
B. Fold inner towel about the head to fashion a turban.
C. Apply towel clips to the corners to hold the turban snugly to the head.
D. With additional clips, attach the bottom towel to a sterile sheet placed over the chest and neck to isolate the entire face, neck, and ears.

The drape also prevents hair from becoming entangled with sutures or falling in the wound.

The technical considerations in application of drapes are as follows:

There should be an opening of adequate size to observe symmetry with surrounding tissues on the contralateral side.
The drapes should be fixed in place so that they can't slide over the operative field and possibly contaminate the wound.

HEAD DRAPES

For a facial wound, the head should be draped as shown in Fig. 2-5. The entire face should be exposed. This allows complete observation for symmetry and for facial movements if injury to the facial nerve is of concern. Moreover, the patient is more comfortable and can breathe without obstruction from the drapes. The very anxious patient may prefer to have his or her eyes either covered or uncovered. If the patient wishes to have eyes covered, a moist sponge is more easily applied and removed than a drape. The sponge placed over the eyes keeps suture ends or debris from contacting the sensitive eye and causing discomfort. Children may become quite agitated if eyes and nose are covered and may prefer to keep a parent in view.

EXTREMITY DRAPES

For any hand injury, even one involving a single digit, the entire hand and forearm should be prepped and the upper arm draped as shown in Fig. 2-6. Draping in the emergency department should not compromise sterile technique or patient and physician comfort. The arm should be in an

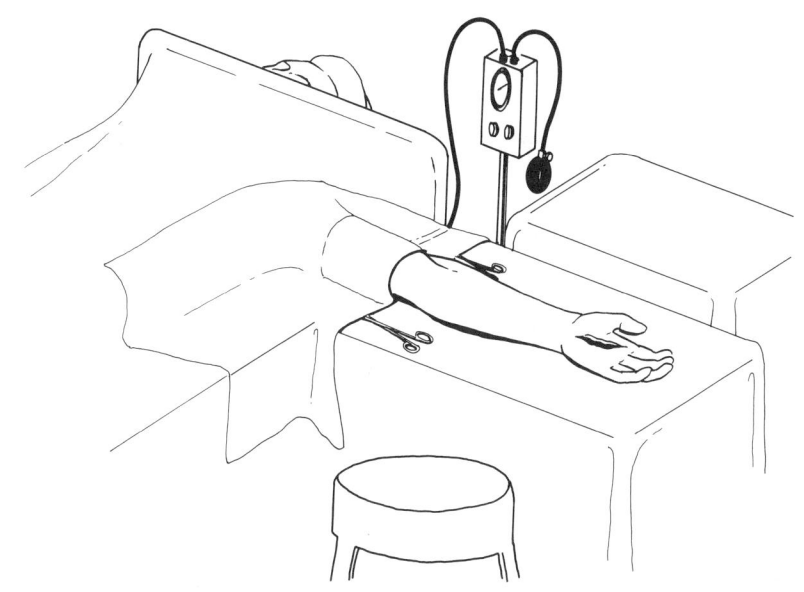

Figure 2-6. Distal extremity prepared and draped to allow examination in its entirety.

abducted position on a stable platform. A hand table, arm board, or even a wooden slat supported beneath the mattress can be used. The arm should be at the same level as the patient's chest to avoid brachial plexus traction.

SURGEON'S PREPARATION

Scrub and Gown

The hands and forearms should be scrubbed. Chlorhexidine and hexachlorophene retard the growth of bacteria under surgical gloves for a longer period than other antiseptic solutions, but are most effective with repeated use, whereas iodophor compounds may be more effective for a single scrub. The first scrub requires 10 minutes. However, a 3- to 5-minute scrub is sufficient for subsequent surgery.

The use of a clean gown, cap, and mask is advised to prevent contamination from organisms on the clothing or nasopharynx, or hair falling into the wound.

Surgical Instruments

Instruments used for soft tissue repair are illustrated in Fig. 2-7.

BASIC INSTRUMENTS
A set of small instruments facilitates rapid and gentle surgical technique. The basic instrument set includes:

(1) needle holder (smooth-jawed)
(2) small skin hooks
(1) curved scissors
(4) clamps (mosquito)
(4) towel clips

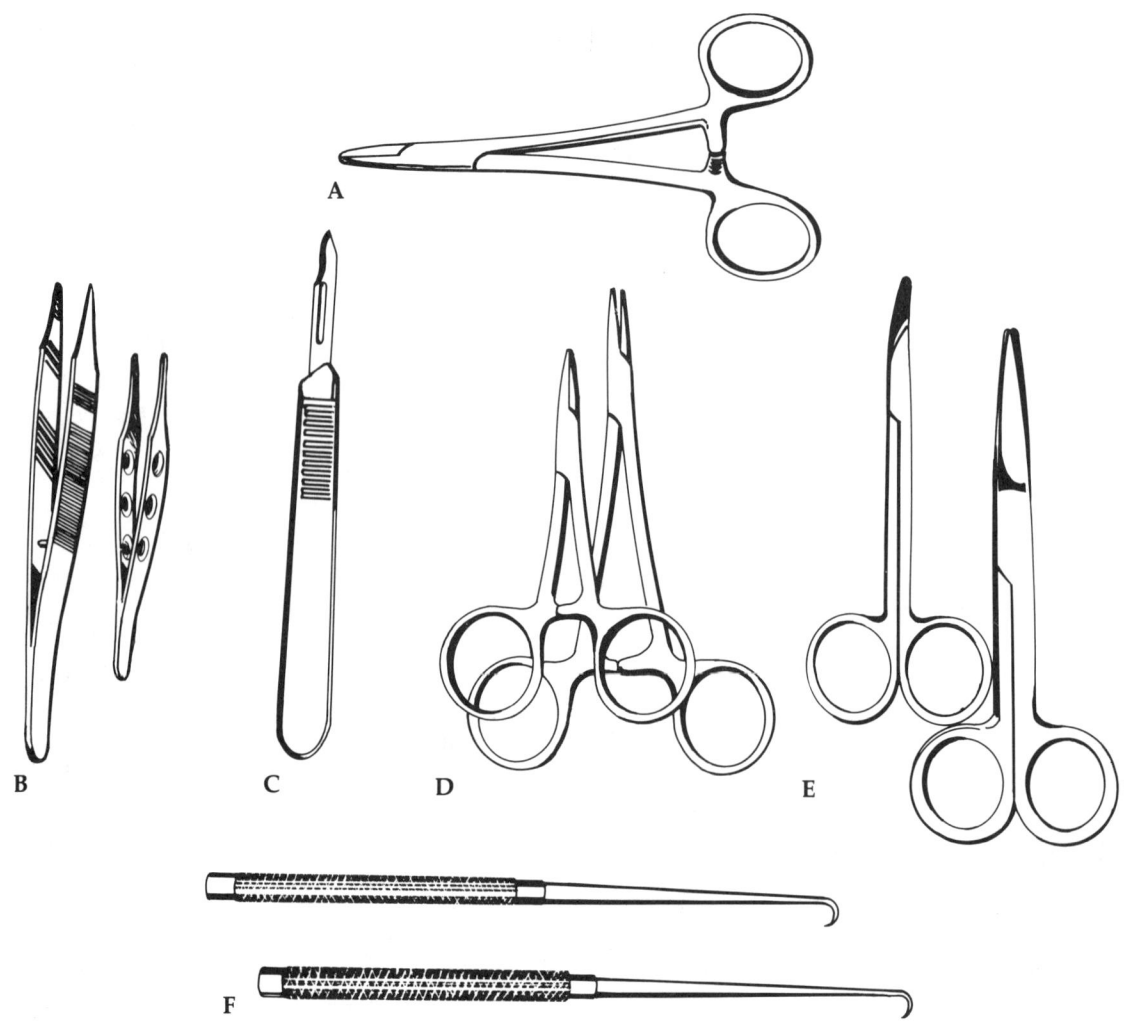

Figure 2-7. Basic surgical instruments for soft tissue repair.
A. Small fine needle holder
B. Fine-toothed forceps: Bishop-Harmon (small); Adson-Brown (large)
C. Scalpel handle and #15 scalpel blades
D. Fine hemostats (mosquito)
E. Fine, curved dissecting scissors and heavier scissors for cutting sutures or dressing
F. Skin hooks

(2) Senn retractors
(2) self-retaining retractors
(1) straight suture scissors
(1) scalpel handle
(1) #15 scalpel blade
(1) forceps (Bishop-Harmon)
(1) forceps (Adson)
(1) cotton-tipped applicator
(1) methylene blue marking ink

SPECIAL INSTRUMENTS

Specific instruments may be required for each anatomic site as seen in the following outline.

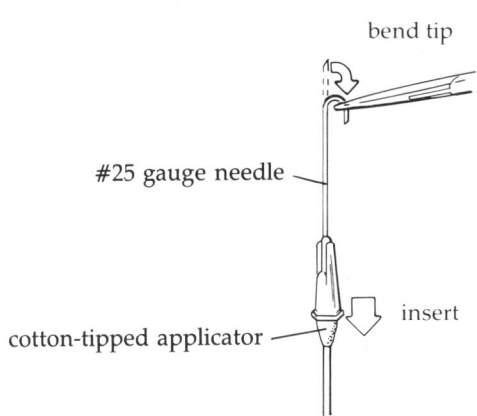

Figure 2-8. Simple method for fashioning a skin hook with a cotton-tipped applicator and a #25 or #22 hypodermic needle.

1. Facial instruments
   a. Periorbital
      (1) Lacrimal probes
      (2) Pigtail probe
      (3) Polyethylene tubes
   b. Nasal
      (1) Speculum
      (2) Periosteal elevator (Freer)
      (3) Asche forceps
2. Hand instruments
   a. Interosseous (Kirschner) wires and a drill
   b. Small rongeur
   c. Periosteal elevator
   d. Dental probes

A skin hook is an effective instrument for atraumatic tissue handling. If there is not a hook in the instrument set, you can make one quite simply (Fig. 2-8).

Sutures

DEFINITION AND HISTORY

A *suture* is a filamentous strand that holds severed tissues in apposition until the healing process has provided sufficient strength to maintain wound integrity.

Unique methods for approximating wounds have been used by ancient cultures. The South American Indians used the head pincers of army ants, and the Greeks used horse-tail hairs threaded into sharpened bones.

TYPES OF SUTURES

1. Materials. Sutures are made from various materials. They can be subcategorized as either absorbable or nonabsorbable and as synthetic or natural.
   a. *Absorbable* sutures are destroyed within days to weeks by a physiologic inflammatory process of cellular phagocytosis and/or enzymatic lysis.

Table 2-3. Strength and diameter of coated multifilament sutures

Size	Knot pull strength (kg)	Maximum diameter (mm)
10–0	0.010	0.018
9–0	0.023	0.038
8–0	0.045	0.064
7–0	0.060	0.089
6–0	0.160	0.127
5–0	0.320	0.179
4–0	0.680	0.241
3–0	1.130	0.318
2–0	1.180	0.406
1–0	2.500	0.495
1	3.400	0.584
2	4.080	0.673
3	5.220	0.762
4	5.900	0.864
5	7.260	0.978

    b. *Nonabsorbable* sutures are not destroyed by inflammatory reaction. (They may be partially degraded over many years.)
    c. *Natural* sutures are made of materials derived from biologic sources. They are predominantly formed from collagen and other proteins.
    d. *Synthetic* sutures are made of materials that do not occur in nature but are synthesized usually as polymers (nylon, Dacron).
2. Physical form
    a. *Monofilament versus multifilament.* A suture can be made as a monofilament nonbraided suture or as a multifilament braided suture. In general, the monofilament sutures are stronger and less reactive and have a lower infection rate, but do not handle as well and are more likely to result in knot slippage. The opposite is true of the braided multifilament sutures. They are generally more reactive and have a higher infection rate, but have superior handling and tying qualities. Of the absorbable sutures, catgut and chromic catgut are nonbraided sutures, whereas Vicryl and Dexon are braided multifilament sutures. Nylon and polypropylene are usually made as a monofilament suture but are available in a woven form. Wire is available either as a monofilament or a braided multifilament.

       For most soft tissue injuries the monofilament or absorbable sutures are preferred because of lesser reactivity and infection. Nonetheless, braided multifilament silk sutures have many advocates and can be used successfully.
    b. *Coated sutures.* Multifilament braided sutures have specific adverse characteristics (increased reactivity and infection because of the interstices between filaments). Therefore, in an attempt to avoid these problems yet maintain the advantages of multifilament sutures (better handling and less knot slippage), many multifilament sutures are coated with Teflon or silicone. The various coated multifilament sutures are listed in Table 2-3.

PREOPERATIVE PREPARATION

Table 2-4. Recommended suture strengths for specific tissues

Tissue	Shear strength (kg)	Recommended suture strength
Tendon (perpendicular)	40.0	4–0
Tendon (longitudinal)	0.5	6–0
Fascia (muscular)	22.0	2–0, 4–0
Dermis	19.0	4–0, 5–0
Muscle	6.0	5–0
Fat (areolar fascia)	1.0	5–0, 6–0
Nerve (epineurium)	7.0	6–0
Nerve (perineurium)	7.0	8–0, 10–0

STRENGTH OF SUTURES

1. **In vitro standards.** The U.S. Pharmacopeia has established minimal standards for strength of suture materials. Separate standards for absorbable, nonabsorbable, and metallic materials have been established. Suture strength is the basis for the number designation (e.g., 4–0) and is measured by the force that is required to break the suture. The weakest suture is designated as 10–0. Furthermore, a minimum and maximum diameter for suture material are also required (Table 2-3). Most sutures for emergency room use are 6–0, 5–0, and 4–0.

2. **In vivo dynamics.** The breaking strength is measured in an in vitro system, and additional consideration therefore must be given to what happens in a healing wound. Four other variables that must be considered are (1) the rate of suture degradation in tissues, and thus, loss of suture strength; (2) the resistance of normal tissues to tearing (shearing); (3) knot slippage; and (4) increasing strength of the wound.

   a. Loss of strength of absorbable suture
      (1) **Catgut.** A distinction must be made between in vivo physical presence of suture material and its actual in vivo strength. For example, catgut may be physically identifiable within the wound many weeks after implantation. However, it loses 50 percent of its strength within 3 to 7 days, and 100 percent of its strength within 10 to 21 days.
      (2) **Chromic catgut.** The method and degree of cross-linking of the collagen with chromic salts is responsible for variability of strength for different trade names of chromic catgut. Reports vary from 5 to 10 percent loss of strength to retention of 70% strength at 14 days.
      (3) **Glycolics.** Contradictory evidence has also been reported regarding longevity and loss of strength of glycolic materials. Between 10 and 70 percent loss of strength has been reported at 14 days.

   b. **Resistance of normal tissues to tearing (shearing).** If a strong force distracts the wound, either the tissue or the suture breaks. Each tissue has a measurable force that it can tolerate before it begins to tear. Table 2-4 lists this parameter for most tissues. The resistance to a shearing type of force depends on the tissue and the relation of the suture to the fiber orientation of the tissue. For example, a tendon (which has a longitudinal fiber orientation) can withstand a force of

20 to 40 kg if the tension is perpendicular to the tendon fibers, but it can only withstand a force of 0.25 to 0.50 kg if the pull is parallel with the tendon fibers.

Sutures of adequate but not excessive strength for the tissues should be chosen. When the strength of specific sutures is compared to tissue shearing, the following conclusions can be made.

(1) Fat will tear before a 6–0 suture will break. Therefore, there is no rationale for using a suture stronger than 6–0 in fat. Nonetheless, it is common to use 5–0, 4–0, or 3–0 sutures in fat. In part, this is because of the relative simplicity of tying larger suture, but primarily it is because the stitch is also being passed through areolar fascia or other layers of the wound closure that permit the use of stronger sutures for approximation.

(2) Muscle will tear before a 4–0 suture will break. Therefore, there is no value using a suture stronger than 4–0 for muscle approximation. However, because the strength in muscle repair is obtained by closure of muscle fascia, a stronger suture can be used in the fascia. We recommend a 4–0 or 5–0 suture for most fascial closures in small muscles or fat that is not under tension, and a 2–0 to 3–0 suture for fascia under moderate tension or around large muscle groups. If tensions of greater magnitude are exerted on a healing wound, other manipulations such as undermining or immobilization may be of greater importance than strength of the suture.

(3) Dermis can withstand a shearing force of approximately 19 kg before it tears. This is approximately the strength of a #1 suture. Nonetheless, we never use a #1 suture for dermal closures. The disadvantages of excessive tissue reactivity and suture marks contraindicate the use of a #1 suture.

For skin closures in which there is no tissue loss and therefore no unusual tissue tension, a 4–0, 5–0, or 6–0 suture has adequate strength.

c. **Knot slippage.** Sutures vary in ease of handling and tendency for knot slippage and unraveling. Knot security is a result of contact friction. The braided multifilament materials are easy to handle, and knots can be tied securely with the least risk of unraveling. This quality has made silk and cotton popular among many surgeons.

Absorbable sutures tend to be less flexible and have a marked tendency to unravel when they absorb water from the wound. Therefore, special care to use only square knots when using catgut, chromic, Dexon, and Vicryl is indicated. Vicryl and Dexon handle more like silk suture because of their multifilament characteristic.

The monofilament nonabsorbable sutures of nylon and polypropylene tend to be quite stiff and difficult to hand tie, but are not more difficult than braided material if an instrument tie is used.

It is essential that a square knot be used if maximum friction is to be achieved and unraveling prevented. For most materials, four throws of a square knot are adequate. Three square knots or two square and two granny (slip) knots reduce the knot security. The method for tying a square knot is described in Chapter 3.

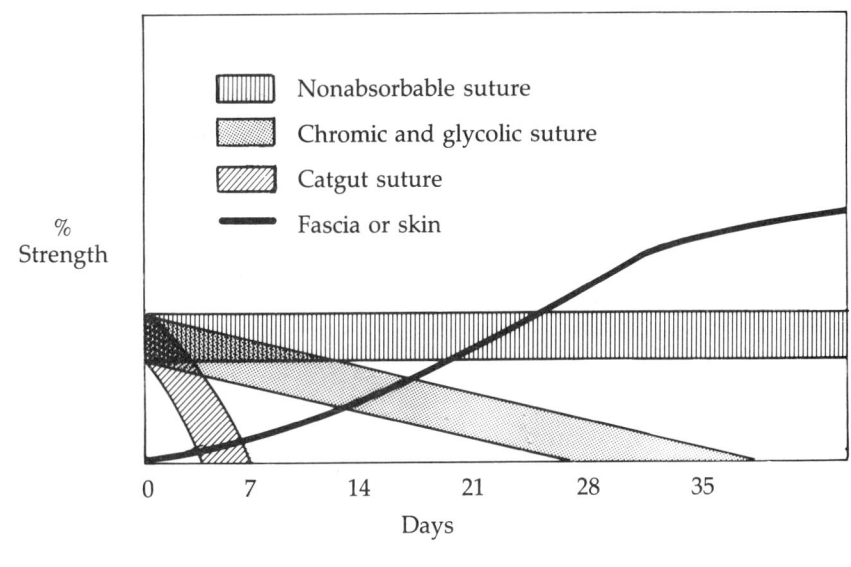

Figure 2-9. Strength of healing wound versus suture over a period of approximately 5 weeks. Approximate variations in percentage of original strength of several categories of suture materials are plotted against length of time in the wound. The strength of catgut suture and chromic and glycolic suture diminishes over a period of time in the wound, the strength of catgut suture decreasing precipitously in the first week. The strength of nonabsorbable suture remains relatively unchanged by contact with the wound. Between the fourth and fifth week of healing, however, the strength of the wound collagen exceeds even the strength of chromic sutures.

d. Increasing strength of the healing wound. All tissues heal at different rates. Skin (dermis), fascia, and tendon are relatively slow healing and never regain the strength of the original unwounded tissue. On the other hand, bowel and bladder rapidly regain their strength and in some instances become stronger than the original normal tissues. Because wound strength is determined from animal studies, variations between animal and human tissues make wound strength studies inexact. The strength curves depicted in Fig. 2-9 are from rabbit or rat skin rather than from human studies.

(1) *Catgut* loses its strength rapidly and is stronger than the wound for no more than 7 days. Thereafter, the healing wound provides greater resistance to disruption than does the suture. Catgut sutures should not be used if movement or tension would disrupt the wound after 1 week. Therefore, catgut is used only when tension is not a major factor. Its primary uses are for ligating blood vessels and mucosal closure.

(2) *Chromic catgut, Dexon,* and *Vicryl* are stronger than the wound until 10 to 21 days. Thereafter, the tensile strength of the wound is greater than the rapidly decreasing strength of these absorbable sutures. Therefore, these suture materials are quite adequate for nearly all dermal and subcutaneous wound closures.

(3) *Nylon, wire,* and *silk* of the recommended strength are stronger than the healing wound for 20 to 30 days. Thereafter, the strength of the wound collagen is greater than the strength of the suture material. If normal wound healing has not occurred by the third or fourth week, the usual result is sutures pulling through the tissue caused by the combination of excessive tension and collagenolysis related to cellular inflammation and infection.

REACTIVITY OF SUTURE

Ideally, a suture material should have minimal reactivity. The importance of suture reactivity to clinical applications is twofold. First, the more intense the foreign body reaction to the suture, the more quickly the suture is absorbed and loses strength. This relation is discussed fully in the section on wound strength. Second, a more intense and prolonged reaction causes more scar formation and greater frequency of extrusion through or around the wound ("spitting").

1. Extremely reactive suture. *Catgut* induces a rapid reaction of a typical foreign body–macrophage type. Strength is lost in 5 to 7 days, and scar formation is extensive; thus catgut should not be used for skin closure except in noncosmetic areas or possibly in children in whom suture removal is a problem.
2. Moderately reactive suture. *Silk, cotton, and linen* are biologic, nonabsorbable sutures that induce a moderately severe foreign body reaction. The reaction is somewhat delayed and less intense than in catgut but persists for many months or years after implantation. The reactivity of these sutures is caused by the greater surface area of the braided filaments. If the sutures are removed within 7 days after skin implantation, the amount of reaction is minimal; therefore this suture is satisfactory for skin closure. However, the high degree of reactivity makes it undesirable for subdermal closure, nerve repair, tendon repair, and vascular repair.
3. Minimally reactive suture. *Chromic catgut, Dexon,* and *Vicryl* show minimal inflammatory reaction for 10 to 30 days. Their behavior is more like a nonabsorbable suture during that time interval. Chromic catgut is then slowly absorbed by a foreign body–macrophage response. Dexon and Vicryl show very minimal foreign body reaction and no observable absorption of suture for 28 to 30 days, despite the fact that suture strength has been greatly reduced. Enzymatic hydrolysis disrupts the cross-linking of the glycolic acid with minimal foreign body reaction. The suture is nearly 100 percent absorbed after 80 to 120 days. The amount of fibrous tissue around the suture site is minimal.
4. Least reactive suture. *Monofilament wire, nylon,* and *polypropylene,* the monofilament, synthetic nonabsorbable sutures, are the least reactive. A minimal inflammatory response is seen at 7 days, and a minimal fibrosis surrounds the suture thereafter.

INFECTION

One of the differences among suture materials is the frequency of "stitch abscess." Suture infection is primarily the result of the multifilament configuration rather than the type of material.

All wounds have some bacterial contamination. Usually the contamination is controlled by the host, and there is no clinical infection. However, suture material can tilt this balance in favor of the bacteria by providing a physical hiding place within the interstices of the suture. The bacteria are capable of filling these interstices, but the larger polymorphonuclear cells and macrophages cannot enter the spaces within a suture. Infection persists until the suture is extruded from the wound or surgically removed. The incidence of suture infection is as follows:

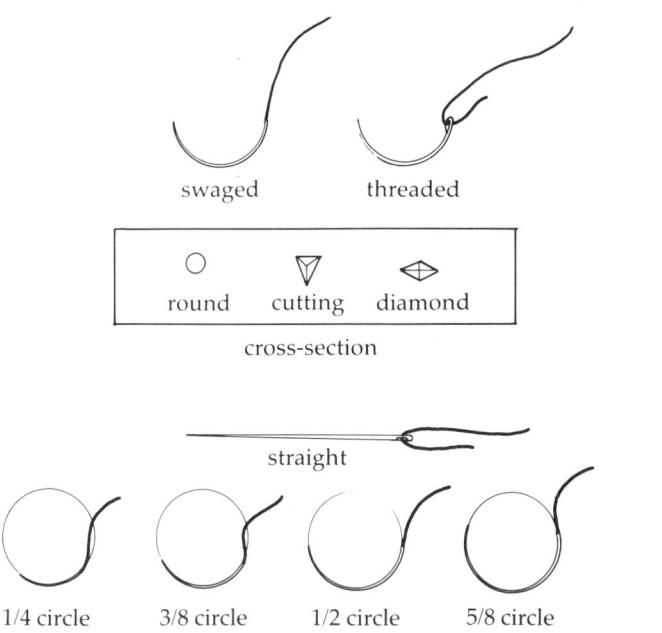

Figure 2-10. Various needles commonly used for introducing suture materials into tissue.

1. Highest infection risk. Multifilament, nonabsorbable sutures present the greatest risk for suture abscess because of the physical characteristics of multifilament suture. Furthermore, because these sutures are not absorbed, the infection persists until the suture is extruded or removed.
2. Intermediate infection risk. The braided absorbable sutures provide a potential nidus for bacterial contamination and growth, but because they are rapidly absorbed by a foreign body reaction, the infection may spontaneously resolve as the foreign material is absorbed and the cellular defenses gain access to the suture interstices.
3. Minimal infection risk. The monofilament, nonabsorbable and absorbable sutures have the least risk of infection. Thus, in areas of potential contamination, absorbable monofilament sutures are most desirable.

CHOICE OF SUTURES

We recommend that suture materials be chosen as follows, on the basis of biologic characteristics.

1. Subcutaneous-subdermal closure
   a. Contaminated—Dexon, Vicryl, or chromic catgut
   b. Noncontaminated—clear monofilament nylon or Dexon, Vicryl, or chromic catgut
   c. Nerves—monofilament nylon, polypropylene
   d. Tendon—monofilament nylon, polypropylene, or wire
   e. Blood vessels—monofilament nylon or polypropylene
2. Skin closure
   a. Facial or other "cosmetic" areas—monofilament synthetic suture (nylon, polypropylene)
   b. Extremities or "noncosmetic" areas—monofilament nylon or silk

c. Genitalia, mucous membranes (oral, nasal, perineal)—chromic catgut, catgut
d. Perioral vermilion, eyelid margin—silk (the softer silk does not irritate cornea or lips)

Needles

Suture materials can be introduced into tissue with various kinds of needles (Fig. 2-10). Decisions must be made regarding the method of attachment of suture to needle (swaged or threaded), type of point (round, tapered, or cutting), shape (straight or curved), and size.

TYPE OF ATTACHMENT

With few exceptions the *swaged needles*, in which the suture is embedded in the needle hub, are preferable. Because they are not resterilized and reused as threaded needles, they tend to be much sharper. Also, the junction of needle and suture is smooth, whereas threaded needles are bulky and tend to tear and pull through tissue.

TYPE OF POINT

The *cutting needles* are much easier to pass through tissue with very little force than are needles with tapered points. With cutting needles, more attention can be directed to precision of placement rather than to forcing the needle through the tissues.

SHAPE

For skin closure, a ⅜ or ½ circle is most effective. *For tendon repair*, the straight needle has distinct advantages for the internal Bunnel, or mattress, technique. (A curved needle is used for the circumferential closure of tendons.) *For vascular repair*, a ¼ circle or straight needle is effective.

SIZE

The choice of needle size is influenced by the size of suture required to maintain tension and the thickness of tissue.

For example, thin skin such as the face or eyelid is best repaired with a small needle. Thick skin of the back or abdomen requires a medium-sized needle. Unfortunately, there is no standard designation of needle sizes. Each company has its own designations, as the following examples show:

Small needles for skin (facial)
    Ethicon P 1–3, PS 2–5, C2–3
    Davis & Geck PRE 1–3, CE 21–23
    Deknatel RE 1–2

Medium needles (trunk)
    Ethicon PS 2–3
    Davis & Geck PRE 4–6, CE 4, 10, T3–5
    Deknatel

LOCAL ANESTHETICS

Local anesthesia can be attained by topical application or injection of medications, cooling, acupuncture, or hypnosis. The advantages of local anesthesia are that the patient maintains a state of mental awareness and cooperation, posttreatment hospitalization is not required, and most techniques are easily mastered.

The most useful technique is the injection of a local anesthetic in and around the wound. The emphasis in this section is on the principles and methods of injectable anesthetics.

Mechanism of Action

Local anesthetics cause a sequential loss of specific sensory modalities. Functions return in the reverse order. Following the injection of a local anesthetic, loss of and changes in sensory function typically proceed as follows:

Two-point discrimination
Pain
Light touch
Paresthesias
Pressure
Proprioception

Thus, the anesthetized patient may be aware of pressure and movement but have no pain. To relieve anxiety, therefore, it is important to tell the patient about this stage.

Classification (Chemical Composition)

All local anesthetic agents have three component parts:

1. An *aromatic acid* (lipophilic portion)—the portion that binds to the lipoprotein membrane
2. An *ester* or an *amide*—the portion of the anesthetic agent that determines its antigenicity and also is a means of classification or grouping
3. A *tertiary amine group*—the hydrophilic portion

Table 2-5 classifies local anesthetic agents and indicates important characteristics.

The Addition of Vasoconstrictors (Epinephrine)

ADVANTAGES
Vasoconstrictors can be a useful adjunct. The advantages of the vasoconstrictive effect of epinephrine include the reduction of bleeding, prolongation of duration of the anesthetic, allowance of a larger volume of anesthetic, and reduction of the possibility of systemic toxic reaction because of reduced absorption.

Table 2-5. Characteristics and applications of available local anesthetic drugs

Chemical and American brand name	Topical	Maximum dosage (infiltration or peripheral nerve blocks)
Esters		
Procaine	Ineffective	
Novocaine		200 ml of 0.5% = 1000 mg
Planocaine		100 ml of 1.0% = 1000 mg
Scurocaine		50 ml of 2.0% = 1000 mg
		(15 mg/kg)
Chloroprocaine	Ineffective	Same as procaine
Nesicaine		
Tetracaine	URT = 2% spray	10 ml of 1% = 100 mg
Pontocaine	2 ml = 40 mg	Do not exceed 200 mg or a 0.25% concentration
Amethocaine		(1.5 mg/kg)
Cocaine	3 ml of 4% = 120 mg	Should not be used
Hexycaine	2 ml of 5% = 100 mg	100 ml of 0.5% = 500 mg
Cyclaine		50 ml of 1.0% = 500 mg
		25 ml of 2.0% = 500 mg
Amides		
Lidocaine	URT = 2% spray	100 ml of 0.5% = 500 mg
Xylocaine	4 ml = 80 mg	50 ml of 1.0% = 500 mg
Lignocaine	2.5% topical ointment	25 ml of 2.0% − 500 mg
	Oral 2% viscous	(7 mg/kg)
	Xylocaine 30 ml	
Mepivacaine	Same as lidocaine	Same as lidocaine
Carbocaine		
Bupivacaine		
Marcaine		
Dibucaine	0.5%–1% topical ointment	
Nupercaine		
Cinchocaine		

DISADVANTAGES

There are numerous disadvantages and specific contraindications to the use of epinephrine, including systemic and local reactions.

1. Systemic reactions. Epinephrine has an adverse systemic effect in specific patients. It is absorbed from the site of local injection and may have a direct cardiac or peripheral vascular effect.
   a. Type of effect
      (1) Because it causes *cardiac irritability*, epinephrine may be contraindicated in patients with cardiac arrhythmias or those having general anesthesia with fluorinated hydrocarbons such as halothane.
      (2) Its peripheral vasoconstrictive effect may cause a systemic labile *hypertension*, which induces additional bleeding.
   b. The symptoms and signs of epinephrine sensitivity or overdose are headache, nervousness, sweating, anxiety, tremor, weakness, pallor, fear, palpitations, nausea, or tachycardia.
      If these signs occur, the following precautions should be taken:
      (1) The patient should be carefully observed, with *ECG monitoring*.
      (2) Frequent *blood pressures* should be taken.
      (3) An intravenous line should be inserted.

Table 2-5. (Continued)

Duration	Onset (local infiltration and nerve blocks)	Uses	Special considerations
30–60 minutes	2–5 minutes	Rare, except in dentistry	Short duration Low potency with occasional ineffective block
30–60 minutes	1–3 minutes	Same as above	Same as above
4–6 hours	15–45 minutes	Spinal anesthesia Topical cornea-conjunctiva	Slow onset but long duration
1 hour	1–2 minutes	Intranasal (it is exceptional vasoconstrictor)	Carefully wring out cotton pledgets
45–60 minutes	5 minutes	Intraoral	
1–2 hours with epinephrine 1.5–3 hours	15–30 minutes	Most local infiltration and nerve blocks	Relatively toxic; can cause CNS convulsions and cardiac depression
Same as above	Same as above	Same as above	
12–36 hours	30–45 minutes	Nerve blocks Long procedure	Very prolonged effect Good for postoperative pain
30–60 minutes	5 minutes	Topical Intraoral Perianal	

2. Local reactions
   a. Tissue ischemia. Epinephrine may reduce the viability of tissue because of its local ischemic effect; tissue of marginal viability is more likely to undergo necrosis. Skin flaps that are elevated using Xylocaine with epinephrine have less tissue survival than comparable skin flaps elevated using Xylocaine alone.

   Epinephrine injected at the site of terminal end-arteries, such as the digits and penis, may have extensive and prolonged vasoconstriction leading to necrosis. Although some sources state that an ischemic effect can occur on the nose and ears, our experience indicates there is no contraindication to epinephrine use anywhere on the face.
   b. Infection. There is a higher incidence of infection in wounds injected with 1:50,000 to 1:200,000 epinephrine than in those injected with Xylocaine alone. However, 1:800,000 epinephrine results in an infection rate comparable to that of Xylocaine alone. These studies were performed in animals; comparable results may not occur in humans.

CONTRAINDICATIONS AND PRECAUTIONS FOR EPINEPHRINE
Epinephrine should not be used in the following patients or situations:

Patients with hypertension
Patients with cardiac ischemic disease or arrhythmias

Contaminated wounds with high risk of infection
Ischemic wounds with marginally viable tissue
Wounds of the digits and penis
Allergy to the preservative in local anesthetics with epinephrine, which in most local anesthetics with epinephrine is metabisulfite

CHOOSING THE BEST CONCENTRATION OF EPINEPHRINE
Concentrations of 1:400,000 epinephrine, and in some circumstances 1:800,000, provide a vasoconstrictor effect without provoking the side effects that may appear with concentrations of 1:50,000 or 1:100,000. It is preferable to add fresh epinephrine without preservative to the local anesthetic rather than use the commercially prepared 1:50,000 to 1:200,000 solutions that must be diluted with saline or plain Xylocaine. The following dose schedule can be used for calculating epinephrine concentrations: 0.1 ml of 1:1,000 epinephrine is drawn into a tuberculin syringe and added to 40 ml of Xylocaine to give 1:400,000 epinephrine.

Reactions to Local Anesthetics

Reactions to local anesthetics are quite common, but most are minor and unnoticed or misinterpreted as nervousness on the part of the patient. The reactions can be categorized in the following manner.

ALLERGY
True allergy to local anesthetic agents is extremely rare and virtually limited to the ester-linked group (procaine, novocaine, tetracaine). Hypersensitivity to the ester group also may be a manifestation of sensitivity to the chemically related paraaminobenzoic acid derivatives used as a preservative. Paraben compounds belong to this group and may be used as preservatives in multidose bottles of amide-linked local anesthetics (Xylocaine) but not in single-dose ampules. In patients with proven ester-group hypersensitivity, therefore, ampules of the amide group rather than bottles should be used.

1. Signs and symptoms. Generalized angioneurotic edema, urticaria, and pruritus are the most common allergic reactions. An anaphylactic reaction with bronchoconstriction and dyspnea or a serum sickness reaction with joint pain and fever may occur.
2. Treatment. If an allergic reaction is suspected, the appropriate treatment includes antihistamines (diphenhydramine [Benadryl] 50 mg IM or IV) and oxygen by mask. If an anaphylactic-type reaction is occurring, use a 1:10,000 solution of adrenaline 0.1 to 0.2 ml subcutaneous plus a steroid hydrocortisone (Solu-Cortef) 100 to 200 mg intravenously.

CARDIOVASCULAR REACTIONS
1. Cause. Xylocaine and other local anesthetic agents are cardiovascular depressants when blood levels reach 7 μg per ml.
2. Signs and symptoms. Bradycardia, hypotension, and cardiovascular arrest are the signs and symptoms of cardiovascular reaction to local anesthetics.
3. Treatment. Initial watchful waiting, careful monitoring, and an intrave-

nous line may be all that is necessary. If bradycardia and hypotension persist, or if there is cardiac arrest, appropriate cardiopulmonary therapy is required.

VASOVAGAL REACTIONS (FAINTING)

1. Cause. The patient may be extremely anxious and, if not adequately sedated, may faint. It is important to distinguish between a vasovagal response caused by anxiety and a cardiovascular collapse from a direct toxic reaction. Because this distinction is not immediately apparent, it is best to prepare for cardiopulmonary resuscitation until the cause can be determined. A bradycardia is more commonly associated with syncope.
2. Treatment. If the patient has fainted, one should use oxygen by mask, lower the head of the table, elevate the lower extremities, and place an intravenous line if one is not already present.

CENTRAL NERVOUS SYSTEM TOXICITY

The principal systemic toxic effect of local anesthetics occurs in the central nervous system. The second systemic toxic effect is a direct myocardial depression. Toxicity is caused by a high blood level. It can be from inadvertent intravenous injection or rapid absorption from highly vascularized areas such as the face or scalp, leading to an immediate type of reaction, or secondary to a slow build-up of a toxic blood level with reaction delayed 5 to 30 minutes following injection.

1. Depressive reactions
   a. Signs and symptoms. Depressive reactions occur with lower blood levels than stimulation reactions. There is decreased blood pressure, slowed respiration, and drowsiness.
   b. Treatment. Give oxygen IV fluids, elevating legs and lowering head. Use a vasoconstrictor if hypotension persists (ephedrine 25–50 mg IV)
2. Stimulation reactions
   a. Signs and symptoms
      (1) Mild stimulation reactions involve talkativeness, increased blood pressure, increased pulse rate, and anxiety.
      (2) Moderate reactions involve restlessness, headaches, blurred vision, irritability, and slight tremor.
      (3) Severe reactions involve convulsions.
   b. Treatment. Mild reactions usually can be treated with oxygen alone and watchfulness for a progression into frank convulsions. During that time, it is important to provide an adequate airway and prepare for possible seizures. If moderate seizures or reactions occur, an initial intravenous injection of 5 to 10 mg of diazepam (Valium) is given. Additional diazepam can be given at 5-minute intervals. If seizures continue, intravenous injection of barbiturate, 100 mg thiopental (Pentothal) or amobarbital (Amytal) can be given. If seizures continue after administration of barbiturates or diazepam, maintenance of an airway and oxygenation are essential. Be sure at this point that there is no associated cardiovascular collapse. If an anesthetist is available, and a status epilepticus has occurred, the use of succinylcholine and endotracheal intubation may be necessary.

This type of reaction requiring intubation and succinylcholine is extremely rare, and these measures should be used only as a last resort.

Avoidance of Reactions to Local Anesthetics

SEDATION
Diazepam prevents convulsions in experimental animals, whereas the barbiturates have little or no effect. Premedication with diazepam is indicated when close to toxic levels of local anesthetics are to be used.

MINIMIZATION OF DOSE
Do not exceed the recommended dose. Remember that toxic doses stated in milligrams represent limits for adult males; most overdoses are seen in children and small adults because of failure to adjust the dose.

AVOIDANCE OF INTRAVENOUS INJECTION
Avoid intravenous injections by aspirating before injection. If injecting in a vascular area, such as into the brachial plexus, aspirate frequently (at least following each 50 mg of injected agent).

AVOIDANCE OF RAPID INJECTION OF LARGE VOLUMES
If possible, inject anesthetics over a prolonged period or inject in divided doses as each area is treated.

Treating Cardiac Complications—CPR

If there is a non–life threatening reaction with minimal symptomatology, careful observation with ECG monitoring, frequent blood pressures, and preparation for potential cardiac arrest are required. The treatment of cardiac arrhythmias or cardiac arrest is the same as for any other cardiopulmonary resuscitation. An outline of the protocol used at the Stanford University Hospital is provided as a guideline to treatment.

INITIAL CARE BEFORE AVAILABILITY OF ASSISTANTS, MONITORING DEVICES, AND RESUSCITATION EQUIPMENT
1. Evaluate patient.
2. Begin CPR and summon help.
3. With absent pulse and blood pressure, patient may be in ventricular fibrillation or asystole; a registered nurse may deliver a single quick light blow to the chest.
4. Apply ECG leads as soon as possible.
5. Start and keep open IV of D_5W.
6. Request blood gas technician.

In the event that resuscitation is not successful after a reasonable period of time and the personal physician is not in attendance, the physician in charge may call for cessation of resuscitation procedures.

When effective heartbeat is established, attention should be given to vital signs, fluid and electrolyte balance, indicated laboratory determinations (e.g., blood gases), and general care. All patients should have a portable chest x-ray done and should be admitted to the hospital, preferably to a specialty unit such as a coronary care unit.

3. SIMPLE LACERATIONS

The management of a simple tidy wound is presented here in four phases:

1. Initial assessment and categorization of wound
2. Preliminary wound preparation
3. Local anesthesia
4. Wound suturing

WOUND ASSESSMENT

Categorization of Wounds

The initial assessment categorizes the wound as a simple tidy wound by its configuration and location. We define a simple laceration by the following criteria:

The laceration is linear, perpendicular to the skin surface, and not complicated by the anatomic site (it is not complex)
It has clean margins that do not require debridement (it is a tidy wound)
There is no damage to other anatomic structures (it is not compound)
The laceration is of recent origin (less than 6 hours) and has no major contamination (it is a clean wound)
There is no tissue loss (there is no amputation)

Although a wound may be a simple, tidy wound in terms of its geometric configuration, special consideration must be given to its location and cause because of risk of unrecognized contamination. A separate assessment for hemostasis is also needed before a decision is made to suture the simple wound.

Assessment of Contamination

MECHANISM OF INJURY
The severity of contamination with debris and bacteria is affected by the mechanism of injury. For example, most home injuries are clean, whereas most injuries from farm machinery and outdoor accidents are contaminated.

Tidy wounds are usually clean, whereas untidy wounds are usually contaminated; yet even the tidiest appearing wound may represent severe contamination. Disastrous infections occur from closing a human bite over a joint. Contaminated wounds must be treated like untidy wounds with debridement of contaminated tissue and/or copious irrigation. For example, an acute animal or human puncture bite of the cheek is best treated by excising the entire contaminated wound and primarily closing the wound.

TIME SINCE INJURY—THE "GOLDEN PERIOD"
The age of the wound is somewhat related to its categorization as clean or contaminated. The concept of the "golden period" developed empirically

as physicians recognized that the incidence of wound infection increased when wound closure was delayed beyond 6 to 8 hours. After 6 to 8 hours, the probability of infection is sufficiently great that many surgical texts recommend that the wound not be primarily closed. It should be debrided and irrigated or allowed to heal by secondary intention (if the wound is small and is in a noncosmetic site), or should undergo delayed closure (3–5 days) if the wound is large or located in a conspicuous area. This golden period represents the time required for bacteria to reach a logarithmic growth rate and high concentration.

Wound preparation by debridement, irrigation, and judicious use of bactericidal antibiotics has extended the golden period of wound closure beyond 6 hours. With these adjuncts, a minimally contaminated tidy wound can be closed up to 24 hours postinjury. At the other extreme, with severe contamination, untidiness, and an unfavorable location, a golden period does not exist. For example, human bites over a joint should never be closed primarily.

CULTURES AND SMEARS

A quantitative relation between wound infection and bacterial contamination has been described. Closure of a wound with a bacterial count greater than 10^5 organisms per gram of tissue frequently results in infection and dehiscence. A tidy wound with less than 10^5 organisms per gram of tissue can be expected to heal. However, the 24- to 36-hour delay for culture results precludes its use in the emergency department setting. The quick method for emergency department use involves biopsy of a small amount of tissue (1–2 mm^3) from the wound and examination of a smear of this tissue under the high-power objective microscope. If greater than one organism per high-power field is found, the bacterial count is greater than 10^5 organisms.

FINAL ASSESSMENT REGARDING CLOSURE

A final assessment should provide the answer to the question, "Should the wound be closed?" Only guidelines can be offered because each instance must be individualized.

1. Tidy clean wounds should be closed primarily.
2. Untidy contaminated wounds that can be converted into tidy wounds can be closed (or covered with skin grafts or skin flaps).
3. Untidy, contaminated wounds that cannot be converted into tidy wounds are best treated with a sterile dressing, or biologic dressing (skin graft, allograft, or xenograft). Early inspection and reassessment may allow delayed closure or coverage.

PRELIMINARY WOUND PREPARATION

Following initial assessment of the injury, treatment of the wound begins. Several general principles govern the initial care of all wounds. The goal is to establish an optimum wound environment to assist the defense mechanisms in preventing infection and to assist wound healing. Proper care of simple wounds includes hemostasis, irrigation and debridement, and the

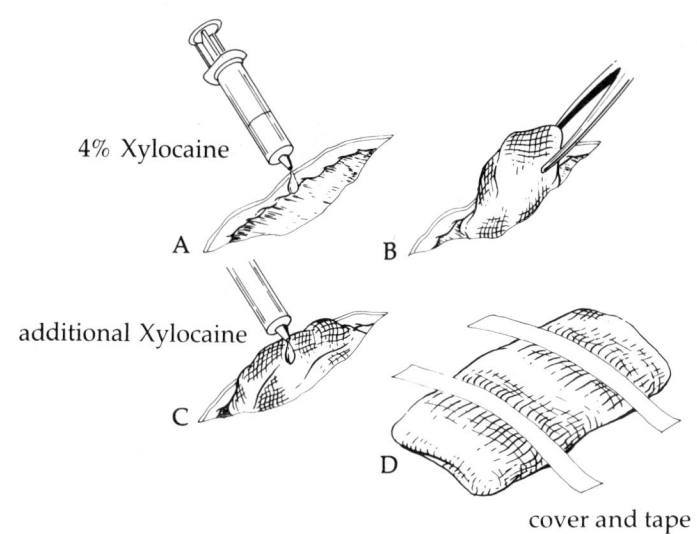

Figure 3-1.
A and B. Topical anesthesia is achieved by instillation of 2 to 5 ml of 4% Xylocaine in the wound saturated in a gauze pack.
C. Additional Xylocaine is added 5 to 10 minutes later.
D. A gauze pad is taped firmly over the wound (or wrap the wound) for 5 to 20 minutes.

decision either to close the wound immediately or to delay wound closure. Failure in attention to detail in these maneuvers leads to a suboptimal wound milieu and a compromised result in even the simplest lacerations. Preliminary topical anesthesia is helpful.

Topical Anesthesia Pack

The open wound can be packed to avoid airborne contamination and achieve topical anesthesia. The packing also helps control persistent bleeding. Topical anesthetics penetrate 1 to 2 mm, allow initial wound evaluation and irrigation, and lessen the discomfort of the wound and later needle injection and infiltration.

Figure 3-1 depicts the steps for application of a topical anesthesia pack. Topical anesthesia is achieved by soaking cotton gauze with a few milliliters of 4% Xylocaine and packing into the wound. Additional Xylocaine should be added 5 to 10 minutes later. Then gauze should be firmly taped in place over the wound, or the wound should be wrapped for 5 to 20 minutes. The anesthetic does not affect intact skin but does penetrate abrasions and lacerations. In fact, most dermabrasions can be carried out with only topical anesthesia.

Hemostasis

For most wounds, bleeding stops spontaneously within 5 to 15 minutes following injury. If bleeding persists, the reason must be determined and specific therapeutic steps undertaken. The principal causes of persistent bleeding may be categorized as either local factors (anatomic or mechanical) with normal clot formation or defects in the hemostatic coagulation systems.

LOCAL FACTORS—NORMAL CLOTTING

If there is no known history of bleeding abnormalities, if blood is forming a normal clot, and if bleeding is localized or pulsatile, there is a presumptive diagnosis of a local mechanical problem, usually caused by one of the following events:

1. Obvious major vessel. Transection or partial transection of a major vessel can cause profuse bleeding from deep within a wound. Hemorrhage from a completely transected vessel may cease as vessel retraction and vascular spasm progress. A partially transected vessel cannot retract and may continue to bleed vigorously.
   Treatment involves:
   a. Direct pressure with a small gauze pad or with the gloved finger, which will control most major vessel hemorrhages. Smaller vessels may cease bleeding following 5 minutes of such pressure.
   b. Ligation or electrocoagulation of vessels that continue to hemorrhage following pressure. This situation requires local anesthesia; surgical exposure of the bleeding site; and either repair, ligation, or electrocoagulation.
2. Multiple small vessels. *Excessive movement* of the injured part may disrupt the platelet plug and clot in small vessels. This may be caused by skin scrub, patient movement, or surgical manipulation.
   Treatment involves immobilizing the wound with a splint or gauze wrap. Do not repeatedly wipe the wound nor frequently remove the initial dressing to inspect the wound.
3. Arterial hypertension. An initially dry wound that later bleeds is frequently associated with an increase in blood pressure secondary to anxiety or pain. Continuous bleeding, especially in elderly patients, is often associated with arteriosclerotic vascular disease and hypertension. The arteriosclerotic vessels do not undergo adequate vasoconstriction, and elevated pressure dislodges the platelet clump.
   Treatment involves:
   a. Simple reassurance to alleviate anxiety
   b. Control of pain with either narcotic analgesics or local anesthetics. Contraindications to the use of analgesics should be identified early in the initial evaluation (e.g., associated neurologic, pulmonary, or abdominal injury).
   c. Prolonged pressure and electrocoagulation for pathologic arteriosclerotic hypertension. Hypotensive medications are rarely if ever required.
4. Venous hypertension. A wound in a gravitation-dependent position may ooze diffusely from capillaries. This usually affects the lower extremity or distal upper extremity. Venous hypertension is treated simply by elevating the bleeding extremity above heart level.

COAGULATION DISORDERS

Although a normal clot may appear in the wound, there may be a failure to form and maintain the intravascular platelet plug or achieve adequate coagulation.

The hemostatic clotting disorder must be evaluated before surgical closure. The methods of diagnosis and treatment of bleeding, although partially described in Chapter 1, are not the subject of this text.* If major

---

*A useful reference is *Clinical Hematology*, 7th ed., by M. M. Wintrobe (Philadelphia: Lea & Febiger, 1976).

bleeding occurs, appropriate consultation should be obtained. A decision must be made either to close the wound or to pack it until the disorder is treated. This is often a difficult decision and must be tempered by the location and type of wound, as well as the severity of the bleeding.

Wound Irrigation

Even simple lacerations require local irrigation to remove foreign material and bacteria.

METHODS

Almost any mechanical cleansing method is useful, although high-pressure methods are most effective. A surgical scrub brush, toothbrush, or sponge may be used in conjunction with mechanical irrigation to facilitate removal of foreign material. The following methods are commonly used:

1. Low-pressure syringes. A bulb syringe or even the same syringe used to inject local anesthesia can be used for irrigation.
2. IV setups. For prolonged irrigation of contaminated wounds, an intravenous tubing can be attached to a bottle of isotonic saline suspended from an IV pole so that gravity provides a forceful stream to irrigate the wound. A pinch clamp controls the flow.
3. High-pressure nozzles. Some emergency rooms are equipped with a device similar to a waterpik that uses pulses of sterile saline to irrigate wounds.

SOLUTIONS

Many antibiotic and antiseptic irrigants are available, but in the open wound all cause some degree of tissue damage or interfere with host defense mechanisms.

1. Antiseptics. A few agents appear to be effective antiseptics (povidone-iodine, chlorhexidine), and if followed by isotonic saline irrigation, they apparently cause little tissue damage.
2. Antibiotics. Antibiotic irrigations are not usually necessary except for severely contaminated wounds, such as human bites. Antibiotics such as polymyxin, bacitracin, neomycin, or a cephalosporin can be instilled in the wound without subsequent saline irrigation.

VOLUME OF IRRIGATION

The amount of irrigation is directly related to the degree of contamination and tissue damage. A clean laceration may require only several hundred milliliters of irrigation, whereas a severely contaminated wound may require many liters of irrigation.

LOCAL ANESTHESIA

Local anesthesia can be achieved by topical application, wound infiltration, proximal nerve blocks, circumferential field block, or intravenous infusion.

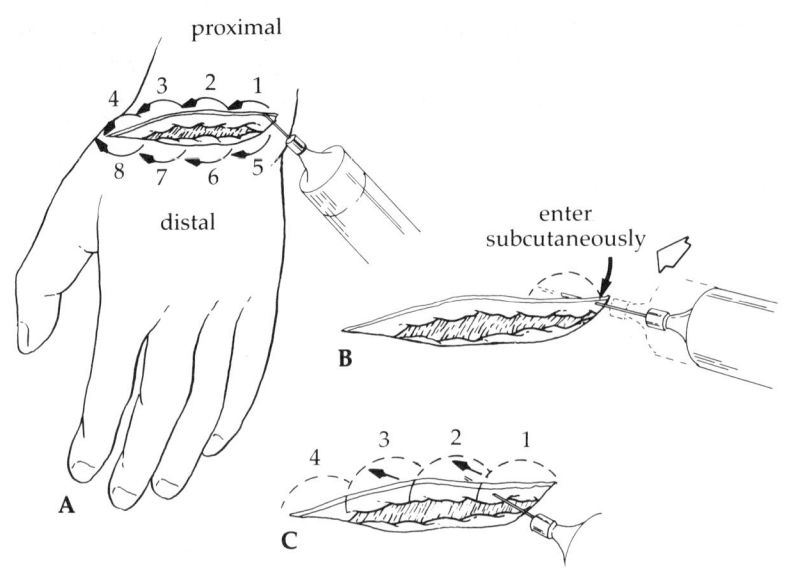

Figure 3-2. Local anesthetic infiltration is achieved by progressive injection around the perimeter of the wound (A), always reintroducing the needle through the subcutaneum that has already been anesthetized (B, C).

Although local infiltration is the most effective method and carries the lowest incidence of side effects, in certain circumstances a field block or nerve block must be used. In the following section the techniques for these alternatives are described and the relative indications for the use of nerve blocks, field blocks, and intravenous infusion are outlined.

General Principles

PSYCHOLOGICAL PREPARATION OF THE PATIENT
The administration of a local anesthetic, regardless of the technique used, should be accompanied by reassurance, explanation, and attempts at diversion of the patient from the injection process.

PHYSICAL PRESSURE
The surgeon or assistant should apply direct pressure around the area to be injected to reduce discomfort during the insertion of a needle. The neurologic explanation is that nonpainful stimuli such as deep pressure and movement are fast-conducting, and pain stimuli are slow-conducting. The fast fibers tend to block the slower conducted stimuli from pain fibers. The area to be injected should be squeezed firmly, before insertion of the needle and during the initial injection.

General Methods of Local Anesthesia

INFILTRATION ANESTHESIA
After choosing the anesthetic agent and concentration, the infiltration proceeds as follows.

1. Use as small a needle as possible. A #30 or #27 needle, and certainly a #25 needle, should be available in most emergency rooms.
2. Inject through the subcutaneous tissue exposed by the laceration (Fig. 3-2). Begin injection in the subcutaneous tissue through the open

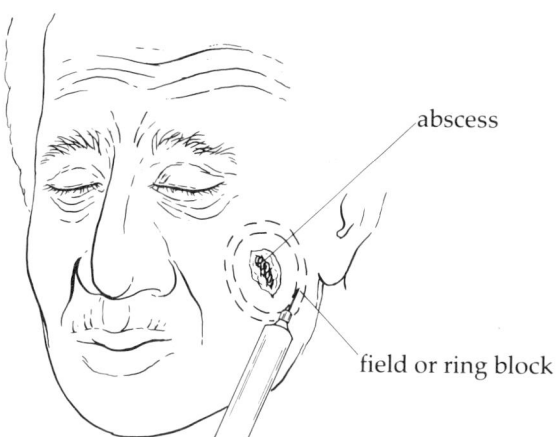

Figure 3-3. Field block anesthesia. The ring of local anesthetic is injected circumferentially around the area of erythema and swelling, several centimeters away.

wound rather than through intact skin. There is less pain when the needle is inserted through subcutaneous tissue.
3. Begin proximally. Begin infiltration on the side of the wound closest to the spinal nerve (cord). If this proximal side is anesthetized first, the distal side may become partially anesthetized through nerve transection, and the initial introduction of the needle may be less uncomfortable.
4. Inject the local anesthetic slowly. Most of the pain from the local anesthetic injection is from the rapid distention of tissues.
5. Advance the needle while injecting. Inject the local anesthetic as the needle is advanced to its full length. Fan out in all directions, without withdrawing the needle from the original puncture site.
6. Aspirate only in the vicinity of large major vessels. Otherwise, aspiration before injection rarely is needed.
7. Withdraw the needle and reinsert it into an area that has already been infiltrated.
8. Repeat the process of injection-withdrawal and reinsertion in a sequential fashion across the open wound.
9. Repeat this process at the distal side of the wound.
10. Wait at least 5 minutes after injection to test the adequacy of anesthesia.

FIELD BLOCK

The field block technique requires the circumferential infiltration of local anesthetic around the wound rather than a direct infiltration into the wound (Fig. 3-3). Field blocks can be used only at anatomic sites in which the cutaneous nerves do not enter the skin from the underlying deep tissue. This technique is used rarely for simple lacerations, but *its primary indication is for local anesthesia in an area of inflammation or infection.* A field block is used for areas of infection because anesthetic solutions are not effective in the acid pH of an inflamed or infected wound, and infection may be spread by repeated local insertions.

The technique of a field block is essentially that described for infiltration except the local anesthetic is injected circumferentially at a distance of several centimeters from the wound rather than into the wound.

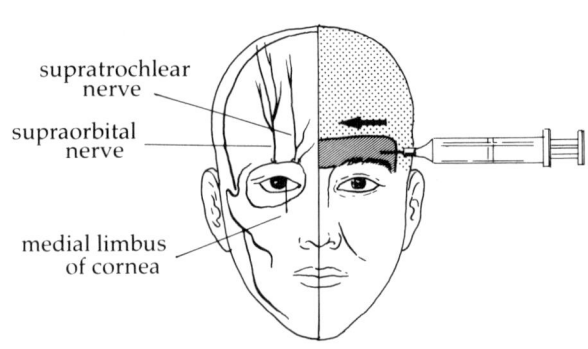

Figure 3-4. Anatomy and method of supraorbital and supratrochlear blocks.

REGIONAL BLOCK
1. General principles. The technique of the regional block requires a detailed understanding of the anatomic distribution of the peripheral nerves. The advantages of this extremely useful method are as follows:
   a. It is effective when there is a large area of injury and the volume of anesthetic agent is to be minimized.
   b. It can be used in situations in which there is local inflammation that precludes direct infiltration or field block.
   c. It is valuable for treatment of injuries to the extremities, especially when a tourniquet is to be used.
   d. Ten to fifteen minutes are required for nerve blocks to diffuse fully and block the major nerve trunk.
2. Types of regional block
   a. Facial nerve block. The sensory nerve patterns of the face are consistent and easily identified. Nerve blocks are useful in the supraorbital-supratrochlear, infraorbital, mental, and dental regions.

   Other nerves supplying the head and neck region can be injected specifically to provide anesthesia in the area innervated. The mandibular and maxillary divisions of the 5th cranial nerve can be anesthetized before operations or manipulations of the upper or lower jaw. These are usually performed for more severe injuries than are comfortably managed in the emergency department. Textbooks of regional anesthesia describe the particular anatomic landmarks and techniques involved in performing these blocks.
   (1) Supraorbital-supratrochlear block—for forehead and scalp anesthesia (Fig. 3-4)
      (a) Anatomy
         (i) The supraorbital nerve exits from the supraorbital foramen at the level of the medial limbus of the cornea (with the eyes in direct forward gaze).
         (ii) The supratrochlear nerve exits from the orbit at the junction of the superior orbital rim and the medial wall of the orbit.
         (iii) The sensory distribution extends over the entire forehead from the eyebrow to the coronal suture and from the midline to the temporal region.

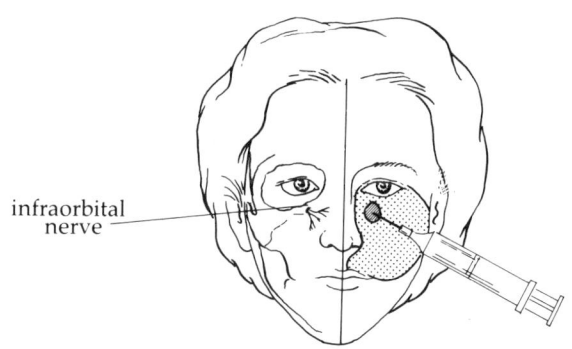

Figure 3-5. Anatomy and method of infraorbital nerve block. The foramen is below the medial margin of the cornea, 3 to 8 mm below the infraorbital rim.

    (b) Method
        (i) Infiltrate subcutaneously completely across the supraorbital rim just above the eyebrow. Do not attempt to infiltrate directly around the nerve or its foramen.
        (ii) Five to ten milliliters of 2% Xylocaine with 1:400,000 epinephrine is infiltrated from the midline of the glabella to the lateral brow.
(2) Infraorbital nerve block—medial cheek and upper lip (Fig. 3-5)
    (a) Anatomy
        (i) The infraorbital nerve exits from the infraorbital foramen within 1 cm below the infraorbital rim.
        (ii) The point of exit is on a vertical line below the medial border of the corneal limbus in primary gaze (straight forward). The foramen can usually be palpated.
        (iii) The nerve supplies the medial portion of the lower eyelid, lateral alae nasi, medial cheek, and upper lip from the midline to the nasolabial crease.
    (b) Method
        (i) Palpate immediately below the infraorbital rim to identify the foramen.
        (ii) If unable to feel the foramen, drop a line from the medial border of the cornea vertically 1 cm down.
        (iii) Infiltrate with 3 to 5 ml of 2% Xylocaine with 1:400,000 epinephrine.
        (iv) A finger on the orbital rim prevents inadvertent intraorbital injection.
(3) Mental nerve block—lower lip and cheek (Fig. 3-6)
    (a) Anatomy
        (i) The inferior alveolar nerve runs in the body of the mandible and exits through the mental foramen as the mental nerve.
        (ii) The mental foramen is on a vertical line just below the second bicuspid tooth.
        (iii) The notch is approximately 1 cm above the mandibular rim.
        (iv) The sensory distribution is to the chin and lower lip to the midline.

Figure 3-6. Anatomy and method of mental nerve block. The foramen is located below the second bicuspid tooth.

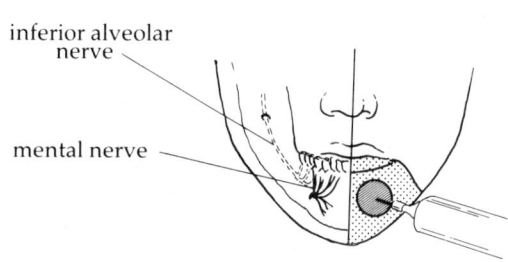

  (b) Method
   (i) Identify the second bicuspid tooth and the approximate point of the mental foramen 1 cm above the mandibular rim. Mark that spot.
   (ii) With either an intraoral approach (transmucosal) or a direct transcutaneous approach, inject 3 to 5 ml of 2% Xylocaine with 1:400,000 epinephrine against the periosteum of the mandible at the predicted site of the mental foramen.
   (iii) A paresthesia is usually not obtained; if it is, back off slightly to reach the correct site.
 (4) Dental nerve block. Anesthesia around individual teeth may be achieved by dental nerve block. This is essentially a field block placed around the roots of the specific teeth to be anesthetized. The surrounding gingiva is also rendered anesthetic. This block is useful if a loose tooth is to be stabilized by interdental wiring to adjacent teeth.
  (a) Anatomy. Each tooth and the surrounding gingiva receive their nerve supply from branches of the mandibular or maxillary nerve.
  (b) Method. One or two milliliters of 1% Xylocaine with epinephrine 1:200,000 or 1:400,000 are infiltrated into the gingiva on the buccal aspect of the tooth root. Diffusion of the agent anesthetizes the tooth and surrounding gingiva.
b. Hand and upper extremity nerve blocks. The anatomic arrangement of sensory nerve supply to the hand lends itself to nerve block. The local anatomy of these nerves will be described.

 For blocks of the radial, median, or ulnar nerve, 1% or 2% mepivacaine (Carbocaine) or 1% or 2% lidocaine (Xylocaine), plain or with epinephrine, is used. Xylocaine with epinephrine prolongs the anesthetic time for extended procedures. For digital nerve blocks, a solution *without epinephrine* should be used.
 (1) Median nerve block (Fig. 3-7). Most median nerve blocks are administered at the wrist level to achieve anesthesia of the median distribution to the hand.
  (a) Anatomy. There is some variability in the distribution of the median nerve.
   (i) In 90 percent of patients, the nerve supplies the radial three and one-half fingers (thumb, index, long, and half of the ring finger).

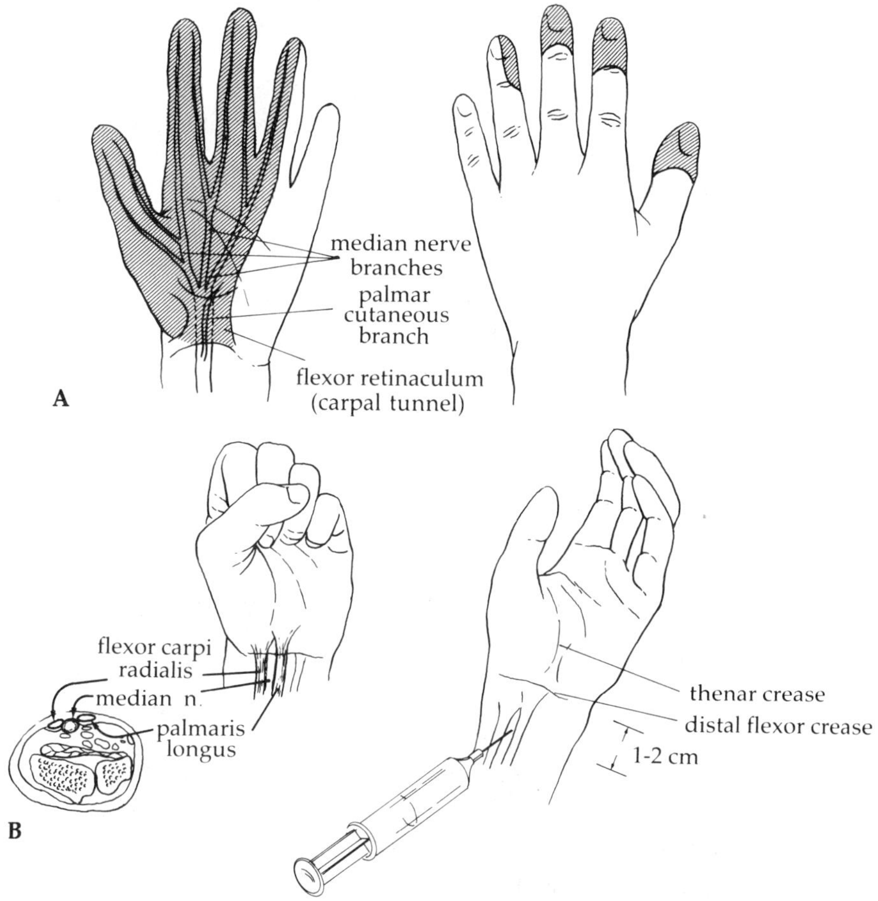

SIMPLE LACERATIONS

Figure 3-7. Anatomy (A) and method (B) of median nerve block.

- (ii) In 10 percent of patients the median nerve supplies the radial two and one-half fingers (up to and including half of the long finger).
- (iii) The median nerve at the wrist is just below the flexor retinaculum and passes through the carpal tunnel.
- (iv) The site of the median nerve can be identified by having the patient make a tight fist and flex the wrist against pressure. This causes the flexor tendons to the wrist and palmaris tendon to stand out visibly.
- (v) The median nerve may lie in the depression between the palmaris longus tendon (if it is present) and the flexor carpi radialis, or slightly under the palmaris longus. It is bounded on its lateral and deep sides by the flexor superficialis tendons.
- (vi) A smaller palmar branch bifurcates proximal to the retinaculum and then travels above the carpal tunnel to supply the area of the proximal palm and thenar eminence.
- **(b)** Method
    - (i) Palpate the space between the large flexor carpi radialis tendon and the smaller palmaris longus tendon.

- (ii) If there is no palmaris longus, identify the site by the flexor carpi radialis and the 1 to 2 cm proximal to the distal flexor crease of the wrist.
- (iii) Introduce a #25 or #27 needle at 45° to the skin, parallel to the course of the nerve. Aim the needle just under the palmaris longus tendon.
- (iv) As the needle is passed through the fascia some resistance may be felt. Inject four to five milliliters of 2% solution. A swelling in the area signifies proper placement. A skin wheal, however, implies that the needle should be advanced slightly deeper. Great difficulty in injecting implies that the needle aperture is probably within the fascia or within the palmaris longus. If paresthesias are elicited, withdraw the needle slightly before injection.
- (v) Following deposition of 4 to 5 ml around the nerve, the needle may be withdrawn until its position is above the antebrachial fascia in the subcutaneous tissue, and an additional 1 to 2 ml injected to block the small palmar cutaneous branch of the median nerve, which supplies part of the palm and thenar eminence. This portion of the procedure should produce a skin wheal as the local anesthetic agent is injected.

(2) Ulnar nerve block (Fig. 3-8)
- (a) Anatomy. Ulnar nerve blocks can be performed at the level of either the elbow or the wrist. The risk of intraneural injection is slightly greater with blocks at the elbow.
    - (i) The ulnar nerve, at the distal wrist crease, lies just beneath the flexor carpi ulnaris.
    - (ii) The dorsal sensory branch comes off approximately 3 to 4 cm proximal to the wrist crease.
    - (iii) This dorsal sensory branch passes beneath the flexor carpi ulnaris to the dorsum of the forearm and continues to the dorsum of the hand and the fourth and fifth fingers.
    - (iv) The ulnar nerve continues beneath the flexor carpi ulnaris to the ulnar tunnel (canal of Guyon).
    - (v) A small palmar cutaneous branch is given off just before the nerve enters the tunnel. The ulnar nerve innervates the ulnar one and one-half fingers and the hypothenar eminence.
- (b) Method
    - (i) The ulnar nerve can be blocked at the wrist by palpating the insertion of the flexor carpi ulnaris on the pisiform. This must be done 3 to 4 cm proximal to the wrist crease if the block is to affect the dorsal branch.
    - (ii) Introduce a fine needle just deep to the tendon on the ulnar side, and insert slightly toward the overlying volar skin so that the needle tip is just on the radial aspect of and deep to the flexor carpi ulnaris.
    - (iii) After aspiration, inject 3 to 4 ml of 2% solution.

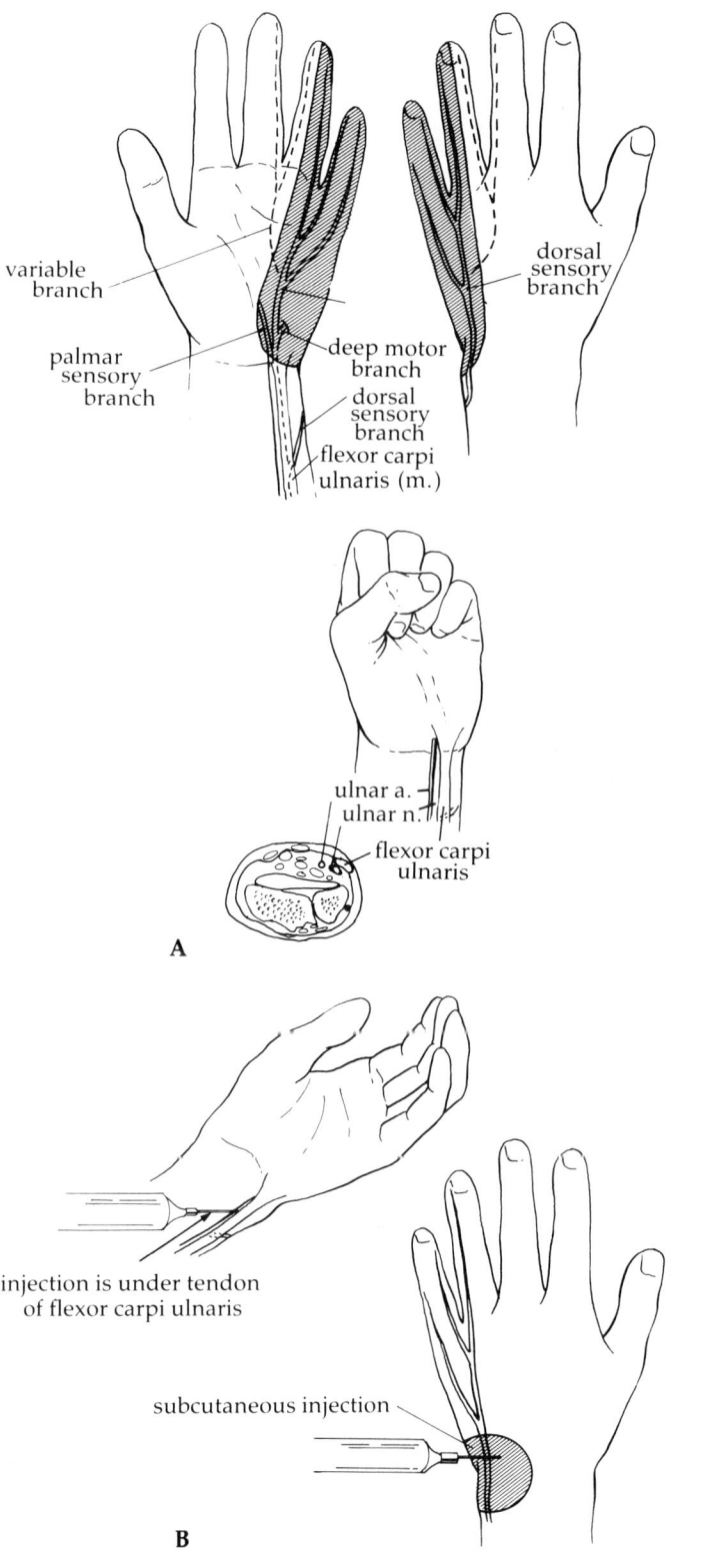

Figure 3-8. Anatomy (A) and method (B) of ulnar nerve block.

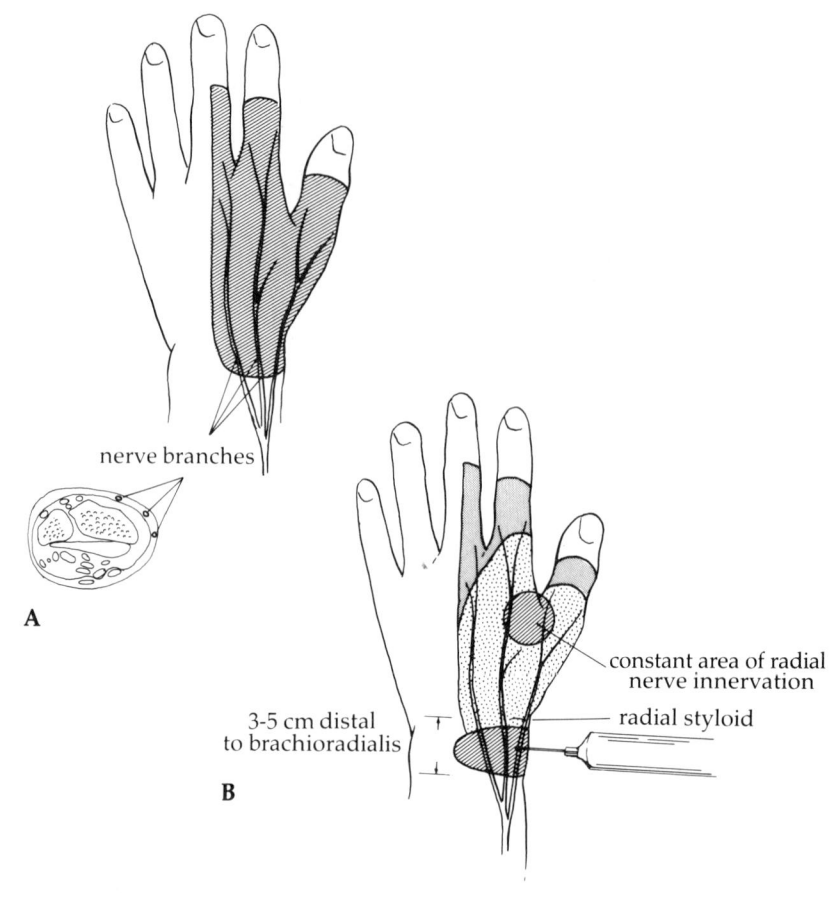

Figure 3-9. Anatomy (A) and method (B) of radial nerve block.

      (iv) Advance the subcutaneous needle dorsally just distal to the ulnar styloid.

      (v) Inject two to three milliliters of 2% solution here to block the important dorsal sensory branch of the ulnar nerve.

  (3) Radial nerve blocks (Fig. 3-9)

    (a) Anatomy

      (i) The radial nerve exits from beneath the brachioradialis muscle approximately 5 cm from the radial styloid.

      (ii) Several branches traverse the soft tissues above the level of the muscular fascia and above the extensor retinaculum.

      (iii) The only absolute area of radial nerve innervation to the hand is in the skin of the dorsal web space between the thumb and index finger.

      (iv) Most commonly the nerve supplies the radial skin of the thumb and index and middle fingers to the level of the proximal or middle phalanx.

      (v) Variable extension out to the level of the distal phalanx of the thumb and index and middle fingers may occur.

    (b) Method

      (i) The radial nerve may be blocked selectively just proximal to the prominence of the radial styloid at the wrist.

SIMPLE LACERATIONS

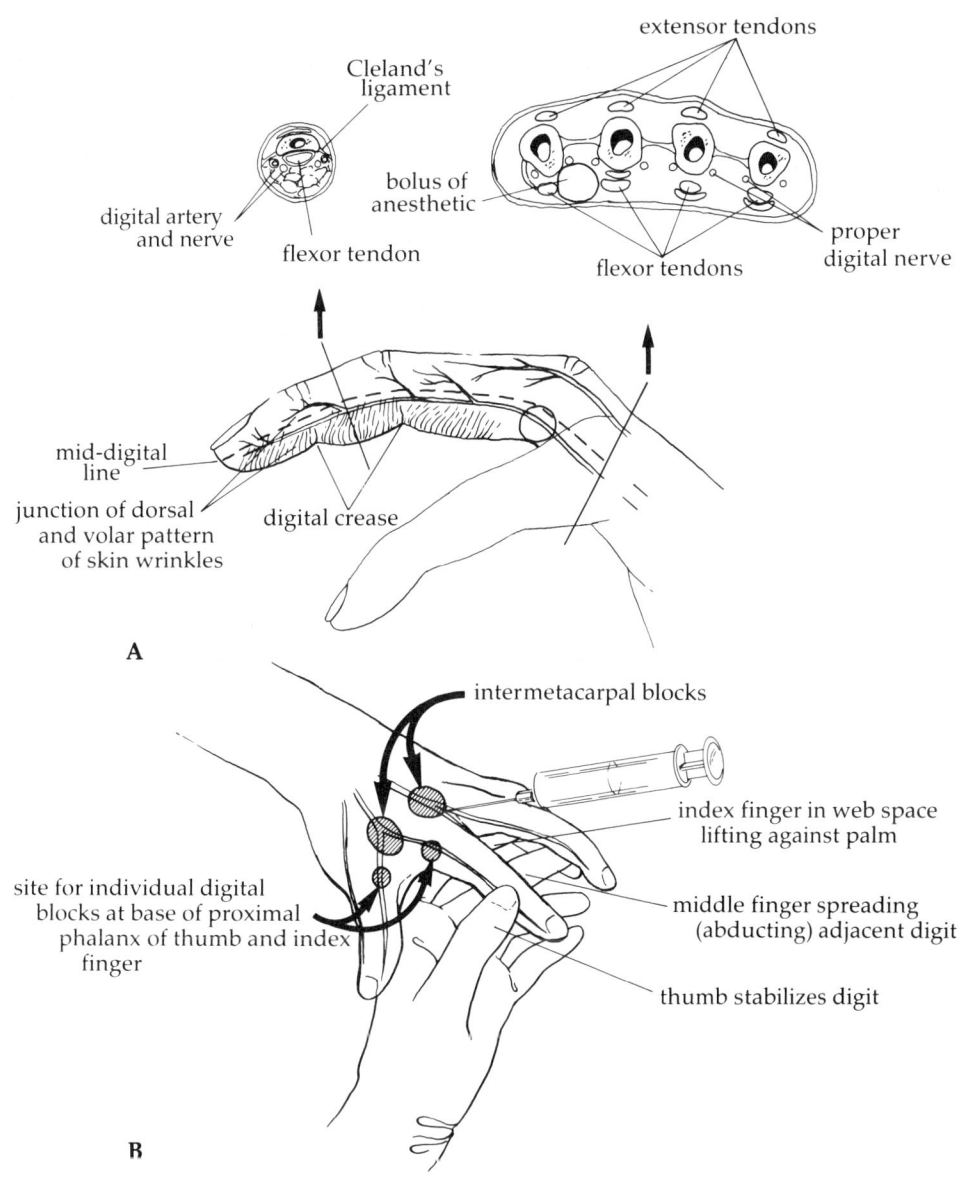

Figure 3-10.
A. Anatomy of digital and intermetacarpal nerve block. Note relation of the digital nerve in the intermetacarpal space between flexor tendons and adjacent to the metacarpals and lumbrical canal.
B. The sites of common digital nerve block are between the metacarpal heads and just below the intermetacarpal ligament.

   (ii) Draw a line from the radial styloid to the lateral epicondyle.
   (iii) Inject three to four milliliters of solution subcutaneously approximately 4 cm or 2 finger breadths proximal to the styloid along this line.
(4) Digital and intermetacarpal nerve block (Fig. 3-10)
   (a) Anatomy
      (i) The digital nerves are the terminal branches of the ulnar and median nerves in the distributions previously described (Figs. 3-7, 3-8).

(ii) The common digital nerve passes volar to the lumbrical canal between the metacarpals to bifurcate into the proper digital nerves to supply the adjacent sides of adjacent fingers. They bifurcate just proximal to the intermetacarpal ligament at about the level of the distal palmar crease.

(iii) The nerves lie very close to the palmar fascia and pass into the individual digits just volar to the midlateral line and adjacent to the phalanges.

(iv) In the digit the nerve is 1 to 2 mm volar to the midaxial line. The midaxial line can be identified by (1) a line joining the apex of the flexion creases of each interphalangeal joint, and (2) the junction of fingerprint patterns: volar = fine finger prints, and dorsal = broad wrinkles.

(b) Method for ring finger, middle and ulnar side of index finger, and radial side of little finger. If only a single digit or several digits are injured distally, complete anesthesia can be obtained by blocking the common digital nerves to these fingers at the intermetacarpal level. This is better than injecting directly into the digital bundle at the base of the finger, where space is limited; the addition of several milliliters of fluid in this relatively closed space may compromise circulation to an already injured digit. An intermetacarpal block is effective and avoids this potential hazard.

(i) Introduce the needle in the dorsal web space (skin is less sensitive here) and direct it volarly between the metacarpal heads.

(ii) Inject two to three milliliters of 2% solution.

(iii) A finger placed on the volar intermetacarpal area should sense the fullness caused by the bolus of liquid.

(iv) If this fullness is not palpable, it may imply that the needle is dorsal to the intermetacarpal fascia and thus above the nerves.

(v) Block the opposite side of the digit in the same manner. For wounds closer to the dorsal base of the digit, a dorsal subcutaneous wheal may be necessary at the base of the finger, because this region may be supplied by dorsal branches of the radial or ulnar nerve.

(c) Method for radial side of index and ulnar side of little finger

(i) The radial digital nerve to the index finger and ulnar digital nerve to the little finger may be blocked at the level of the distal palmar crease.

(ii) The needle should be introduced at the junction of dorsal and volar skin and 1 to 2 ml of 2% solution injected.

(d) Method for thumb

(i) The proper digital nerves to the thumb may be blocked at the level of the most proximal thumb flexor crease.

(ii) The nerves are very superficial and lie immediately adjacent to the readily palpable flexor pollicis longus tendon.

(iii) Introduce the needle to a depth of 2 to 3 mm in a slightly proximal direction along either side of the thumb flexor tendon. Inject one to two milliliters of 2% Xylocaine, and note subcutaneous fullness.

(5) Axillary nerve block (Fig. 3-11)
  (a) Anatomy. The entire arm can be anesthetized by blocking the contents of the brachial plexus at the axilla. This block requires some practice to develop proficiency, but it is very useful and safe if certain precautions are followed. Precautions include the presence of a functioning IV line and the availability of resuscitation equipment should complications such as overdose develop.
    (i) The terminal nerves from cervical roots C5 through T1 are contained in a common sheath along with the axillary artery and axillary vein. The axillary sheath is a continuation of the prevertebral fascia. Therefore, *injection into the sheath effectively blocks all nerves to the upper extremity, and specific blocks of the radial, ulnar, or median nerve are not required.*
    (ii) The sensory supply to the upper arm in the region of the tourniquet comes primarily from the intercostobrachial cutaneous nerve—a terminal branch of the 2nd intercostal nerve—and the medial brachial cutaneous nerves, which arise high up in the brachial plexus. This nerve may have left the sheath proximal to the region of the axillary block. Therefore, there may be normal feeling in the upper arm unless special attention is paid to the technique of achieving retrograde flow of the anesthetic to the more proximal brachial plexus.
    (iii) The terminal portion of the musculocutaneous nerve to the thenar eminence—the lateral antebrachial cutaneous nerve—also leaves the sheath above the axilla. Therefore, there may be sensibility of the volar side of the hand. The musculocutaneous nerve and the intercostobrachial cutaneous nerve are blocked by injecting a subcutaneous ring of anesthetic agent circumferentially above the tourniquet level.
  (b) Method. The type of anesthetic agent may be determined by the anticipated length of the procedure. The usual agents are 1% lidocaine (Xylocaine) or 1% mepivacaine (Carbocaine). Bupivacaine (Marcaine) may be used for longer action.
    (i) Forewarn the patient that there may be paresthetic "tingling" or an "electric shock" felt in the arm, hands, or fingers, and when these are felt, the patient should hold absolutely still.
    (ii) Place the patient on an operating table in a supine position with the arms extended on an arm board—the shoulder abducted 90° and the elbow flexed 90°.
    (iii) Attach a #25 or #27 needle to a 2- to 3-foot IV tubing extension or a #25 pediatric scalp vein, which is in turn connected to a syringe containing the local anesthetic.

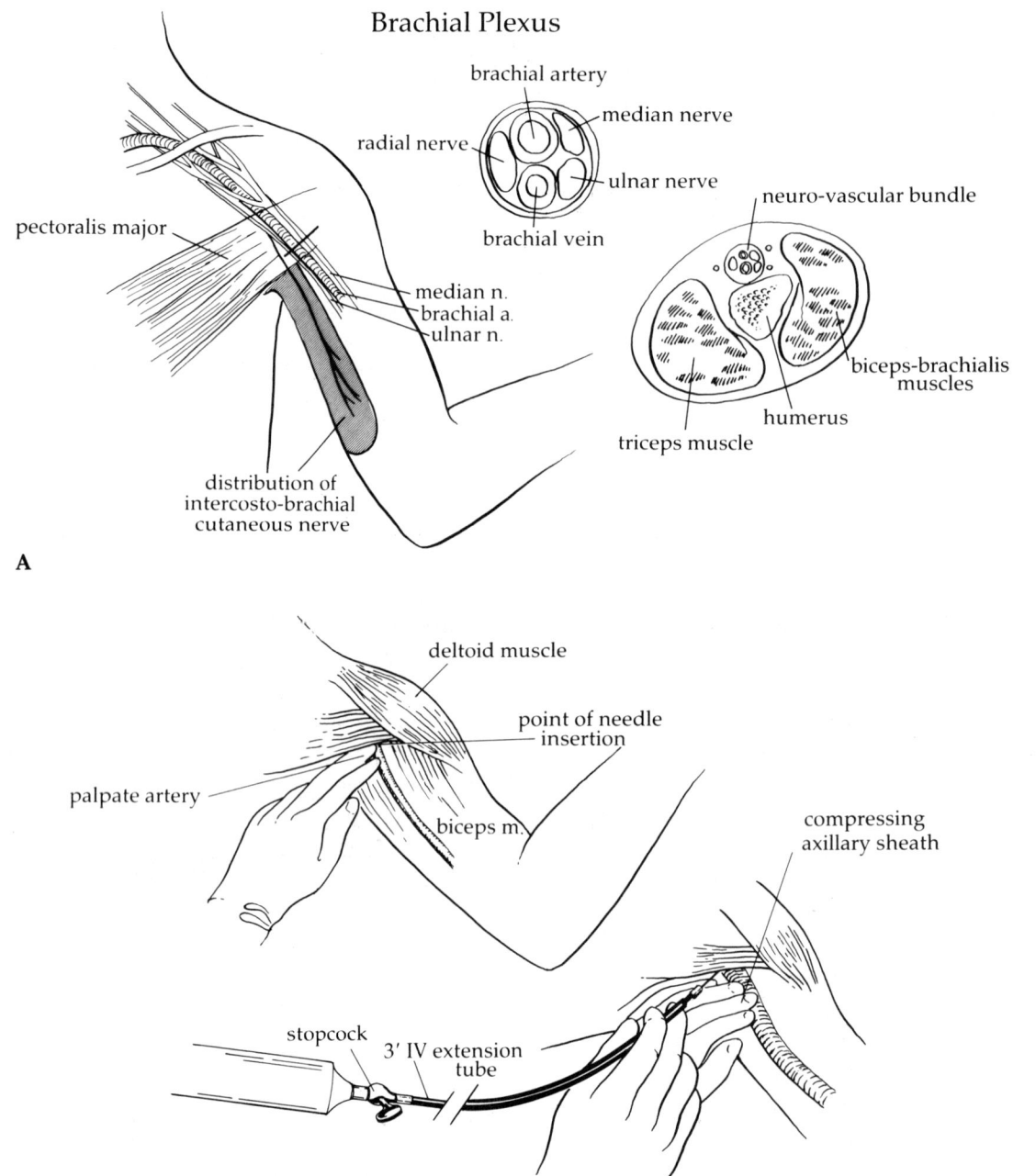

Figure 3-11.
A. Anatomy of axillary nerve block. Note that all the major nerves are contained within a single sheath along with the artery and vein.
B. Technique of axillary block. The most important aspects as described in the text are careful introduction of the needle to avoid leakage from the sheath and distal compression to force as much anesthetic as possible into the proximal portion.

This extension tubing alows the physician to insert the needle and stabilize it while an assistant injects the anesthetic. Inadvertent movement of the needle can withdraw it from its desired position within the sheath or irritate the surrounding nerves.

(iv) The axillary artery can be palpated as high as possible in the axilla. The artery is located at the level of the pectoralis major insertion and in the interseptal space between the biceps and triceps muscles.

(v) With index and long fingers directly on the axillary artery, insert the needle on the superior side of the artery if one is seeking to elicit median nerve paresthesia and on the inferior side for ulnar nerve paresthesia. Since it is easier to elicit a median nerve paresthesia, the needle is usually inserted superior to the artery. However, if the surgical procedure involves only ulnar nerve innervated areas, the inferior side of the artery may be chosen.

(vi) Slowly advance the needle 1 to 1.5 cm. A frequent mistake is to advance the needle too far and pass through the axillary sheath.

(vii) As the needle is advanced, two signs confirm that the position is correct. There may be a slight popping sensation as the axillary sheath is encountered and the needle suddenly passes through the tougher collagen of the axillary sheath. The patient may experience paresthesias, which he or she may describe or which may be recognized by the patient's reaction.

(viii) Stop as soon as the paresthesia occurs or the axillary sheath has been entered. The best blocks occur when the needle enters the axillary sheath on the first attempt. Otherwise, anesthetic agent may leak through the perforations from repeated punctures.

(ix) Maintain the position of the needle, but ask the assistant to aspirate. This ensures that the needle is not in the axillary artery or vein.

(x) Place pressure on the axillary sheath just distal to the site of the needle insertion. This prevents diffusion distally and forces the anesthetic agent proximally.

(xi) Slowly inject 20 to 30 ml of 1% or 40 to 50 ml of 0.5% Xylocaine. A sausage-shaped mass may develop below the fingers from the distention of the sheath by the local anesthetic.

(xii) Apply the tourniquet if it is to be used and *wait 20 minutes* while the operative area is prepped and surgical scrub performed. Do not begin testing to see if an anesthetic block has been obtained until the full 20 minutes have passed and the tourniquet has been applied. The injured area can then be cleaned and more thoroughly examined without discomfort to the patient.

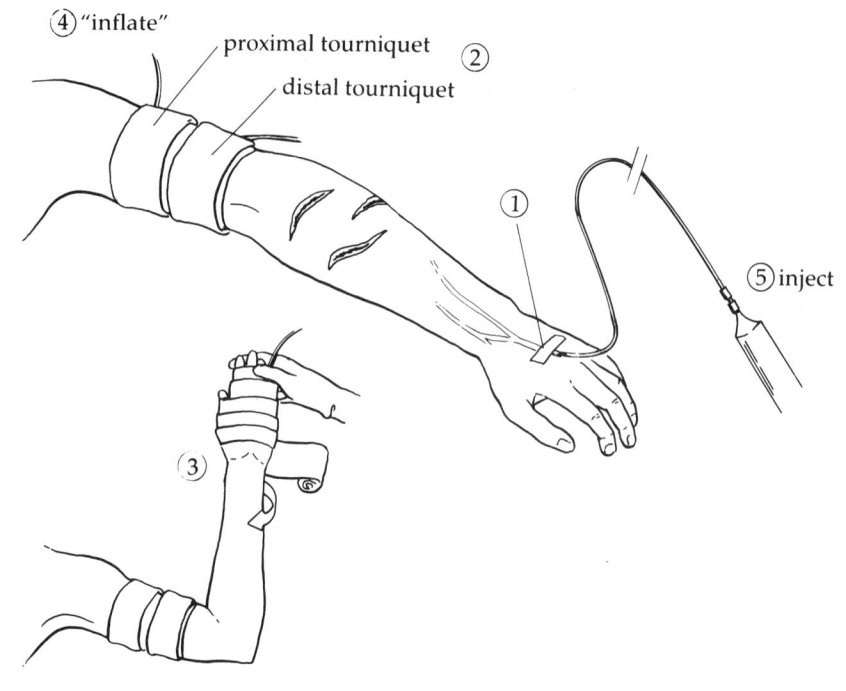

Figure 3-12. Method of regional intravenous nerve block. The importance of two tourniquets is emphasized. (1) Insert a 19- or 21-gauge scalp vein into a dorsal vein; (2) place two padded tourniquets about the upper arm; (3) exsanguinate the limb and inflate the proximal tourniquet 75 to 100 mm Hg above systolic pressure; (4) inject an appropriate volume of anesthetic agent; (5) when discomfort from the proximal tourniquet is experienced, inflate the distal tourniquet and deflate the proximal.

REGIONAL INTRAVENOUS ANESTHESIA

This technique is used for the upper extremity on the rare occasion in which infiltration and regional blocks are not feasible (Fig. 3-12). Usually it is used for an extensive injury of the forearm or fractures that are not located within the distribution of a specific cutaneous nerve, and it can be used instead of an axillary block. The method is simple and can be used by those not practiced in axillary blocks. The same precautions mentioned for the axillary block apply here. *Two (2) well-tested, reliable tourniquets must be used!* The method is as follows:

1. Insert a #25 scalp vein needle into a hand vein.
2. Place two tourniquets on the upper arm. This is for protection against tourniquet failure, which would allow a large volume of anesthetic solution to enter the systemic circulation.
3. The arm is elevated and exsanguinated with an elastic bandage.
4. The proximal tourniquet is inflated 75 to 100 mm Hg above arterial pressure and carefully checked to ensure that it is functioning. This is done by feeling for pulses, observing the wound, and directly palpating the tourniquet.
5. After functioning of the tourniquet has been confirmed, a 20-ml bolus of 1% Carbocaine or 1% Xylocaine (plain) is injected.
6. Thirty to sixty seconds later the distal tourniquet is inflated and rechecked for function, and the remaining 20 ml of anesthetic is injected.

The sequence of tourniquet inflation and anesthetic injection allows anesthesia to occur at the site of the distal tourniquet. Thus, if severe tourniquet pain develops after 30 to 60 minutes with both tourniquets inflated, the pain can be relieved by deflating the proximal tourniquet. By 30 minutes most of the anesthetic diffuses out of the venous system

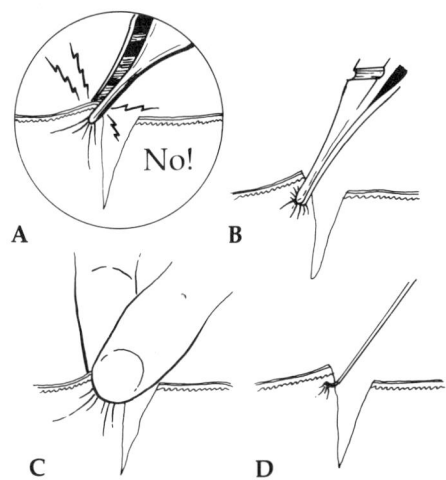

Figure 3-13. Nontraumatic surgical technique is achieved with a forceps blade (B), fingers (C), or hook (D). Squeezing tissue with two forceps (A) leads to necrosis, infection, and excess scarring.

and is fixed to the tissue. The risk of toxicity is extremely minimal after 30 minutes even if the tourniquet is released.

7. If the procedure is completed in less than 30 minutes, the tourniquet must be left in place. Slow deflation does not allow slow release of anesthetics. When the tourniquet pressure drops below venous pressure, there is an immediate bolus, regardless of the rate of deflation.

ALTERNATIVES TO LOCAL ANESTHESIA

Acupuncture and hypnosis are reported to be extremely effective means of obtaining anesthesia. The limitations of these techniques are presently under study. They are ideal anesthetics for the physician who is familiar with them and for appropriate patients, because many of the potential complications from injection of local anesthesia are eliminated.

BASIC SUTURING PRINCIPLES

Tissue Handling

NONTRAUMATIC MANIPULATION

All physicians should use nontraumatic technique (Fig. 3-13). The wound should be handled with gloved fingers, skin hook, or side of the forceps. The forceps should be used gently to manipulate the tissue, because grasping or squeezing tissue with forceps is likely to cause tissue necrosis, resulting in excessive fibrosis or infection.

NATURAL HEMOSTASIS

Bleeding is best controlled by applying direct pressure and allowing time for the natural hemostatic processes. A clamped vessel with a suture ligature, or a cauterized vessel, causes inflammation that could result in additional fibrosis or establish a nidus for infection. Only "large" subcutaneous vessels require ligation or cautery. The bleeding dermal edges do not require surgical hemostasis.

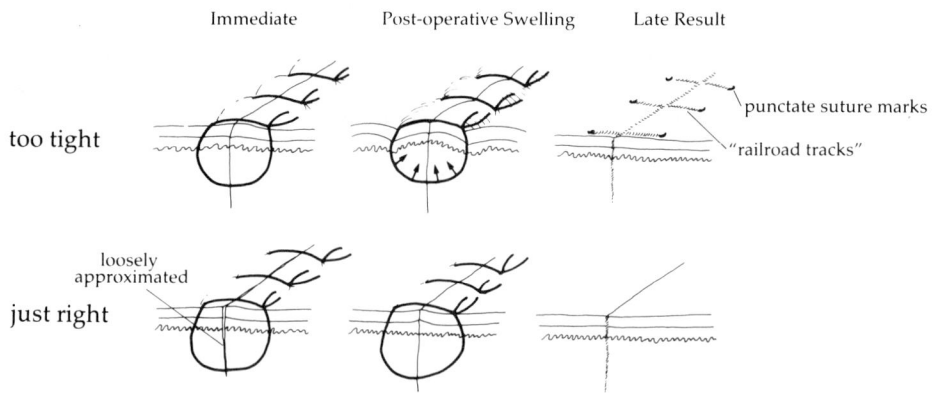

Figure 3-14. Correct versus incorrect suture tension. Loose approximation of the skin edges of even a small gap is important. Tight sutures become even tighter because of edema and tissue necrosis, and suture marks can occur.

ATRAUMATIC NEEDLE PLACEMENT

The needle should be passed through the tissues one time. Each misplacement and withdrawal of the needle causes additional tissue damage.

APPROXIMATING SUTURES

Sutures should be tied with just enough tension to approximate the edges of the wound (Fig. 3-14); a slight gap between the wound edges will be obliterated by the postoperative swelling. If sutures are tied too tightly, ischemic necrosis of the interposed tissues results. The dictum is, "Approximate, don't strangulate."

Wound Approximation

Careful approximation of the wound surface results in a flat, minimally noticeable scar. Overlapping, step-off, or sunken edges are to be avoided because they cause shadows that make the scar more apparent.

MATCH THE LENGTH OF BOTH SIDES OF THE WOUND

A laceration that is parallel or perpendicular to a natural skin wrinkle (Langer's lines) has balanced forces acting on each side. A laceration oblique to a natural crease has unbalanced forces that shift the skin alignment. These shifts must be realigned carefully to avoid "dog-ears" at the ends of the wound. Matching the lengths of the sides can be achieved with skin hooks, reapproximation of anatomic landmarks, or direct measurement (Fig. 3-15). Most commonly, a *visual estimation of equal distances* is required.

The sequence of suture placement is sometimes determined by the need to match the length of both sides. "Splitting the difference" is a method for matching length when skin hooks are used (Fig. 3-16), whereas a sequential end-to-end method can be used for easily aligned lacerations.

MATCH DEPTH OF SIDES

The depth of suture placement must be equal on the opposite sides (Fig. 3-17). If the depth of placement is unequal, the side with the more deeply

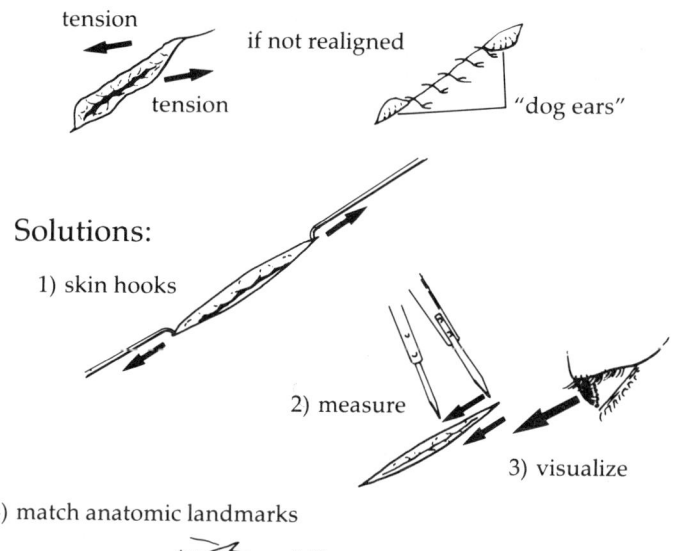

Figure 3-15. Malalignment creates excess tissue at the opposite sides of both ends of the wound ("dog-ears"). The wound length alignment can be achieved by any of these methods, but hooks or visual approximation is most efficient.

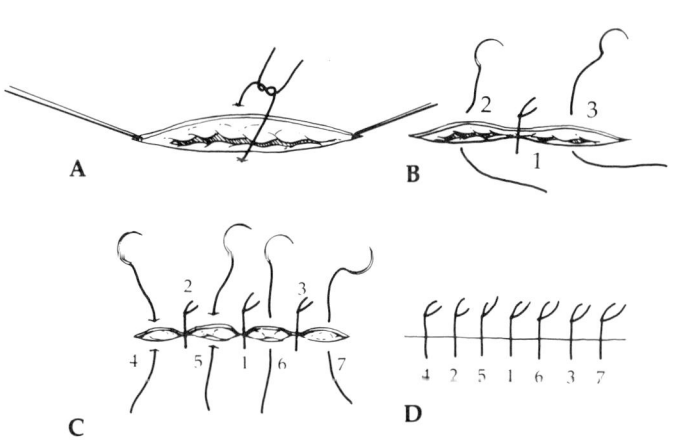

Figure 3-16. The "split the difference" method of suture sequencing is most useful for malaligned wounds.
A. Align the wound with skin hooks. Place the initial suture (1) at the middle of the laceration.
B. Place the next sutures (2 and 3) on both of the remaining halves of the wound.
C. Repeat the sequence with sutures 4, 5, 6, and 7.
D. Final position and sequence.

placed suture tends to ride higher and overlap the opposite side. The higher side casts a shadow onto the opposite lower side.

EVERT EDGES

Slight eversion of the skin edges is essential to achieve a flat skin surface. Any edge inversion at the time of surgical repair leads to a depressed scar. A depressed scar is quite noticeable because of the shadows cast into the contour (Fig. 3-18). Wound eversion can be achieved by the following methods:

1. Subcutaneous and subdermal sutures. These sutures approximate the deeper tissues and prevent the skin margins from collapsing into the underlying dead space.

Figure 3-17. Matching depth of sides.
A. Unequal depth of bites causes elevation of one side of the wound. The deeper side overlaps and casts a shadow on the lower side, or the side with the more shallow bite.
B. Equal depth of placement avoids overlapping and can be achieved by careful visualization.

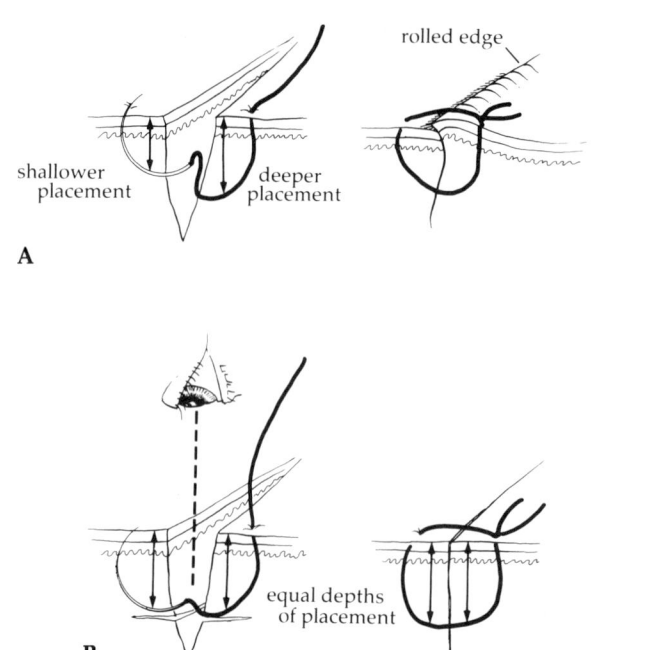

Figure 3-18. An inverted skin edge results in a depressed, wide scar caused by nonhealing of the epidermal contact. The surface inversion may be deceptively inapparent and must be carefully achieved.

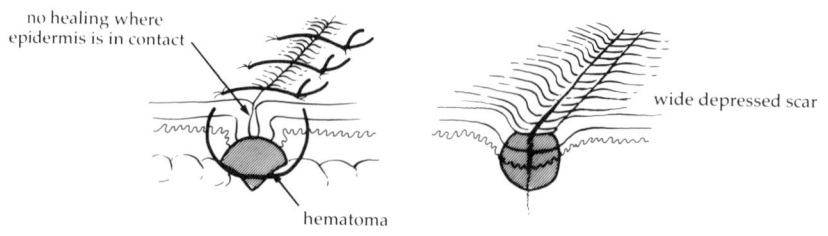

2. Skin sutures. A careful technique with simple skin sutures or horizontal or vertical mattress sutures everts the edges (Fig. 3-19). A detailed description of how to evert edges with a simple, horizontal, or vertical skin suture is described in this chapter.
3. Scoring (Fig. 3-20). Scoring involves a 1- or 2-mm incision into the subcutaneous tissue parallel to the skin surface. It usually is done in the dermis-subcutaneous junction or just below the dermis in the fat of an older, scarred wound. Scoring allows a more accurate depth of suture placement and wound eversion by unrolling the scarred edge. Scoring does not relieve tension on the wound or allow tissue mobilization.

   A distinction should be made between *undermining* and *scoring*. Undermining requires extensive surgical separation of the superficial skin from underlying subcutaneous tissue, muscle, or bone. Undermining is often required for advancement of wounds with tissue loss that are difficult to close because of tension. Undermining is usually done in a fascial plane, but it can be in the subdermis.

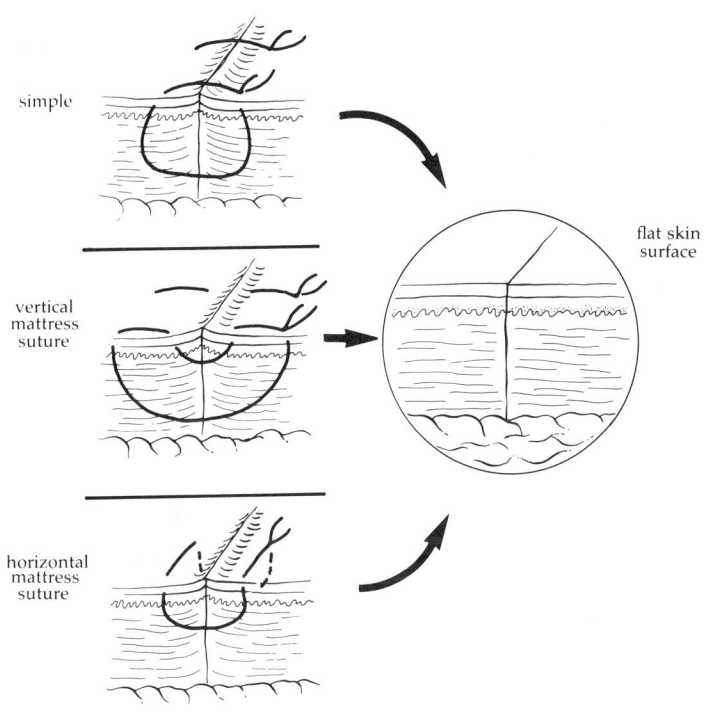

Figure 3-19. Slight eversion of wound edges eventually results in a flat skin surface. A simple suture is most commonly used, but in difficult areas a mattress suture can be effective.

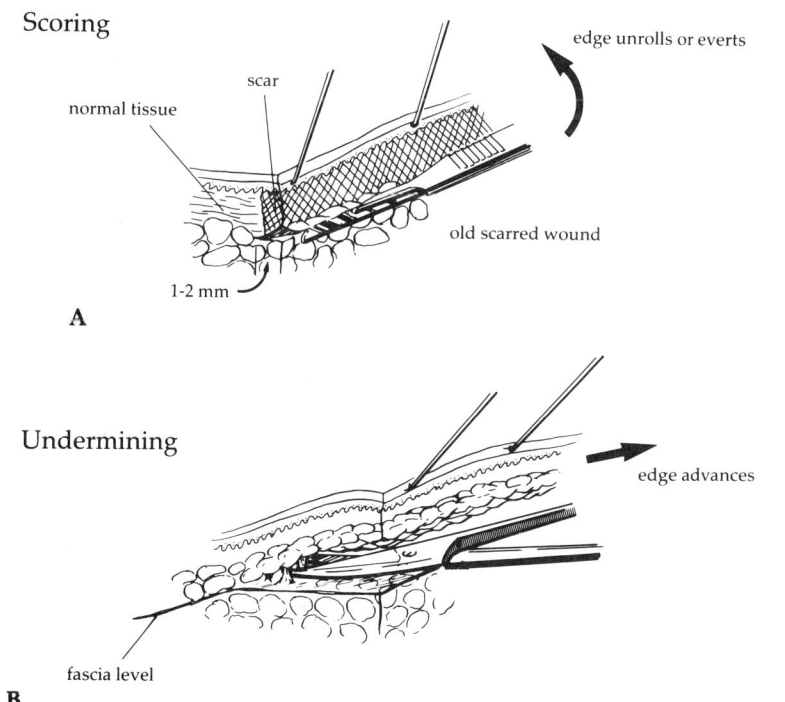

Figure 3-20. Scoring and undermining.
A. Place skin hooks at each end of the wound or about 2 to 3 cm apart. With the skin under tension, lightly sweep a #15 scalpel blade in a plane parallel with the skin surface.
B. Undermining is usually done at the level of the superficial fascia or within the superficial subcutaneous fat.

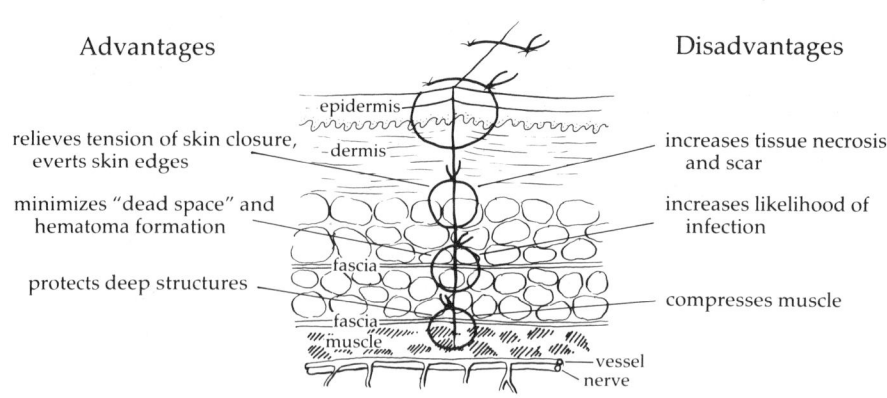

Figure 3-21. Advantages and disadvantages of layered closure. As a general rule layered closures are indicated in wounds with excessive tension and contraindicated in unhealthy, untidy, contaminated wounds or very simple shallow wounds without tension.

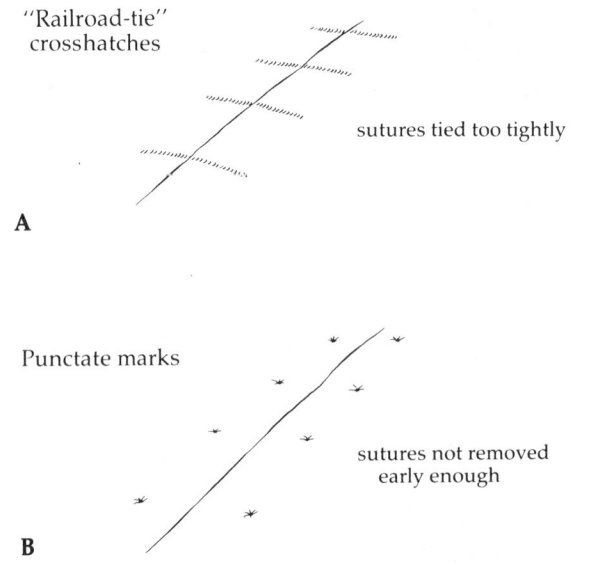

Figure 3-22.
A. Railroad-tie cross-hatch marks are caused by sutures tied too tightly (wound edema).
B. Suture marks caused by sutures left in the wound too long, suture infection, and reactive sutures (catgut) are punctate.

Subcutaneous and Dermal Layered Closure

Because layered closure has advantages and disadvantages, judgment is required to determine when layered closure should be used (Fig. 3-21).

ADVANTAGES OF LAYERED SUBDERMAL CLOSURE
1. Distribution of tension. With layered closure, tension can be distributed throughout the deep dermis and fascia rather than concentrated at the surface. Sutures are placed in the strong collagenous layers of the dermis, subcutaneous fascia, and muscle fascia. (Fat should not be sutured because of its low tensile strength.) Without layered closure, excessive tension on skin sutures can occur and cause wound separation and suture marks. Tension can occur with the following circumstances:
   a. Movement from the pull of underlying muscles
   b. Laceration parallel with extensor or flexor surface of a joint
   c. Skin loss caused by the injury or surgical debridement
2. Avoidance of suture marks. Layered closure allows earlier removal of sutures and thus avoidance of suture marks (Fig. 3-22). There are two

types of suture marks: punctate marks, in which the suture enters the skin, and cross-hatch or "railroad-tie" marks, in which the suture crosses the laceration. These marks can occur separately or in combination. Suture marks are usually unwarranted and can be avoided with appropriate precautions. They are caused by the following problems:
   a. Sutures left in the wound longer than 7 days (punctate marks). If wounds are not repaired with a layered closure, there may be excessive tension at the wound margins requiring the continued presence of skin sutures. When skin sutures are present for longer than 7 days, epithelium and scar form around the suture, resulting in a punctate suture mark. Deep, layered closure allows earlier removal of skin sutures without additional risk of wound separation.
   b. Sutures tied too tightly (railroad crosshatching). If wounds are not repaired with a layered closure, there may be excessive tension at the wound margins. To overcome this tension the sutures may be tied too tightly, thus compressing the intervening skin, causing ischemia, and resulting in railroad-tie marks.
   c. Several factors unrelated to layered closure, including:
      (1) Unusual postoperative wound edema. Swelling of the tissue can cause railroad-tie marks from tissue compression and ischemia just as sutures tied too tightly can.
      (2) A reactive suture in the epidermis. Plain catgut and, to a lesser degree, natural multifilament sutures, chromic catgut, and the glycolics may cause an excessive inflammatory reaction that results in punctate suture marks.
      (3) Suture infection. Multifilament sutures are a nidus for bacterial growth and wound infection and can result in punctate marks.
3. Obliteration of dead space. "Dead space" occurs under the skin where there is no tissue-to-tissue contact. Such spaces, filled with serum or blood, increase the susceptibility to infection, depressed scars, and hypertrophic scars. Subcutaneous sutures minimize infection only if they obliterate the dead space. Otherwise, they increase the risk.
4. Eversion of edges. A layered closure prevents retraction of the subcutaneous layers and the resultant inversion of the epidermal margins. Instead, the layered closure maximizes subsurface volume and wound eversion.
5. Protection of vital structures. A layered closure should cover nerves, joints, major vessels, or tendons with an intact skin and subcutaneum.

DISADVANTAGES OF LAYERED SUBDERMAL CLOSURE
1. Increased infection rate. Sutures in the dermal and subcutaneous layers increase the risk of infection because bacteria can accumulate around the foreign material. Multifilament nonabsorbable sutures are particularly unsuitable for subcutaneous closure.
2. Increase in scar deposition. Additional sutures in the dermal and subcutaneous layers increase the foreign body inflammatory reaction and thus the amount of scar deposition.
3. Necrosis of ischemic tissue. Tissue with marginal viability may become ischemic. The additional wound tension and obstruction of vascularity caused by a suture may cause necrosis of the tissue. Dehiscence and/or infection are then likely to occur.

4. "Spitting" of sutures. If the dermal sutures are very close to the surface of thin skin and there is inflammation with delayed absorption of the suture, the suture will extrude ("spit"). This leaves a slight wound separation and additional scar.

INDICATIONS FOR LAYERED CLOSURE
1. Dermal closure may be used to:
   a. Relieve excessive tension in a healthy wound. Excessive tension may be caused by skin avulsion, debridement, movement from adjacent muscles, or movement across extensor surfaces.
   b. Evert a wound that has edges rolled inward
2. Subcutaneous closure (areolar fascia) may be used to:
   a. Close potential dead space
   b. Protect vital structures, such as nerves, tendons, joints, and vessels
3. Muscle fascia closure may be used to:
   a. Relieve tension on the overlying wound
   b. Prevent herniation of muscle

CONTRAINDICATIONS TO LAYERED CLOSURE
1. General contraindications
   a. Wounds without tension
   b. Wounds with poor vascularity
   c. Wounds with a high risk of infection, bacterial contamination, or foreign bodies.
   d. Wounds in noncosmetic areas.
2. Contraindications to dermal closure
   a. Partial laceration of dermis without extending into fat
   b. Wounds in specific anatomic sites, such as the:
      (1) Scalp (Deep sutures may destroy hair follicles and cause bald spots.)
      (2) Nasal tip (Subcutaneous sutures have a high risk of infection or reaction in sebaceous nasal skin.)
      (3) Ear cartilage (increased risk of chondritis)
      (4) Palm of hand (There is never enough dead space or tension to warrant layered closure here. If there is, the wound should be packed open, not closed.)
      (5) Fingertip (increased risk of tender scars)
3. Contraindications to layered closure in muscle fascia
   a. Inability to close completely, leaving muscle hernia. If the muscle fascia cannot be completely closed, a small painful muscle hernia can occur.
   b. Damaged underlying muscle (crush). The damaged muscle in a sutured closed space is more susceptible to swelling and may cause a "compartment" syndrome with nerve and/or vascular compression.

SUTURING TECHNIQUE

Once preliminary wound care and anesthesia have been achieved and a decision is made regarding the need for subcutaneous sutures, the actual suturing can proceed. In this section we describe various technical maneuvers that can be used.

Knot Tying

A method of knot tying to produce a square knot is described (Fig. 3-23). As mentioned before, the knot should be placed to approximate the edges lightly. After completion of the knot, it should be shifted to the side rather than left overlying the laceration. This reduces inflammation and crusting and simplifies suture removal.

Methods of Layered Closure

1. Repair the deepest tissue first, then work toward the surface.
2. Use absorbable, long-duration sutures, such as glycolic or chromic sutures. Monofilament, nonabsorbable nylon can be used for the deep closure of fascia.
3. Place subcutaneous and dermal sutures so that the knot is deepest in the wound. This is called the "buried" subcutaneous suture. The knot is buried to avoid the cut ends of the knot extending through the skin surface (Fig. 3-24).
4. Place the suture in the layer of areolar fascia or dermis rather than in the fat, which has little tensile strength.
5. Stagger the spacing of layers. The subcutaneous dermal and epidermal sutures should not overlie each other.
6. Use the minimal number of sutures that is effective.

Skin Surface Approximation—Types of Sutures

SIMPLE SUTURES—DEPTH AND POSITION

We have discussed the objectives of the skin surface approximation: matching length, matching height, everting edges, and avoiding suture marks. These objectives can be achieved with layered closure or with skin sutures alone.

Ideally, the surface suture should be confined to epidermis (the epidermal suture) to avoid suture marks and to obtain the most precise surface approximation. However, wound strength would be inadequate because epidermis cannot hold sutures. Moreover, it is technically very difficult to limit the sutures to the epidermal layer.

Thus, the usual method of surface approximation involves the epidermal-dermal suture. This suture is placed in the epidermis, all or part of the dermis, and the most superficial fat. This is also referred to as the "skin" suture.

How far from the cut edge, how deep, and how far apart should the skin sutures be placed? The depth and distance between sutures are functions of the anatomic site; the patient's age, sex, and state of general health; and the quality of the local tissue. Therefore, there is no absolute measure. Suture placement must be individualized for each patient and for different regions of the same wound. Although there is no absolute answer to these questions, there are some helpful guidelines.

Figure 3-23. The instrument tie.

A. After placement of suture, "reel in" needle and excessive length of suture to palm of hand. Don't let needle dangle; it can accidentally injure the eye or other structure. The remaining "free" end is 1 to 2 cm long.

B. Place the needle holder over the wound between two suture ends.

C and D. Loop the suture around the needle holder (or the needle holder around the suture), and grasp the free end with the tip of the needle holder.

E. Pull the free end across the wound while the long end is being pulled across in the opposite direction.

F to J. Repeat this sequence three times but alternate positions of the free end and suture end.

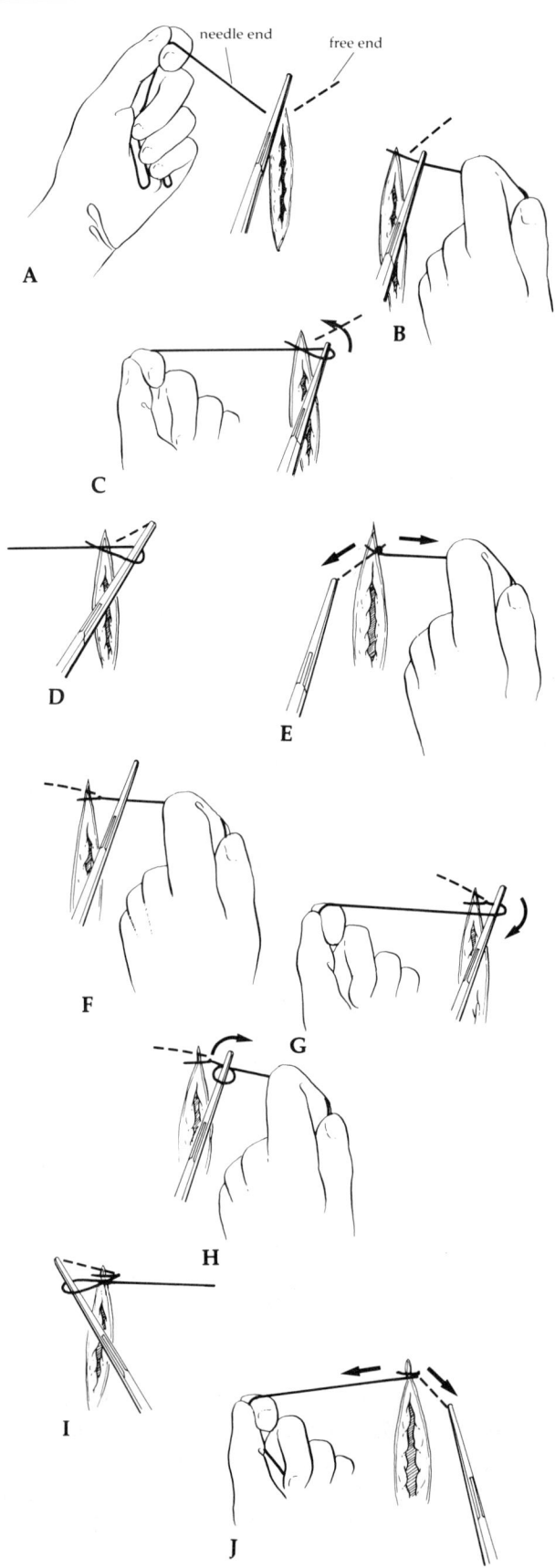

SIMPLE LACERATIONS

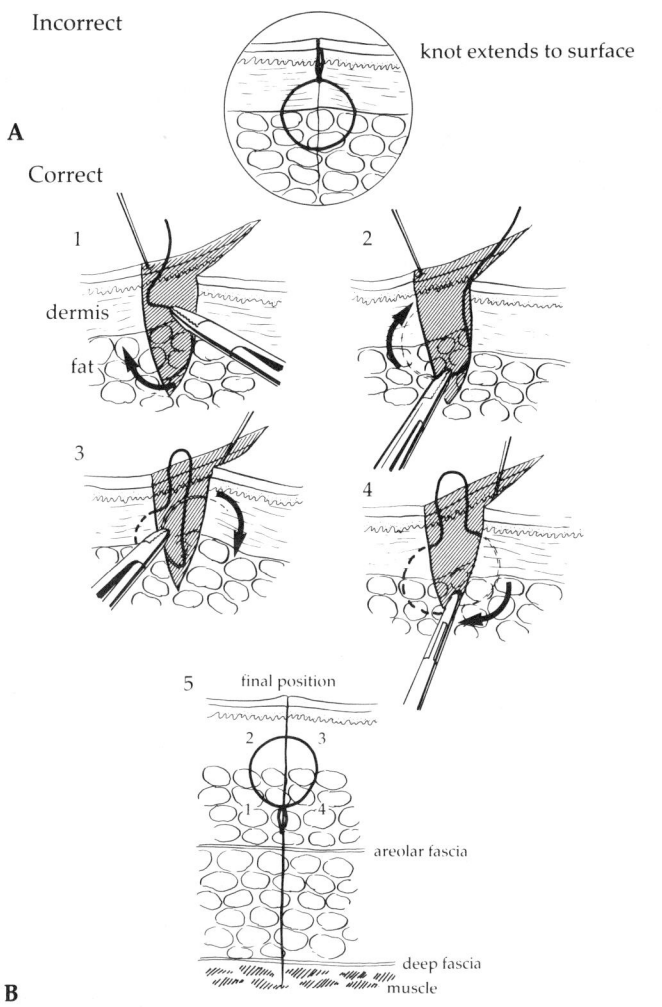

Figure 3-24. The subcutaneous suture.
A. The incorrect method would leave the knot at the surface.
B. Correct method. 1. Introduce the needle in the subcutaneous fat 1 or 2 mm below the dermis. 2. Advance the needle upward into the dermis while everting the skin with a skin hook. There is less likelihood of exposure of the suture and eventual extrusion if the needle is placed deep in the dermis. 3. Reintroduce the needle on the opposite side of the wound at the same level. 4. Exit the suture through the fat and lightly tie. 5. Final position, with knot ends extending downward in the subdermal layer.

1. Without layered closure—deep laceration. If there is not a layered closure, the skin suture must close the "dead space" in the subcutaneous fat and approximate the surface (Fig. 3-25A). Therefore, the skin suture includes not only the dermis but also a considerable amount of lacerated subcutaneous fat.
2. With layered closure—superficial laceration. If a layered dermal closure is used because of tension or tissue loss, the skin sutures are not placed as deeply (Fig. 3-25B). Only the dermis and minimal fat are included in the depth of the suture. The skin sutures should be staggered so that they do not directly overlie the dermal-subcutaneous suture.

In either situation, the placement of the suture requires that skin edges be everted. This necessitates incorporation of more tissue in the depth than at the surface.

To determine how far from the wound edges to place the suture, estimate the thickness of the skin from the top of the epidermis to the desired depth (Fig. 3-26). For most lacerations this is the dermis and 1 or 2 mm of underlying subcutaneous fat. Examples of average thickness in adult males

Figure 3-25. The depth of skin suture placement is also determined by the presence or absence of layered dermal closure.
A. Deep laceration without a dermal layer. Some additional subcutaneous fat may be included to avoid a dead space.
B. Deep laceration with a dermal layer, only the dermis is included in the skin suture.
C. Superficial laceration. Only the epidermis and dermis are included in the suture.

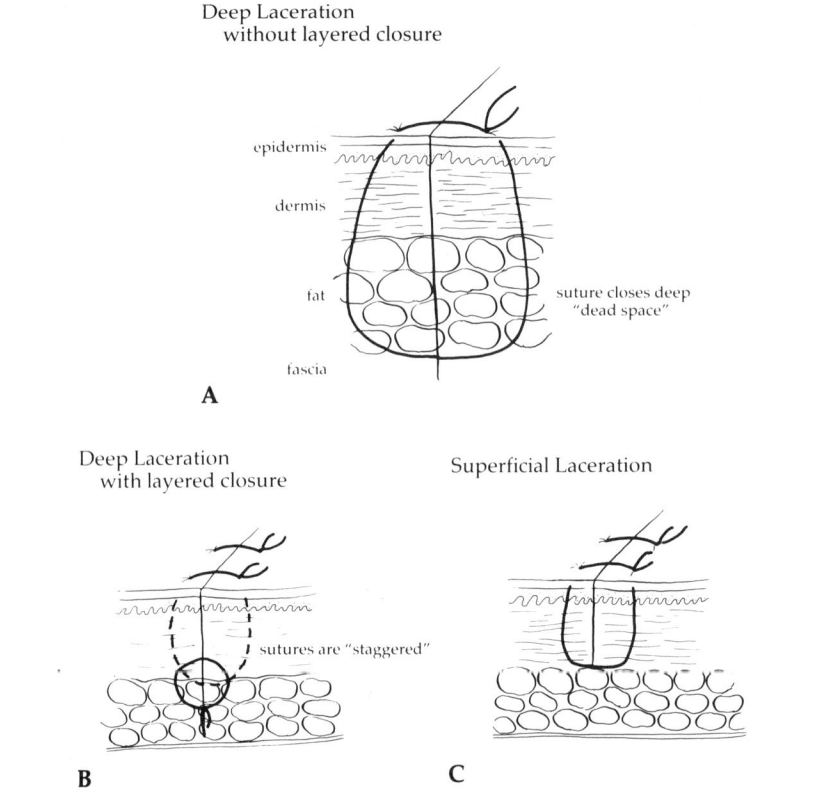

Figure 3-26. The needle entrance site relative to the wound edge is estimated as one-half of the depth of the dermis.

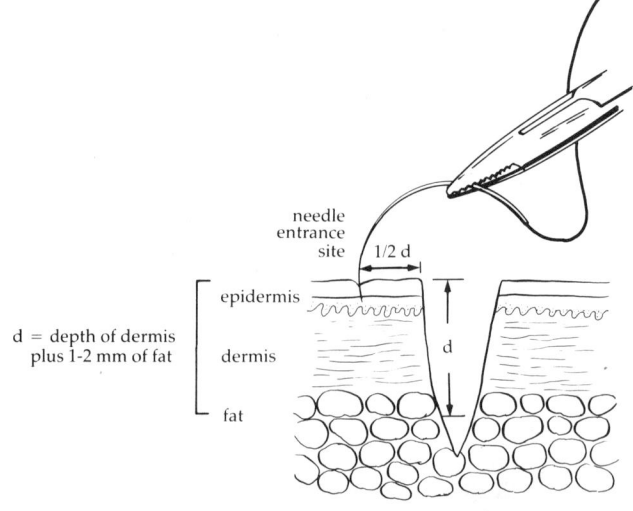

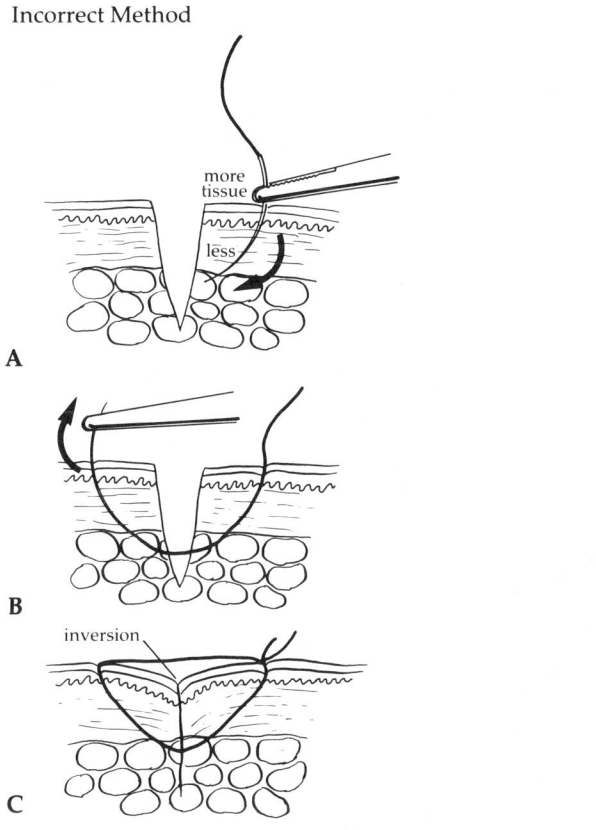

Figure 3-27. Incorrect needle positioning results in an inverted wound because of inadequate dermis in the depth of the wound.
    A. The needle incorporates more superficial than deep tissue.
    B and C. A similar "bite" on the opposite side causes inversion of the wound edges as the suture is tied.

are as follows (these are approximations, and there may be considerable variation):

Eyelid	1–2 mm
Face	2–4 mm
Nose	3–4 mm
Scalp	10–15 mm
Forehead	4–6 mm
Trunk	6–10 mm
Extremities	5–8 mm
Volar hand	3–5 mm
Dorsal hand	2–4 mm

The distance from the lacerated edge to the needle entrance site is about half this estimated thickness:

Eyelid	0.5–1 mm
Face	1–2 mm
Nose	1.5–2 mm
Scalp	5–7.5 mm
Forehead	2–3 mm
Trunk	3–5 mm
Extremities	2.5–4 mm
Volar hand	1.5–2.5 mm
Dorsal hand	1–2 mm

The incorrect method, which leads to edge inversion, is shown in Fig. 3-27. Edge inversion is a result of guiding the needle directly across the

Correct Method

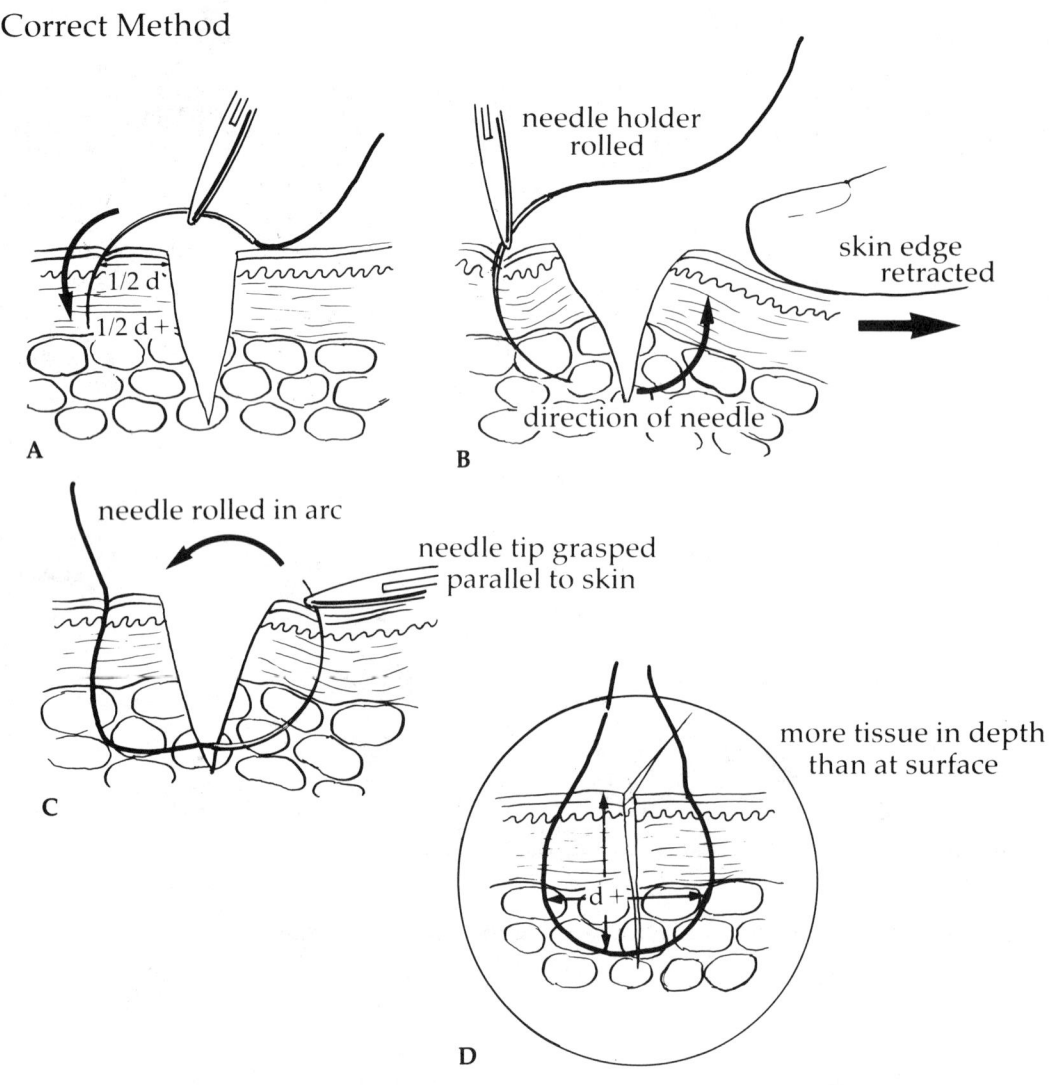

Figure 3-28. The simple suture.
A. Hold the needle upside down by excessively pronating the wrist, so that the needle tip moves farther from the laceration as the needle penetrates deeper into the skin. Thus there is more dermis in the depth of the wound than at the surface. Drive the needle tip downward and away from the cut edge, into the fat.
B. Advance the needle into the laceration. The needle tip can be advanced directly into the opposite side. This can be achieved by rolling the needle holder as the needle enters the opposite side at the same level, and the arc pathway of the needle is controlled by retracting the skin edge. This causes more dermis to be incorporated into the depths than at the surface. As an alternative, if a small needle is used in thick skin or the distance across the wound is great, the needle can be removed from the first side, remounted on the needle holder, and advanced to the opposite side.
C. Advance the needle upward toward the surface so that it exits at the same distance from the wound edge as on the contralateral side of the wound. Grasp the needle behind the tip and roll out in the arc of the needle.
D. The final position, with more tissue in the depth than the surface. The distance from each suture exit to the laceration is one-half the depth of the dermis.

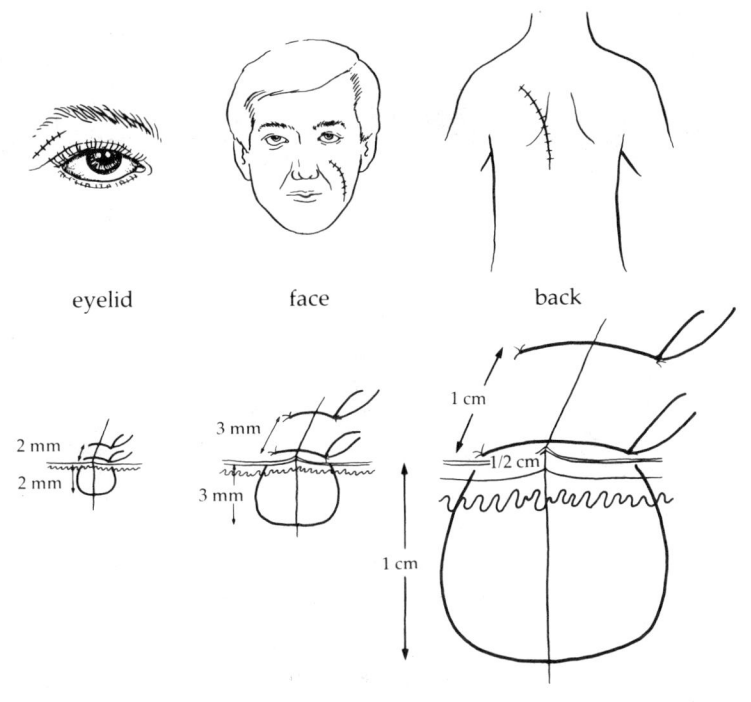

Figure 3-29. Correct distance between sutures on various parts of the body. The distance between sutures is approximately the same as the depth of the suture. This distance is also approximately equal to the distance between suture exit and entrance sites.

wound, thus including more tissue at the surface than in the depths. When the knot is tied, the extra tissue at the surface is forced to roll inward.

The method for skin suture placement to achieve edge eversion is shown in Fig. 3-28. The objective is to include an excess of deep dermis relative to superficial dermis.

The simplest criterion for determining the *distance between sutures* is to use the smallest number of sutures that achieves coaptation along the length of the wound. As a guide to making this determination, the distance between sutures is usually comparable to the depth of suture placement (Fig. 3-29).

When the suture is tied, the ends should be cut so that the loose ends do not become entangled in the adjacent suture.

CONTINUOUS (RUNNING) SUTURES—TYPE OF SUTURE

Sutures that are separately placed, tied, and cut are called interrupted sutures. If the next series of needle placements is made without tying and cutting, this is called a continuous, running, or over-and-over suture (Fig. 3-30). When using a continuous suturing technique, the same principles are used as described earlier for interrupted sutures. The advantages of continuous sutures are rapid repair and ease of suture removal. The disadvantages include (1) greater difficulty in achieving accurate edge approximation in height and length, (2) greater danger of wound ischemia caused by constricting sutures, (3) inability to use them for contaminated wounds that may require suture removal for drainage, and (4) the fact that unraveling of the knot at either end may loosen the continuous suture and result in wound dehiscence.

Figure 3-30. The continuous, running, or over-and-over technique is a rapid method of closure because knots do not have to be tied and cut at each site.
  A. Place the first suture and tie in the usual manner, but do not cut the knot.

B and C. Make the second and subsequent placement in the usual manner. Pull the suture very loosely in position. A suture that is too tight can cause constriction and ischemia.

  D. Leave the final loop very loose so that the knot is made with the loop (there is no suture end).
  E. The final arrangement.

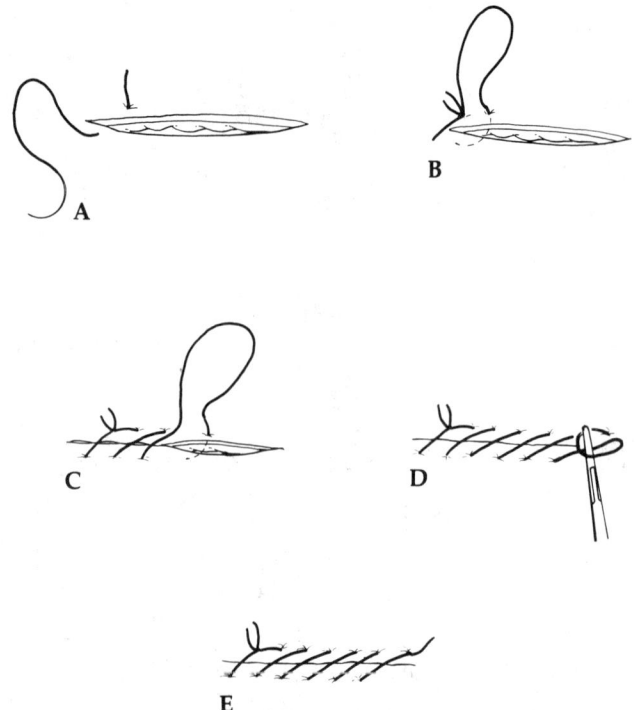

1. Vertical mattress sutures.

    The advantage of vertical sutures is that they ensure wound eversion (Fig. 3-31). The disadvantages are that
    a. They tend to compress the tissue and therefore have a higher risk of causing local ischemia.
    b. They are more difficult to remove.
    c. Because four suture exits are made, and they are farther from the laceration, secondary scar revision is more difficult if suture marks develop.

2. Horizontal mattress sutures. The horizontal mattress suture is placed the same distance from the wound edge as a simple suture (Fig. 3-32); thus secondary wound revision is not difficult should suture marks develop. Otherwise, the advantages and disadvantages are similar to those of the vertical mattress suture.

    The most common use of the horizontal mattress suture is in the palms and soles, because vertical mattress sutures pull through the thick keratin layer in these anatomic sites.

3. Half-buried mattress sutures
    a. Advantages. This suture is used when one skin margin is ischemic, such as the tips and margins of flaps. The buried horizontal dermal suture is less likely to compress the subdermal vessels.
    b. Disadvantages. There is greater risk of mismatch in the height and length of the wound margins because of the technical difficulty of placing the suture. Considerable skill is required for proper placement of the half-buried horizontal mattress suture (Fig. 3-33).

SIMPLE LACERATIONS

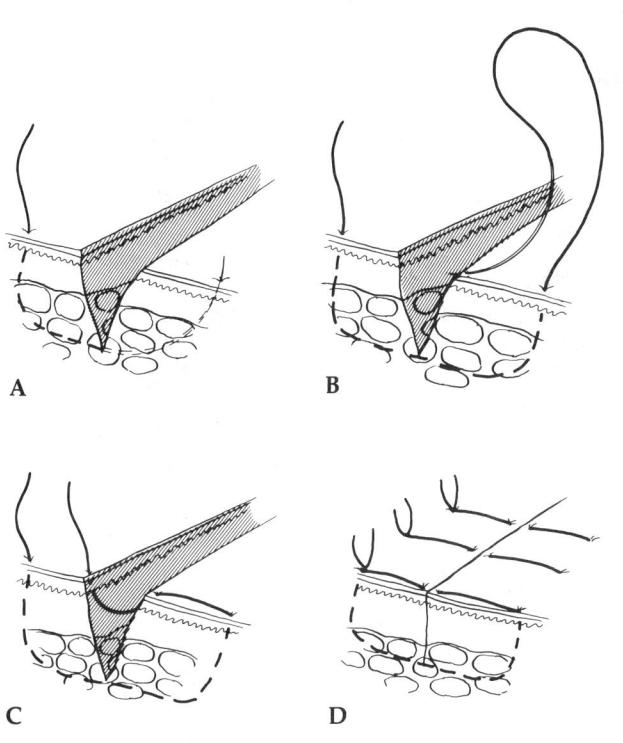

Figure 3-31. The vertical mattress stitch.
A. Make the needle entrance point about twice as far from the skin edge as it is in the simple interrupted technique. The needle does not have to be turned so that the needle enters at an angle greater than perpendicular to the skin, as in the simple suture.
B. Have the needle exit the opposite side at the same distance.
C. Withdraw the needle. By everting the skin with a hook or forceps, enter the needle almost perpendicularly approximately 1 mm from the margin. Pass it across the wound to exit the other edge at the same level. If these last two bites are placed too far from the edge, excessive eversion occurs.
D. The final arrangement.

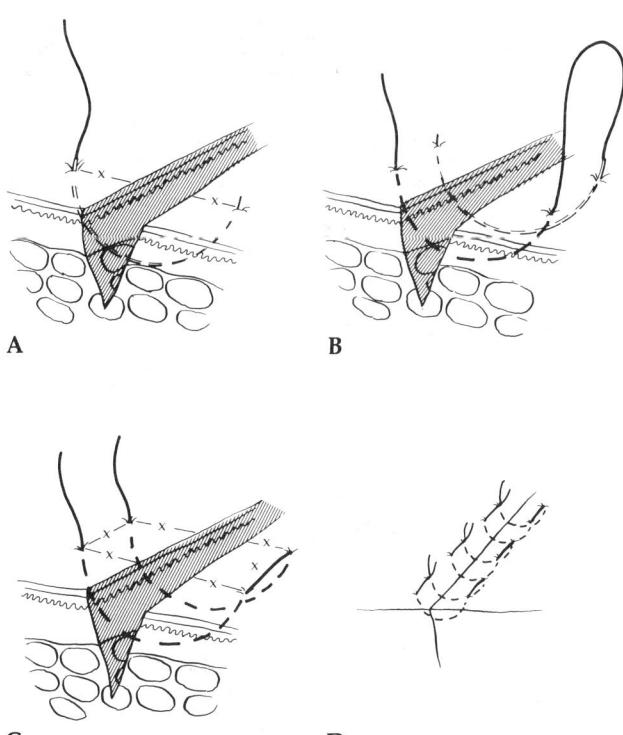

Figure 3-32. The horizontal mattress stitch.
A. Introduce the needle as in a simple suture, although less effort need be made to take a larger bite of deeper tissue. Bring it out through the surface on the opposite side, reversing direction.
B. Have the needle reenter the skin surface, approximately equidistant from the wound edge and its exit point and traverse the wound again in a manner similar to that of a simple suture.
C. Cause the needle to exit the skin on the opposite side, again equidistant from the wound margin and the original starting point of the stitch.
  If the two limbs of the stitch are too widely spaced when the suture is tied, the center of the wound may separate.
D. Tie the knots very loosely to avoid ischemia.

Figure 3-33. The half-buried mattress stitch.
A. Introduce the needle into the skin of the margin with the richer blood supply (nonflap side), pass it vertically downward, and bring it out in the upper dermis.
B. Introduce the needle into the upper dermis of the flap side and pass it several millimeters horizontally.
C. Bring the needle out and return it through the nonflap dermis; pass it vertically through the skin to exit.
D. Tie the sutures loosely; interrupted sutures can be used away from the flap tip.

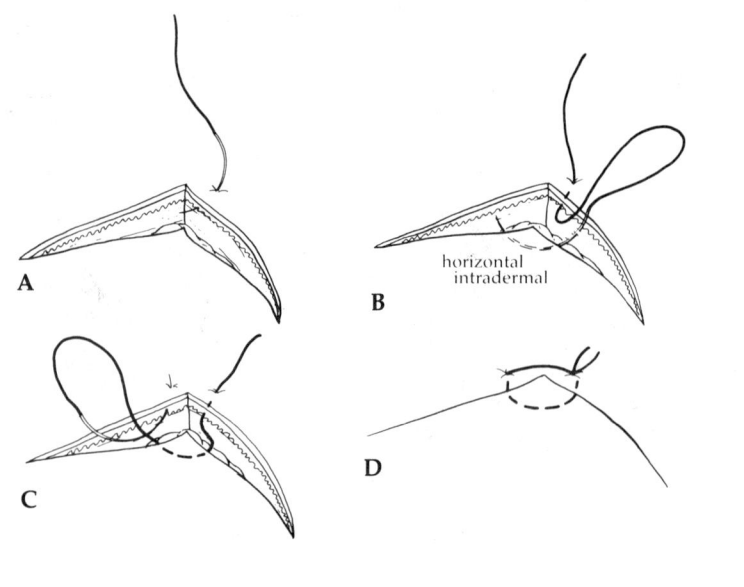

4. Intradermal (cuticular) "pull-out" sutures
    This suturing technique is extremely effective and has many uses (Fig. 3-34). It is important to use a strong monofilament suture, such as polypropylene, nylon, or wire, to have adequate strength and to allow easy sliding out of the suture.
    a. Advantages
        (1) Skin suture marks can be avoided except for the entrance and exit sites at the end of the wound.
        (2) The suture can be left for long periods of time in areas of wound tension or underneath a cast, with minimized problems of suture reaction and skin irritation.
        (3) Suture removal is simple, rapid, and with minimal pain. This is a major advantage for laceration in children.
    b. Disadvantages
        (1) The technique is somewhat more difficult than that of the simple interrupted skin sutures.
        (2) It is difficult to achieve accurate edge approximation on curved or irregular lacerations. Gaping of the edges of the wound and inequality of matching the height or length of the wound can easily occur.

SKIN TAPING
Tape can be used to approximate skin edges in lieu of or as an adjunct to sutures (Fig. 3-35).

1. Advantages
    a. The method is rapid, and local anesthesia is not required. Therefore, it is particularly useful in children.
    b. There is less foreign material within the wound and therefore a lower risk of infection.
    c. Suture marks can be completely avoided.

SIMPLE LACERATIONS

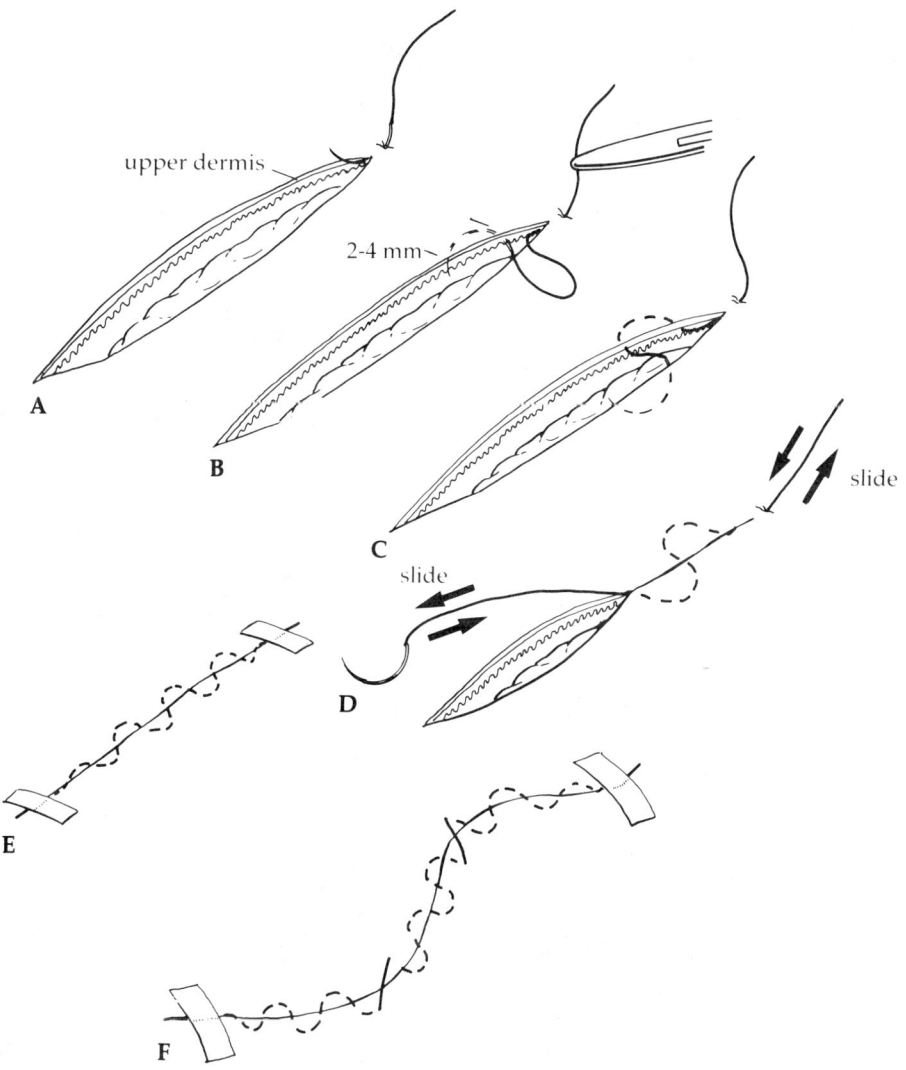

Figure 3-34. The intradermal stitch.

A. Introduce the needle through the skin a few millimeters from one end of the laceration and bring it through the end of the wound in the superficial dermis. Hold the end in place with a clamp.
B. Hold the needle parallel to the skin surface and reintroduce it into the dermis adjacent to the initial suture site. Advance the needle through the dermis 2 to 4 mm parallel to the skin surface. Stabilize the skin with a finger, skin hook, or forceps.
C. Directly across on the opposite side, introduce the needle at the same height. Again, advance the needle through the dermis parallel to the skin plane another 2 to 4 mm.
D. After several needle passages, grasp the suture ends and pull in one direction parallel with the laceration and then pull back to the original position to make sure the suture can slide.
E. At the end of the laceration pass the suture through the dermis and out through the skin, and make a final check of the ability of the suture to slide back and forth. Fix the suture in position with adhesive tape, a Steristrip (3 mm), or by tying a loop at each end.
F. The suture may not pull through long or curved wounds because of excessive friction. In these anticipated situations, bring the suture through the skin surface and across to the opposite side as a simple skin loop suture. When the suture is to be removed, cut the simple skin loop suture and remove the suture by pulling on both ends. Then continue the subdermal suturing technique. Any gaps can be approximated with skin tape.

Figure 3-35. Skin taping.
A. Apply benzoin or Ace adherent around the periphery of the wound.
B. Pinch the wound together so that the edges tend to evert and are accurately approximated.
C. Lay the tape across the wound and repeat this process along the length of the wound.

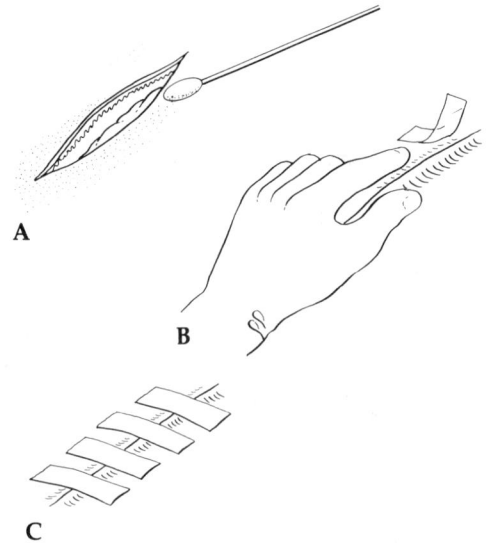

    d. Tape removal is painless, and therefore the postoperative discomfort of suture removal can be avoided.
2. Disadvantages. Although the advantages are highly desirable features, skin taping has not achieved acceptance because of technical problems, including the following:
    a. *The tape can separate* from the skin because of tension or movement, causing the edges of the wound to dehisce. This is particularly common in wounds around the face, where there is extensive movement, or wounds close to joint surfaces that are not adequately immobilized.
    b. The tape may be difficult to apply or may separate spontaneously because of sweat, discharge, or blood on the skin or hair.
    c. There is a marked tendency for skin taping to cause wound inversion rather than eversion. Inversion can be avoided by use of subcuticular sutures, but sutures partially negate the advantages of skin taping.

STAPLES

Staples have not been used extensively for closure of traumatic lacerations except for attaching large skin grafts or closing simple lacerations in noncosmetic areas. Their advantages are that they are rapidly applied, that the wound everts easily with them, and that they are less reactive than sutures. Their disadvantages are that accurate skin edge positioning is difficult and they require special equipment.

4. COMPLEX LACERATIONS

The simple laceration is tidy, linear, and superficial and can be closed without additional surgical manipulation. In contrast, the complex laceration presents unusual problems that require special management to achieve optimal results. The complexity of the wound may be caused by adverse wound conditions, the anatomic location, or the geometric configuration of the wound.

This chapter describes lacerations that are complex because of the adverse condition, location, or configuration of the wound. Considerable experience is required to make appropriate decisions and plan surgery. When confronted with a complex laceration, do only what you are confident can be achieved. Otherwise, simply close the wound or obtain consultation.

ADVERSE WOUND CONDITIONS

Untidy Wounds

Untidy wounds usually result from forceful impact, crush, bites, or tissue avulsion. The wound edges are irregular and of reduced viability and must be debrided. Several decisions must be made, including:

1. How to identify nonviable tissue, and amount of tissue to be debrided
2. The direction and configuration of the debridement
3. The technique to be used

IDENTIFICATION OF NONVIABLE TISSUE
How do you identify the limits of necrotic and marginally viable tissue in an untidy wound? In areas of critically important tissue that cannot be easily reconstructed, such as the eyelids and digits, a very conservative limited debridement and delayed closure may be preferable. The following methods are helpful in making the decision regarding tissue viability.

1. Color. Viable tissue has a healthy pink color. Either extreme pallor or cyanosis is suggestive of necrosis.
   Exceptions: anemia, shock, and local vasoconstrictors may cause unusual pallor. Polycythemia and dependency may cause cyanosis.
2. Blanching-flushing. Elevation or light pressure causes the blood in the capillary bed to empty (blanch). If circulation is adequate, the area will refill (flush). The area must be tested in a position level with the heart and/or without pressure. Assessment of the flush of hyperemia following release of a proximal tourniquet is an excellent test of tissue viability.
   Exceptions: Capillary refill is not necessarily a valid indicator unless compared quantitatively to a normal area. Blanching-flushing can occur slowly in an excised piece of skin sitting on the operating table or in tissue that has inadequate circulation from passive capillary refill not dependent on active circulation.

Furthermore, refill may not be seen in vasoconstricted areas because of epinephrine use or traumatic vasospasm.

3. Bleeding. Viable tissue bleeds from the arterioles after debridement.

    Exceptions: Pooled blood may ooze from nonfunctional vessels. However, the bleeding quickly stops and is nonpulsatile, cyanotic, and more likely to be seen in fat than dermis.

4. Muscle contraction. Viable muscle contracts and relaxes when gently squeezed, cut, or electrically stimulated. Questionable muscle contractions should be compared to obviously normal muscle.

    Exceptions: Local anesthesia may invalidate this phenomenon and give a false-negative interpretation. Recently injured nonviable muscle retains the capacity to contract, giving false-positive information.

5. Sensibility and pain. Pain (pinprick) and tactile (light touch) stimuli can be elicited from viable skin.

    Exceptions: Pressure on skin may be transmitted to deeper proprioceptive nerve endings in muscle and tendon, thus giving a false impression of skin sensation. Local nerve injury may induce a transient unresponsiveness to normal stimuli (neuropraxia) even though the skin is viable.

6. Turgor. Viable tissue is firm and supple, whereas nonviable tissue is rigid or "mushy."

    Exceptions: This is a subjective judgment without clear-cut standards of normality and may vary with patient age, mechanism of injury, and time elapsed since injury.

7. Injection of fluorescein dyes. Intravenous injection of 500 to 1000 mg of fluorescein stains viable perfused tissues. The characteristic yellow-green color is also easily identified with an ultraviolet Wood's lamp. Vigorous fluorescence, as evidenced by random dots of fluorescein, indicates that this tissue is viable at this time and will probably survive, and lack of fluorescence indicates devitalized tissue that should be debrided. This test is inconclusive when epinephrine has been used or in patients with inadequate perfusion from shock. There have been no deaths reported from its use in this manner, but anaphylactic reactions occur rarely. Therefore, the resources to treat such reactions must be available (e.g., IV line, epinephrine 1:1000, and other supportive measures). More commonly, some nausea is associated with injection.

8. Configuration. The configuration of the tissue can predict viability. Large pieces of tissue with a small pedicle or base have compromised flow. Thus, small irregular fragments and narrow pedicled tissue should be excised.

9. Type of injury. Certain causal mechanisms have a high likelihood of producing tissue necrosis. Therefore, more aggressive debridement is indicated. The following are examples of such mechanisms:

    a. Prolonged pressure or crush
    b. High-velocity missiles (see section on missiles)
    c. Chemical, electrical, and thermal burns
    d. Severely contaminated injuries such as bites, because of potential infection, toxins, and enzymes
    e. Shearing injuries in which the underlying blood vessels may have been damaged in addition to direct tissue trauma

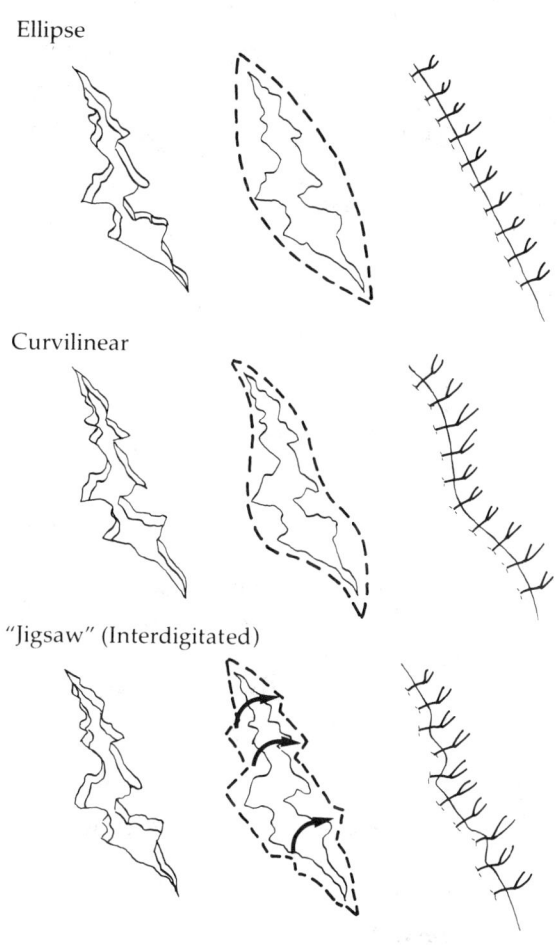

Figure 4-1. The alternative geometric shapes of debridement. The simple ellipse is most commonly used, but the curvilinear or interdigitation method can be used by the experienced surgeon in circumstances that require tissue conservation or when the line of the scar is perpendicular to the natural skin lines or cross concavities.

10. Location. The site on the body relative to blood flow may alter survival. Facial and scalp tissue is highly vascularized and survives better than comparable lower extremity tissue. Retrograde flaps, which have their pedicles in the opposite relation to normal arterial and venous flow, survive less well than antegrade flaps.

CONFIGURATION OF EXCISION

After the presence and distribution of nonviable tissue and thus the need for debridement is identified, the next decision is to determine the configuration of the excision (Fig. 4-1). Should it be excised in its exact distribution or should a specific geometric shape be used (e.g., by elliptical excision)? The jagged, irregular-shaped laceration can be debrided in various geometric patterns. Additional problems of excision are discussed in this chapter, such as crossing natural landmarks, small flaps, oblique flaps, and undermining and distortion of adjacent structures. The choice of geometric shape for the debridement is determined by:

1. Relation of wound to natural skin creases. The simple ellipse is preferable when the wound is parallel to natural wrinkle lines. The curvilinear or jigsaw interdigitation is preferable when crossing natural landmarks.

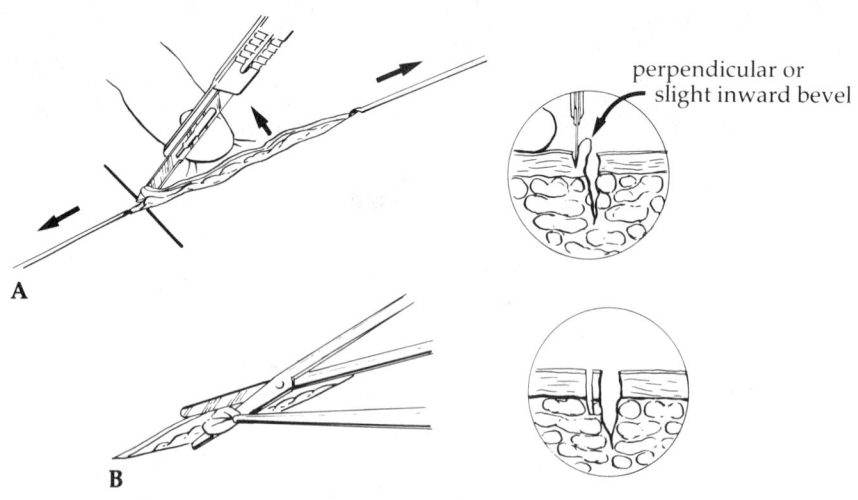

Figure 4-2. Skin debridement.
A. Stabilize the skin surface by hooks and incise with a knife, with fingers pressing away from the wound to prevent inward rolling.
B. Debride the fat and muscle with a pair of scissors.

2. Availability of sufficient adjacent tissues. The ellipse or curvilinear excision is used where there is surplus skin that can be excised without causing excessive tension when the wound is sutured closed. Because more normal tissue is removed with this method, the jigsaw configuration which conserves tissue is recommended for critical anatomic sites, such as the eyelids, nose, and lips.
3. Skill of the surgeon. Ellipses should be used by most surgeons. If irregular configuration is indicated, the procedure should be performed by experienced surgeons only because additional adverse scar can occur.

TECHNIQUE OF DEBRIDEMENT

Skin debridement, depicted in Fig. 4-2, proceeds as follows:

1. Establish a pattern of debridement. Debride in a specific direction rather than haphazardly. Begin at the wound end rather than in the middle of the wound or carrying out random debridement. This systematic approach ensures that all devitalized tissue is removed. Debridement results in small pinpoint areas of active bleeding denoting viable tissue.
2. Irrigate loose fragments. Minimally attached bits of fat can be floated away with irrigation. Fat and muscle, which offer little resistance to the pressure of the scalpel, can be debrided sharply with a pair of small forceps and scissors. The forceps and scissors can also be used to test muscle contractility and viability.
3. Stabilize wound edges. There is a tendency for the skin edges to roll under when being debrided. Unless care is taken to stabilize the dermis, an irregular, beveled edge will be produced. Stabilization is achieved by manual manipulation and skin hooks.

Knife cuts should be perpendicular to the surface.

Tension

GUIDELINES FOR UNDERMINING
1. *Problems with wounds closed with tension.* Debridement of devitalized tissue creates a tissue deficit. Wounds that are closed with excessive ten-

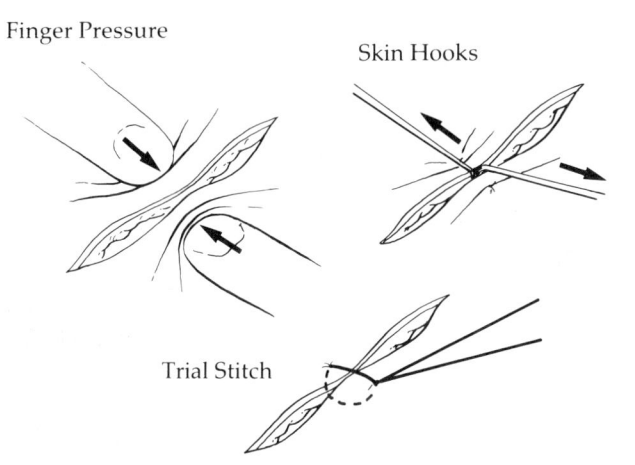

Figure 4-3. Testing for tension. Determine if the wound can be closed by one of three methods shown; a temporary trial suture may be the only definitive test.

sion because of tissue deficit are susceptible to dehiscence, infection, wide unsightly scars, and slough of wound edges.

2. *Testing for tension.* Wounds with tissue deficit should be tested to see if they can be closed without tension (Fig. 4-3). If the wound is too tight as determined by blanching of tissue or failure of wound edges to approximate, a choice must be made between undermining with advancement of the wound edges and/or adding tissue with a flap or graft.

3. *Problems with undermining.* Wound tension can be minimized by undermining and advancing adjacent skin. However, undermining itself can cause complications. Hematoma under the skin flap, additional scar, and damage to cutaneous nerves can result from undermining. Therefore, undermining should be performed only when necessary.

4. *Indications for undermining.* There are several guidelines for determining the need for undermining. Undermining should be performed when there is only minimal tightness so the edges can be brought close enough to be sutured. If the gap is so wide that it cannot be closed even with undermining, and a graft or flap is required, then undermining is contraindicated. Making this decision requires considerable experience. The scalp, face, extremities, and back can be undermined. The abdomen rarely requires undermining because of its laxity.

5. *Areas not to be undermined.* Another clue to the need for undermining after debridement is the anatomic area. The palms, soles, and pretibial area should not be undermined because no additional tissue advancement is gained by undermining the skin in these regions.

LEVEL FOR UNDERMINING

The level of undermining is determined by the anatomic area and level of the injury (Figs. 4-4 and 4-5). Each anatomic structure has a best or natural plane for undermining. In general, the areolar fascial planes are best because of natural lateral mobility and minimal disruption of normal vascular patterns. However, superficial lacerations into fat are sometimes better managed by undermining in the fat at the deepest level of the laceration rather than deepening the cut to an anatomic fascial plane. There is danger of injuring an underlying cutaneous nerve if a deeper plane is sought. Intradermal and intramuscular undermining should not be done.

Figure 4-4. Differing levels of undermining: head and neck areas.

A. Scalp should be undermined below the hair follicles to prevent bald spots. The loose areola below the galea is the natural plane. Scoring of the galea may relieve tension.

B, C, and D. Facial and neck skin should be undermined above the facial muscle or parotid fascia to avoid damage to the facial nerve. The appropriate level is in the fat just below the dermis.

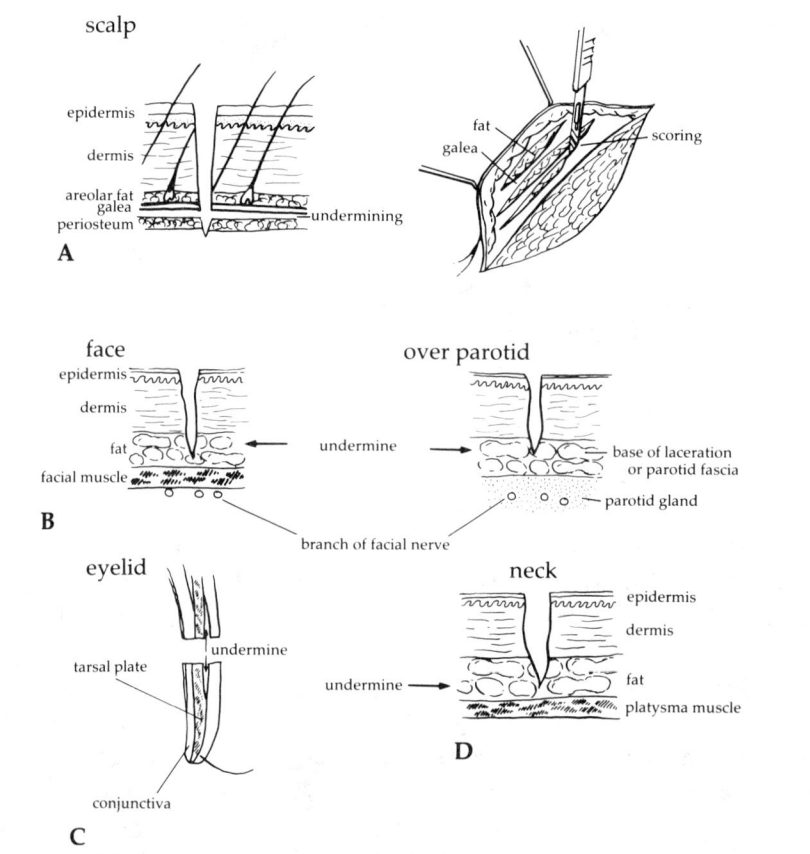

Figure 4-5. Differing levels of undermining: bone, cartilage, trunk, and extremity.

A and B. Skin overlying bone or cartilage should be undermined above the perichondrium to prevent cartilage exposure and infection.

C. Skin of the trunk and extremity should be undermined in the areolar fascia of the fat or on muscular fascia, depending on the depth of laceration.

D. Skin of hand or foot dorsum should be undermined on fascia overlying the tendons. DO NOT undermine palm or sole.

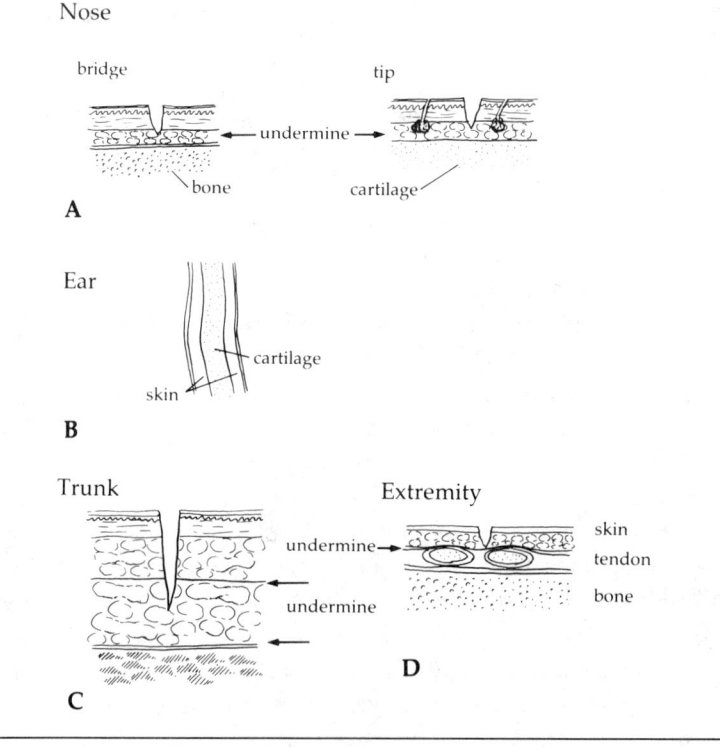

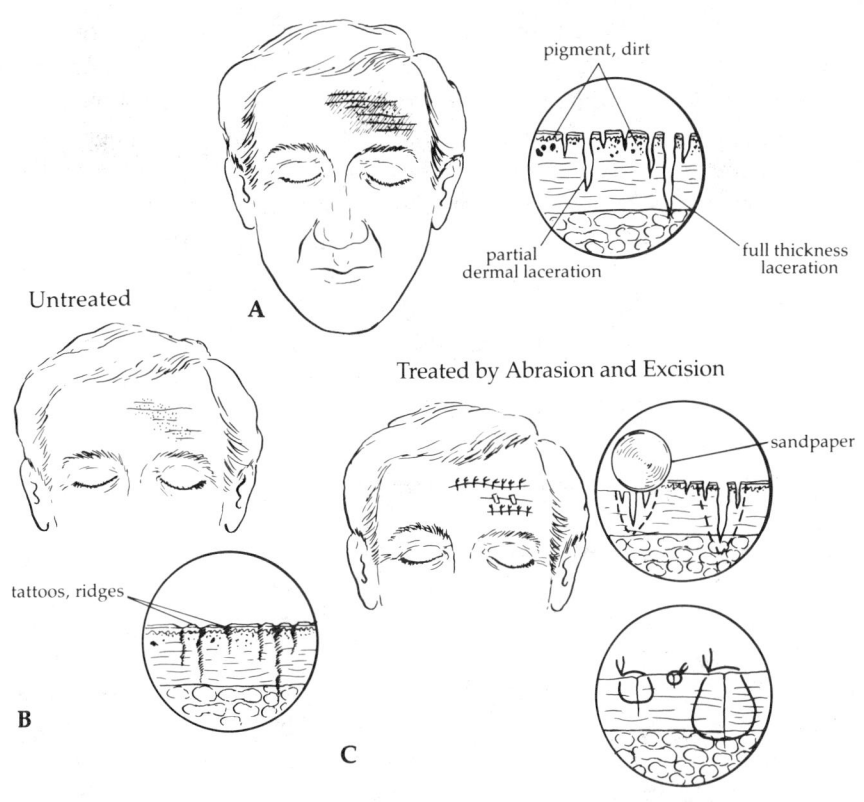

Figure 4-6. Abrasion-laceration.
A. The wound has multiple lacerations, foreign material, and abrasions.
B. The untreated wound heals with residual ridges and tattoos.
C. The abrasion-laceration must be treated by a combination of therapeutic dermabrasion of the skin and excision of clusters of abrasions that extend into the fat. Isolated dermal lacerations need not be sutured.

Abrasion–Dermal Laceration

The abrasion-laceration is a dual problem caused by scraping on a rough surface. A fall from a bicycle, motorcycle, or skateboard can result in a skid across dirt and asphalt. The skin is partially abraded and has many parallel lacerations (Fig. 4-6). Some of the lacerations are deep, but most are superficial. Superficial lacerations do not completely transect the dermis and thus no fat can be seen in the base of the wound. More importantly, the intact deep dermis maintains the skin continuity.

Specific problems that require treatment include traumatic tattoos, multiple superficial unsuturable lacerations, and skin deepithelialization.

1. Pigment. Road dirt, grease, and grass are partially embedded in the skin. These pigmented particles are phagocytized by tissue macrophages and thus remain intracellularly at the site of the injury. Phagocytosis occurs within 72 hours of injury. Thus, if permanent intracellular tattooing is to be avoided, *dermabrasion must be performed as soon after injury as possible.*
2. Multiple superficial lacerations. Many lacerations are so closely arranged that sutures cannot be used. The lacerations must be approximated to avoid parallel ridges, which cause shadows to be cast into the depressions.

TREATMENT
1. Anesthesia. Topical anesthetics can be absorbed through traumatic abrasions if most of the epithelium has been lost. Our drug of choice for

topical use is 4% Xylocaine. Maximum anesthesia is obtained in 15 to 20 minutes. The depth of anesthesia obtained is only a millimeter or more into the soft tissue; hence, care must be taken to proceed slowly and not work beyond the limits of the absorption, unless an infiltration or regional block is administered in addition to the topical anesthetic. The area is covered with a dry 4 × 4 gauze pad, which is in direct contact with the wound. The 4% Xylocaine is then applied to the gauze. Irrigation and superficial sandpapering can be achieved with topical anesthesia. However, areas requiring sutures or deep sandpapering must be anesthetized with infiltration or regional block methods.

2. Irrigation. All pigment and foreign material must be removed by irrigation, mechanical debridement, and sandpapering. Irrigation with a high-velocity pulsatile water stream such as the Waterpik or Surgilav is very effective.

3. Dermabrasion. Dermabrasion not only aids the removal of foreign particles but also removes the most superficial dermal lacerations. The depth of dermabrasion depends on the thickness of the dermis and depth of the wound.

4. Suturing and excisions. Full-thickness lacerations are sutured or excised in the appropriate manner. This may require debridement of untidy wounds or excision of closely clustered multiple adjacent lacerations. Converting four or five small lacerations into one somewhat longer or larger laceration results in a better scar. A fuller discussion of the management of multiple lacerations is contained in the next few sections.

5. Taping. Superficial dermal lacerations can be treated best by surface taping. It is not always possible to tape the dermal lacerations individually because blood or abrasions may prevent the tape from sticking to the skin. If so, the lacerations must be sutured individually.

6. Dressing. The dressing is part of the therapy. (An open dry wound is maintained so that any residual dermal lacerations and pigment can be removed.) The dry dressing causes desiccation of the superficial dermis, and a reepithelialization occurs at a subsurface level, thus entrapping pigment in the eschar, which later sloughs off. A closed dressing with antibiotic ointment allows for a more superficial level of reepithelialization.

Multiple Adjacent Lacerations

PROBLEM: MULTIPLE SCARS AND SLOUGH OF INTERVENING SKIN
Clustered lacerations result in necrosis of intervening skin bridges and poor scars (Fig. 4-7). Standard window glass and automobile safety glass result in different types of lacerations. The new safety glass does not break into large chunks, but shatters into small fragments. The closely arranged fragments cause relatively shallow adjacent lacerations and small U-shaped flaps. Narrow bridges of tissue are isolated between lacerations. These bridges have compromised blood supply and are susceptible to necrosis particularly when sutures are placed on each side. Multiple lacerations leave multiple scars, with a tendency to form depressions and ridges.

TREATMENT: GROUPED EXCISIONS
Clusters of lacerations with narrow skin bridges should be surgically excised, thus converting a grouping into a single laceration. The number,

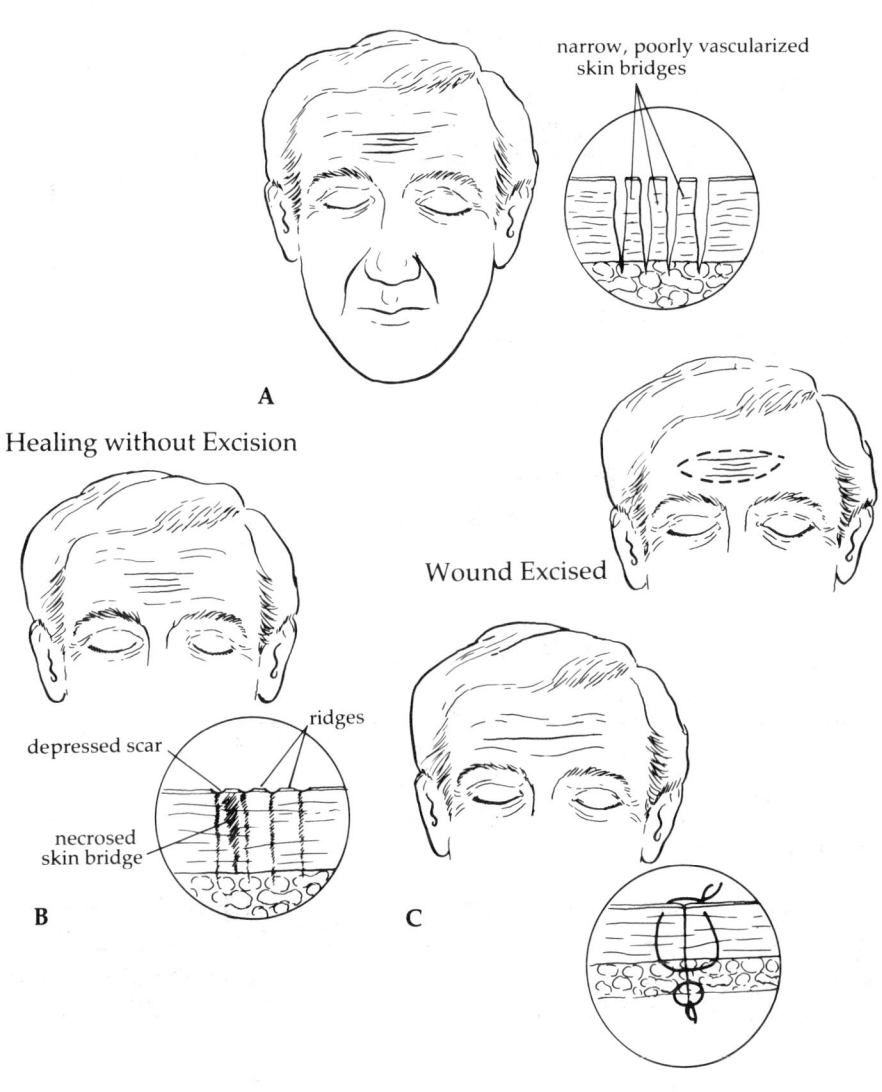

Figure 4-7. Multiple adjacent lacerations.
A. The multiple lacerations cause narrow skin bridges.
B. If sutured without excision, skin necrosis and multiple depressed scars can occur.
C. The excision of multiple adjacent lacerations as a single grouping results in more favorable scarring. Care must be taken not to excise too much tissue.

dimensions, shape, and depth of excision are challenging puzzles. Various combinations of grouped excisions can be conceptualized, and several guidelines are available:

1. Always choose to excise a safe, limited amount. Overzealous surgery can create a defect that is too large to close by approximation and thus requires a skin graft. *Be conservative* with excisions. The amount of excision depends on the anatomic site and relative tissue excess.
2. *Determine the ideal and acceptable directions for scar placement* (parallel with skin wrinkles and creases).
3. Identify anatomic borders that cannot be entered without problems (e.g., hairlines, lid).
4. Debride and *close the worst areas first* and proceed serially with additional cluster excisions until the smallest numbers of lacerations remain or until a highly acceptable set of individual wounds is achieved. Each area of excision must be closed before proceeding to the next so that the limits of tissue tension and availability can be assessed.

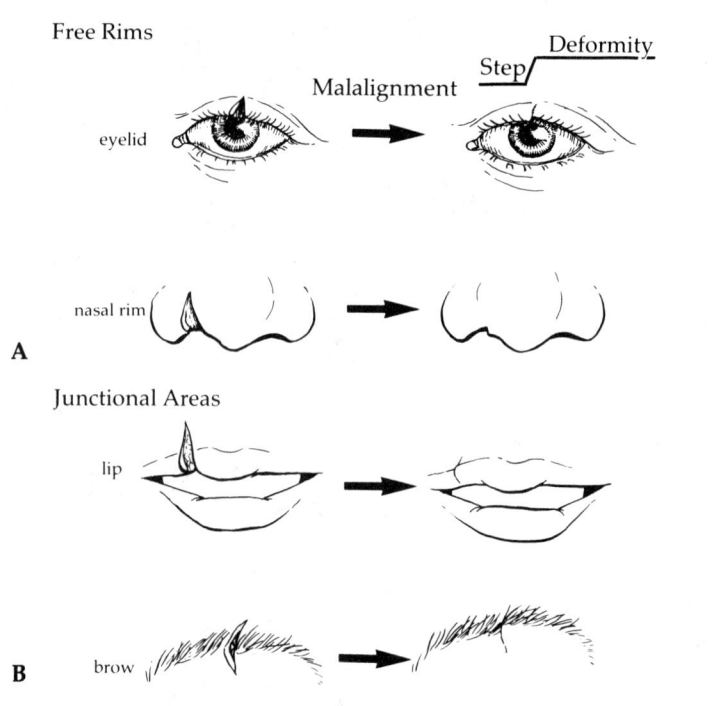

Figure 4-8. Malalignment causing step deformity.
A. A step deformity of free rims of the eyelid, nose, and ear can occur if precise alignment is not achieved.
B. The anatomic junctional areas also must be precisely realigned.

LOCATION

Anatomic Borders

Certain wounds are complex because they border distinct anatomic regions, such as hair-bearing skin, vermilion, or free margins. Exact anatomic repositioning and avoidance of crossing into another tissue type are the objectives of treatment.

THE PROBLEM: STEP DEFORMITY
There are numerous areas of the face that have characteristic colors, textures, shapes, or hair. The border between the unique anatomic areas must be repaired with absolute precision. Malalignment of the border results in a step deformity (Fig. 4-8). These anatomic borders are characterized as either free rims (prominences) or junctions of two distinct anatomic areas.

Free rims include the eyelid, ear helix, and nasal ala. Junctional areas include the borders between lip vermilion and skin, eyebrow and skin, and hairline and skin.

TREATMENT
Surgical repair is directed primarily at precise realignment of the border and underlying tissues (Figs. 4-9 and 4-10). This can be achieved most accurately using *ocular loupes for magnification*. Alignment is ensured by identification and *marking of the anatomic border*. On the vermilion the ink identification should be made before injection of local anesthesia. Other sites can be defined adequately afterward.

A layered closure is used, *beginning with a key stitch to align the anatomic border* of the free rim or junctional area. After the key alignment stitch is placed, a layered closure is completed.

COMPLEX LACERATIONS

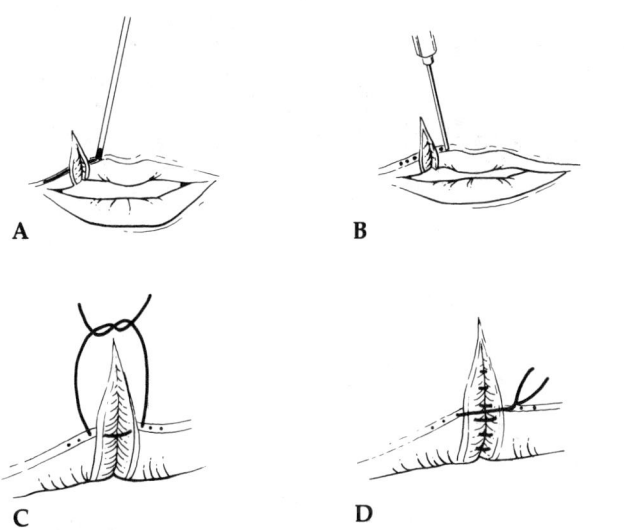

Figure 4-9. Avoidance of step deformity.
A. Identify the anatomic border using a magnifying loupe when available.
B. Mark it with an ink line or inked needle punctures.
C. Place the key stitch.
D. Close the remaining layers.

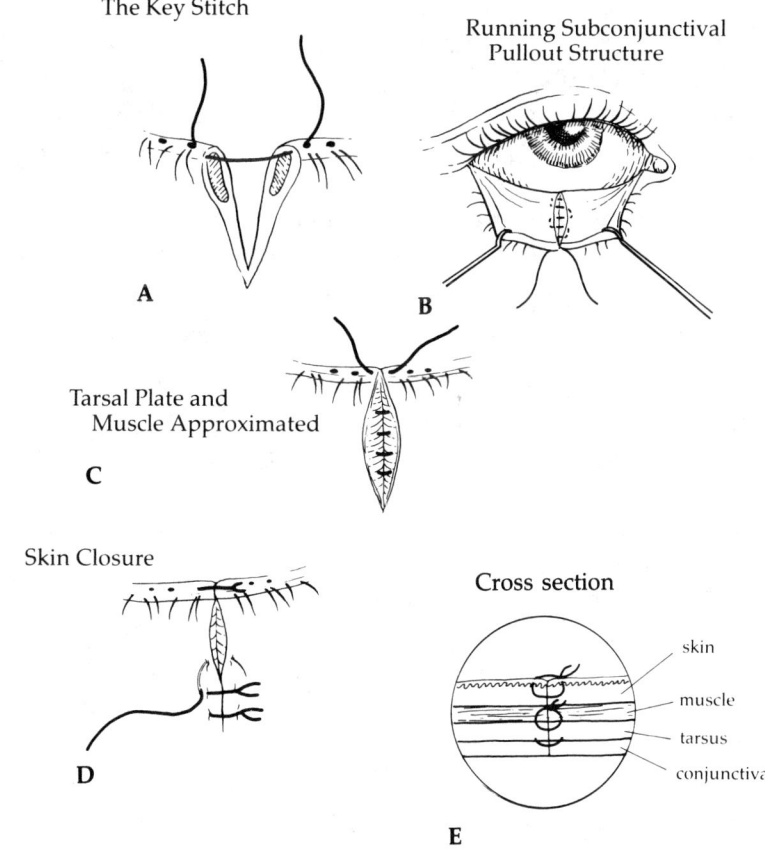

Figure 4-10. Closing eyelid lacerations. Note that a submucosal suture is used on the conjunctiva to avoid having suture ends rubbing on the cornea.
A. Place the first or "key" stitch at the junction between eyelid and conjunctiva (gray line). A fine silk suture is usually used. Nylon is too stiff and the suture ends may irritate the conjunctiva. Align this gray line carefully.
B. Place a running pullout suture subconjunctivally.
C. Use several interrupted simple sutures of 5–0 Dexon or Vicryl to approximate the tarsal plate and orbicularis muscle.
D. Close the skin with fine nylon sutures.
E. A three-layered closure is achieved.

Figure 4-11. Incorrect method for debriding eyebrow lacerations.
A. A laceration across the eyebrow injures obliquely growing hair follicles.
B. Debridement of the wound edge perpendicular to the margins destroys additional follicles, resulting in a hairless area after wound closure.

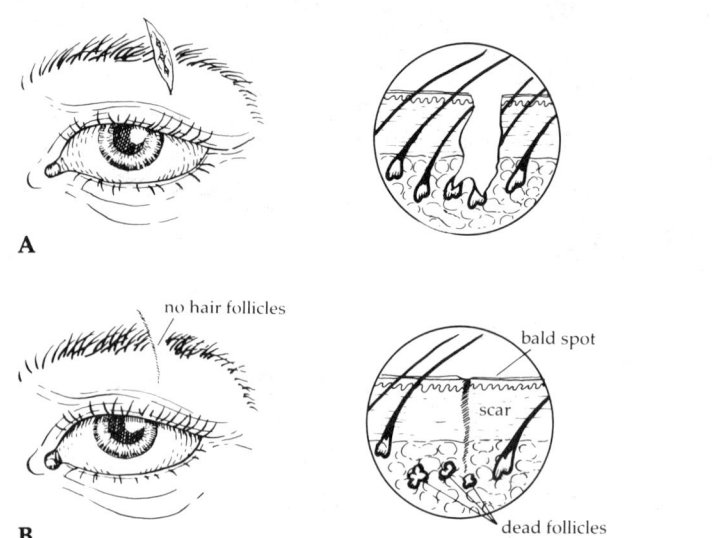

Hair-Bearing Skin

THE PROBLEM: BALD SPOT

In addition to malalignment at a junctional border, a bald spot in hair-bearing skin can be quite noticeable even if there is a perfect scar (Fig. 4-11).

The normal hair follicle grows at an oblique angle, rarely perpendicularly. If the laceration is not parallel with the follicle, the hair bulb can die and leave a bald spot.

TREATMENT

Excise the laceration at an obliquity parallel to the hair follicles and not perpendicular to the skin surface (Fig. 4-12). This difficult technique may cause an irregular scar, but the scar will be hidden by the hair.

1. Carefully examine the hair follicles to determine the growth angle relative to the skin surface.
2. Cut with a knife blade to create an oblique wound parallel to the hair follicles.
3. Do not use absorbable sutures and carefully avoid injury to the bulb with the needle. Use subcutaneous sutures below the hair bulb and skin sutures above, but no intradermal sutures.

Concavities, Convexities, and Flexion Creases

THE PROBLEM: BOWSTRING SCARS

Certain anatomic sites have a concave or convex surface (Fig. 4-13). Scars crossing a concave or convex surface follow the shortest, straightest course, resulting in either a bowstring scar in a concavity or a scar depression in a convexity (Fig. 4-14). Examples of concave and convex surfaces follow.

COMPLEX LACERATIONS

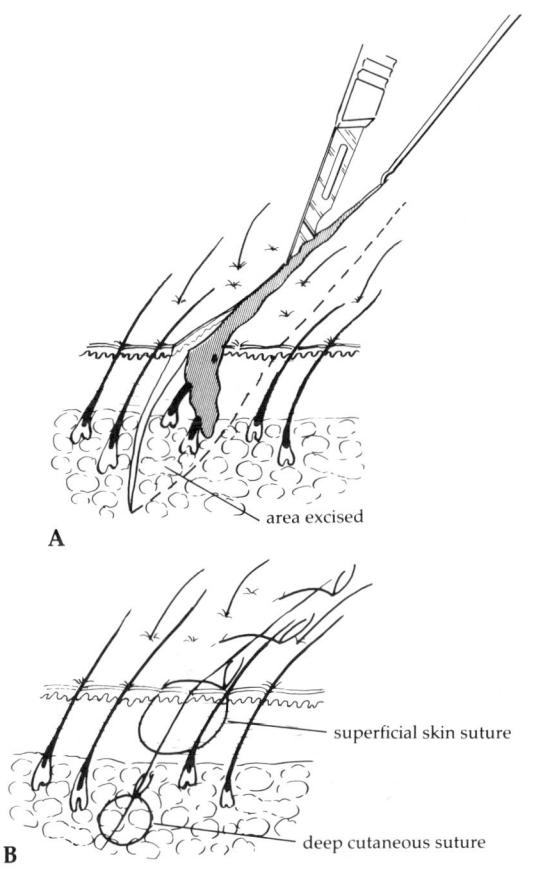

Figure 4-12. Correct method for debriding eyebrow lacerations. The wound edges are debrided in an oblique manner that parallels the direction of the hair follicles (A). As a result, fewer hair follicles are damaged.

This avoids a bare area about the closure (B).

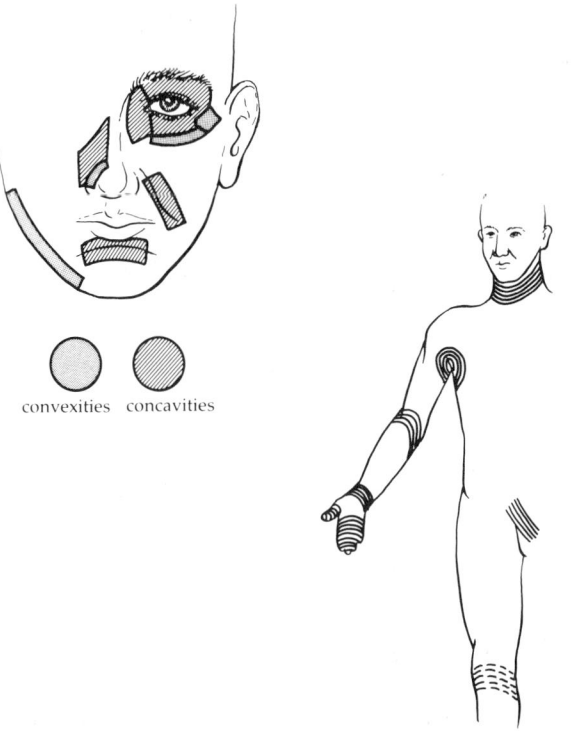

Figure 4-13. The concavities, convexities, and flexion creases of the body surface.

Figure 4-14.
A. Several lacerations directed perpendicular to natural concavities.
B. With healing and contracture, the scar "bowstrings" across the concavity.

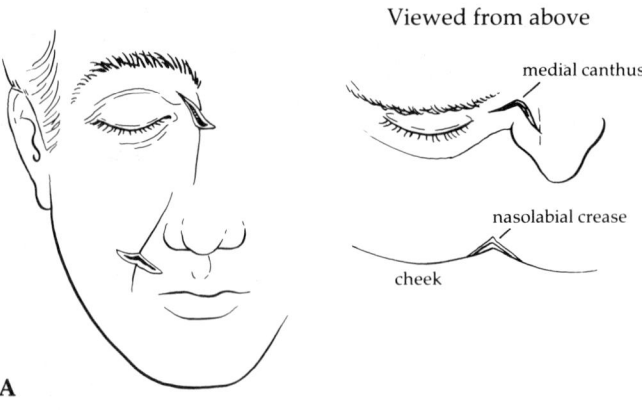

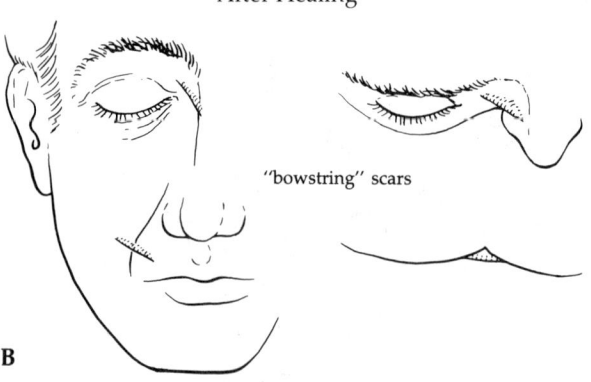

1. Concavities
    a. Medial canthal region, junction of nose with eyelids
    b. Upper lid sulcus (vertical laceration)
    c. Lower lid sulcus (vertical laceration)
    d. Lateral canthal (vertical laceration)
    e. Nasolabial crease (horizontal laceration)
    f. Junction of neck and chin (vertical laceration)
    g. Junction of nose and cheek (horizontal laceration)
    h. Mentum (vertical laceration)—junction of lip with chin
    i. Junction of posterior ear and skull
    j. Finger web spaces
    k. Thenar-palmar junction
2. Convexities
    a. Mandibular rim
    b. Malar rim
    c. All joint flexion surfaces

TREATMENT: Z-PLASTY
Caution! If you are not sure of the method of Z-plasty and no one is available for consultation, close the wound as a simple laceration. Tell the patient that a thick noticeable scar will probably form, and revisional plastic surgery will be

needed. Do not attempt primary Z-plasty unless you are adequately familiar with the principles and methods, because if it is improperly performed a worse scar will form, which may not be correctable.

The tips of a Z-plasty flap (or any traumatic flap) are susceptible to necrosis because of reduced flow to the tip; this is compounded by the constricting devascularizing effect of excessive simple sutures. The flap stitch (half-buried dermal mattress) is used because it has less effect on the flap circulation than a simple stitch or standard mattress suture. Figs. 4-15 and 4-16 depict the procedure for performing Z-plasty.

CONFIGURATION OF THE LACERATION

Even though a laceration is tidy and in a favorable location, it can be adverse because of its configuration. An unfavorable appearance occurs because of elevation of a skin surface, which appears as a bulge with adjacent shadow. Wounds that produce noticeable scars because of flaps of skin, oblique cuts, and unequal lacerations can be altered at the initial injury to achieve optimal results.

Small U-Shaped Flaps

The new laminated safety glass in automobile windshields has eliminated most major deep lacerations from shattered windshields during automobile accidents. However, impact with safety glass causes multiple small cuts that tend to form flaps with a U-shape. Fragments of glass may be embedded under the flap. The glass must be removed, and after that the flap laceration should be altered.

THE PROBLEM
Small oblique skin flaps bunch up to form a raised "biscuit deformity" or "trap door" as they heal (Fig. 4-17). This is caused by a semicircular scar contracting and bunching the central tissue. A glass fragment can cause additional fullness and scar.

TREATMENT
Treatment consists of excision of the flap and conversion into a linear wound. The principles of using natural skin lines, 3:1 ratios (see page 112), and avoiding concavities, convexities, and natural borders must be observed and are discussed in this section.

1. Glass removal. Each flap must be examined separately for an underlying glass fragment. These are identified and removed with small forceps or a clamp. The glass usually can be visualized, felt with the finger, or heard when scraped with a forceps blade.
2. Determining the best direction for excision. Flaps should be excised as an "ellipse" or curvilinear S parallel within the skin wrinkles or other anatomic contours (Fig. 4-18). Wrinkle lines are perpendicular to facial muscle (Fig. 4-19) and can be accentuated by exaggerated facial animation. Contour sites occur at the junction of anatomic areas, such as cheek-nose, ear-cheek, lip-chin, chin-neck, and nose-lip.

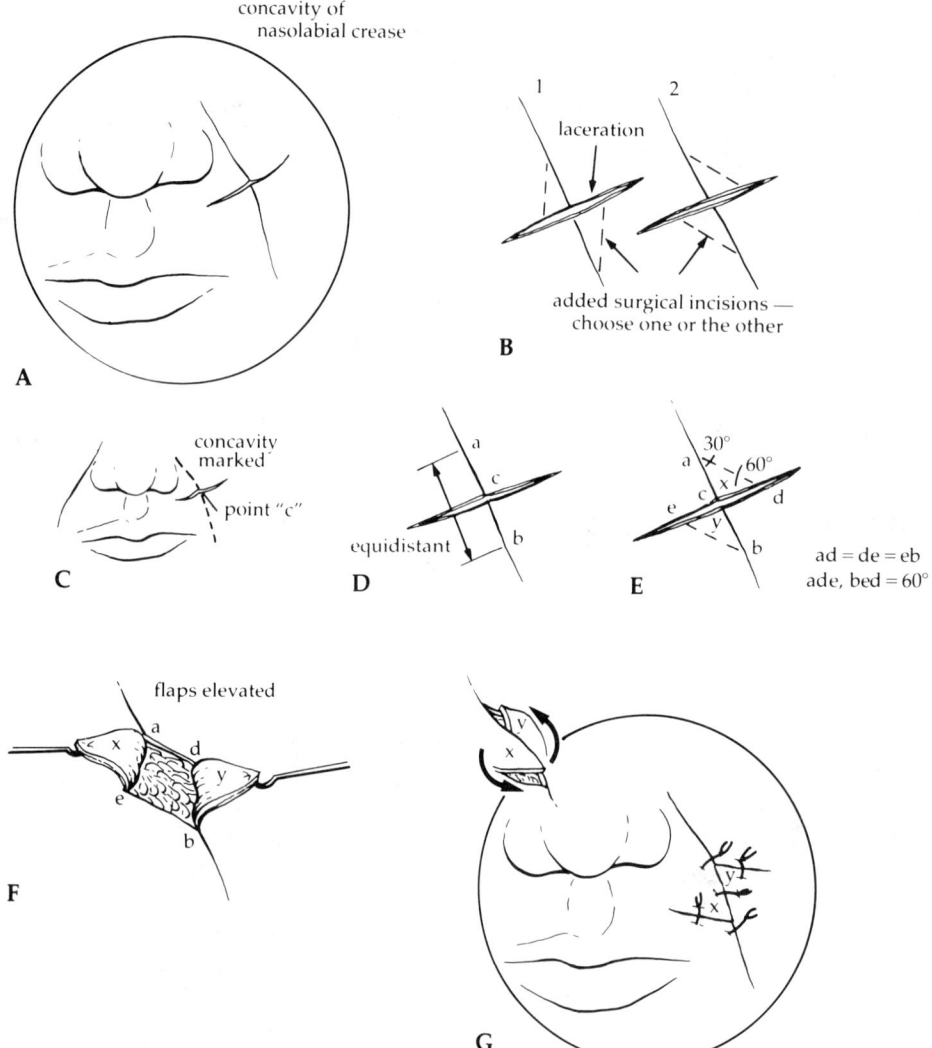

Figure 4-15.
A. The laceration is the central oblique limb of the Z.
B. Two additional horizontal limbs must be cut so that two flaps are formed. The choice of limb direction depends on local circumstances, such as adjacent scar and adjacent anatomic structures (see step E).
C. Dot the concavity of flexion crease with marking ink. The junction of the laceration and the crease is called point c.
D. From the point at which the laceration crosses the concavity, pick equidistant points (a, b) on both sides of the concavity line. The distance should be less than the length of the laceration (i.e., ca = cb). The actual length of ca and cb may vary from 0.5 cm to 1 cm.
E. If the laceration is at an angle of approximately 90° to the concavity, draw a line from the equidistant points a and b to form a 30° angle with the concavity line, and continue the line until it meets the laceration (at points d and e). Double check that the following criteria are met: 1. The lines ad, de, and eb are approximately the same length. 2. The angles ade and bed are approximately 60°. 3. There are no scars or lacerations at the bases of these triangles (i.e., across ae or bd).
F. Incise the lines (ad, eb) that extend from equidistant points to the laceration and elevate the flaps (x) and (y) in the plane that you would normally undermine in that particular area, or in the plane at the base of the wound.
G. Transpose the flaps. Note that the scar line now is a Z, but the central limb of the Z lies within the concavity rather than crossing it.

Incorrect

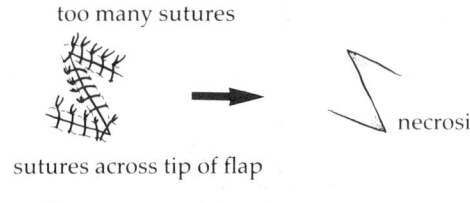

A

Correct

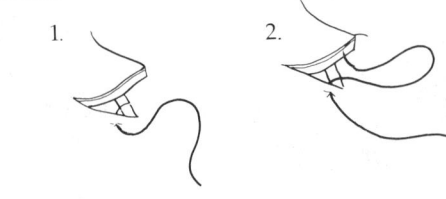

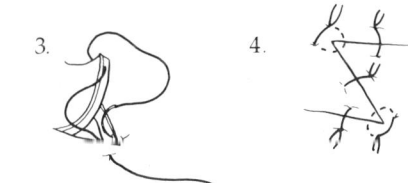

B

Figure 4-16.
A. The incorrect method for suturing Z-plasties. Too many sutures, too closely placed embarrasses the circulation of the flap, especially the tips.
B. The correct method: Use a half-buried horizontal mattress suture (tip-stitch) to approximate the tip of each limb of the Z-plasty. (1) With the first bite, enter the skin and exit within the deep dermis. (2) Make the needle enter and exit the dermis of the tip of the flap at the same level (the buried portion of the stitch). (3) Enter the dermis of the far side of the wound, again at the same depth as the two previous bites, and exit the skin at the same distance from the wound margin as the initial bite. Tie the suture just tight enough to pull the tip of the flap into the angle. Achieving the proper tension is important because excessive tensison bunches the tip and may necrose the skin, while insufficient tension leaves a gap that must heal by epithelialization and contracture. Approximate the remaining edges by the method of "halving" the wound, using just enough suture to achieve precise closure.

3. Will the excision close? Before excising any skin flap, be certain that the defect created by excision of a flap or group of flaps can be closed without excessive tension and distortion of normal contours (Fig. 4-20). The amount of skin that can be excised is variable. The age of the patient, site on the body, and orientation must be considered.
4. Will the excision cause distortion? The major facial problem areas are around the eyelids and mouth. Around these orifices, excessive skin excision causes distortion (Fig. 4-21). Although temporary distortion is acceptable for the purpose of achieving a healed wound, it is not acceptable to cause eyelid ectropion. Ectropion causes excessive tearing (epiphora) and can lead to corneal ulcers. Therefore, if the cornea is

Figure 4-17. Biscuit deformity.
A. The "biscuit" or "trapdoor" flap occurs with small U-shaped wounds in which the laceration has scythed and undercut the skin or contains foreign material.
B. The healed wound is noticeable because of the shadows cast by the bulging flap.

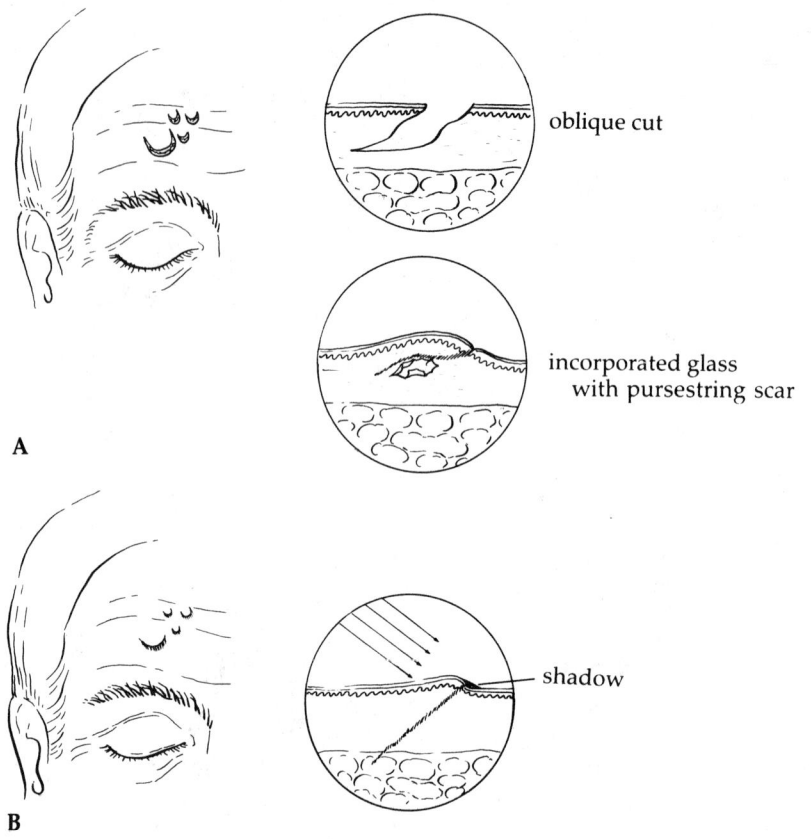

Figure 4-18. Direction of excision.
A. Elliptic excision paralleling skin creases is the preferred method of removing multiple small U-shaped flaps.
B. Curvilinear excisions can be designed to encompass groups of flaps.
C. Multiple separate excisions may be necessary if the other methods cannot be applied, e.g., for widely spaced or separated flaps, but is not acceptable for this example.

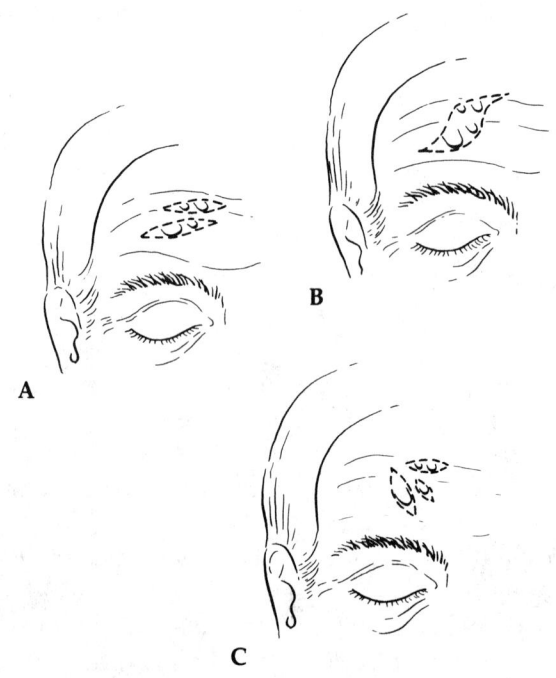

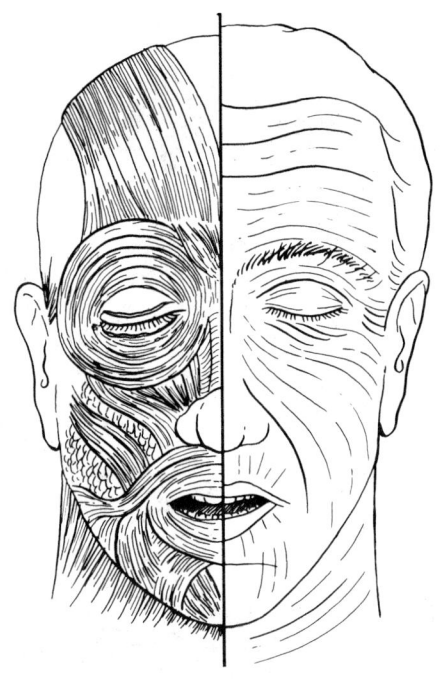

Figure 4-19. The natural wrinkle lines and their relations to underlying facial muscles. The junction of two distinct facial areas usually has a fold or shadow that hides a scar. These are the contour lines.

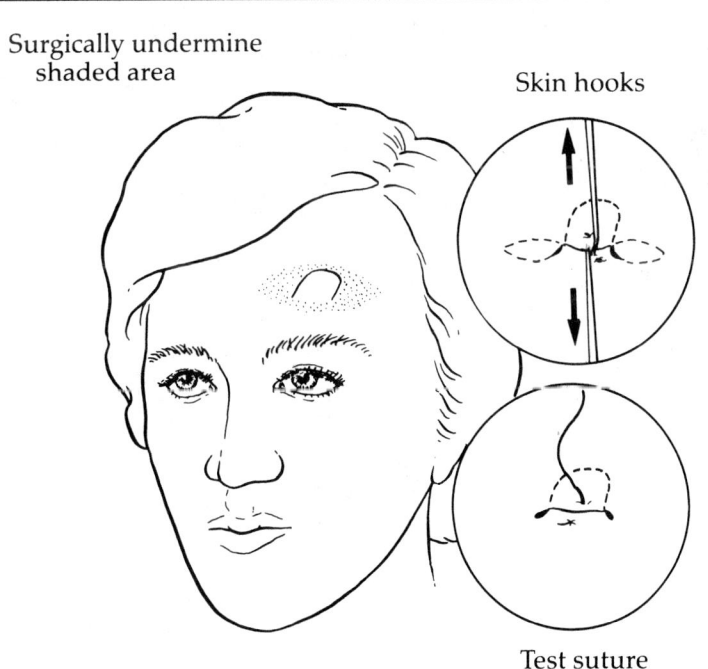

Figure 4-20. Testing for wound closure. Before excising a relatively large flap, the surgeon must be sure the wound will close. The use of hooks or a test stitch is helpful.

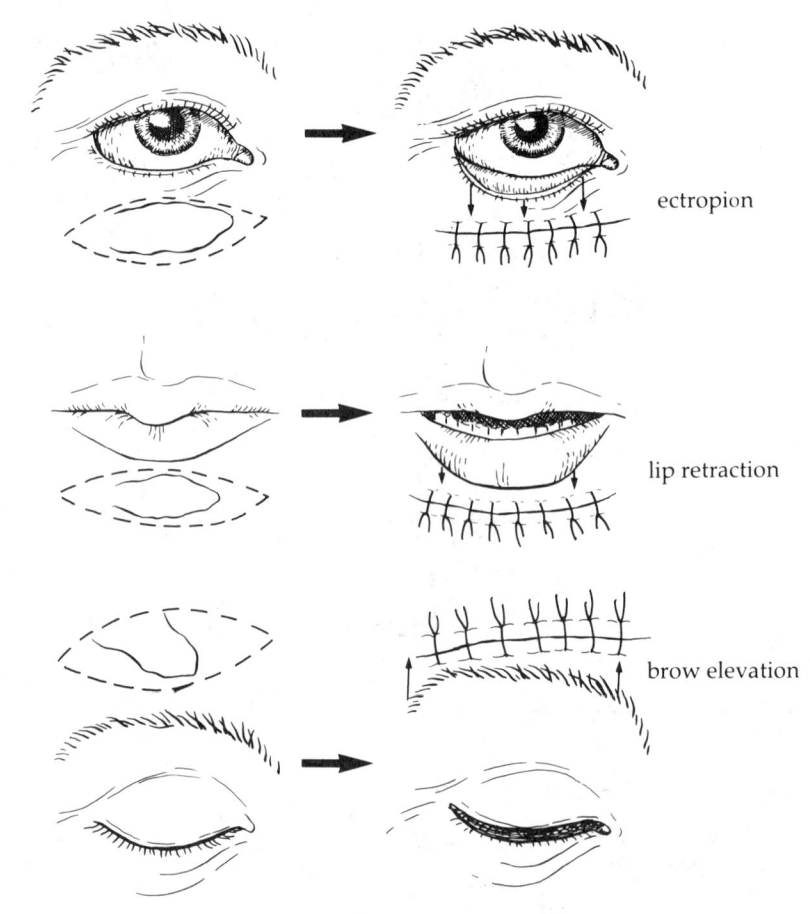

Figure 4-21. Distortion of the lids, lips, and brow caused by injudicious, excessive excision.

exposed by flap excision or wound debridement, a skin graft, flap transfer, or tarsorrhaphy must be used.

5. How much can be excised from the face? The following figures represent maximums in the adult patient, *not minimum safe excisions*. Considerably less can be excised from children's faces. Excisions of greater than these dimensions are more likely to cause noticeable distortion.
   a. 1½ cm of forehead in either direction
   b. 2 cm of scalp
   c. 1 cm of cheek
   d. ½ of lip—2-cm vertical wedge, 5-mm horizontal wedge
   e. ¼ of an eyelid—1-cm vertical wedge, 3- to 4-mm horizontal wedge
   f. 1 cm of nose

   If the flap is too large to excise, another treatment must be used. Either use the method described in the next section for large C flaps or fill the defect with a skin flap or skin graft.

6. Design an elliptic 3:1 excision. After the desired direction has been determined, the flap should be excised. The "ellipse" should be at least three times as long as it is wide (Fig. 4-22). This 3:1 ratio of length to width applies for any skin excision. If a lesser ratio is chosen, a "dog-

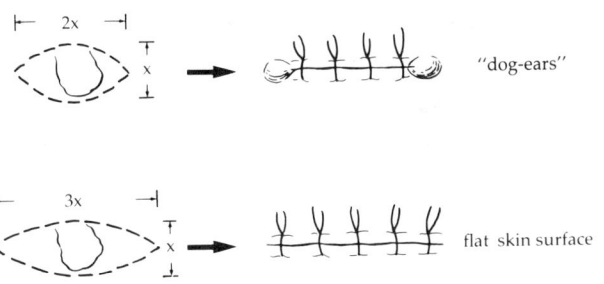

Figure 4-22. Elliptic incisions. The elliptic design usually requires that the length be three times as long as the width. Shorter ellipses result in skin bunching (dog-earing) of the ends of the wound.

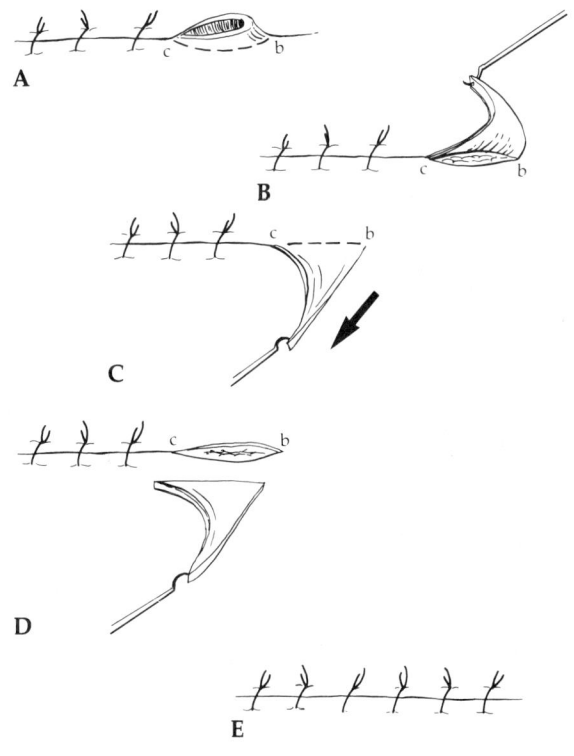

Figure 4-23. Removal of the dog-ear.
A. Mark the junction of the plane of the normal skin and the flap (c–b).
B. Incise it, and elevate the resultant flap.
C. Overlap the flap as shown, and draw another line corresponding to the underlying incision line (c–b).
D. Incise this, and discard the excess skin (dog-ear).
E. Close the remaining wound by the "halving" technique.

ear" may form at either or both ends. Sometimes dog-ears form even though this guideline has been followed. They should be removed, using the method described in Fig. 4-23.

7. Flaps with an unfavorable long axis (Fig. 4-24). If the long axis of the skin flap is oriented across a natural wrinkle, or if the ellipse would cross a natural border or concavity, an alternative skin excision can be designed. The alternative methods are more complex and must be performed properly. It may be better simply to debride necrotic untidy edges and resuture rather than excise the flap.
   a. Flaps on cheek, forehead, or chin. If the flap cannot be excised in a natural line without distortion, it should be excised in its long axis. In these areas a scar that is not in a natural wrinkle will heal adequately, and simple excision is adequate.

Figure 4-24. Excision of flap with long axis.
A. If the flap were excised parallel to its long axis, the resultant linear scar would be unfavorable because it would cross the lateral canthal concavity and because it would be perpendicular to the natural wrinkles.
B. If the flap were designed in the other direction, a very wide and long excision would be required, and excess tissue would be excised.
C. An appropriate alternative is the curvilinear S-excision, which places the limbs in the natural crease.
D. Another alternative would be a Z-plasty after simple vertical excision.

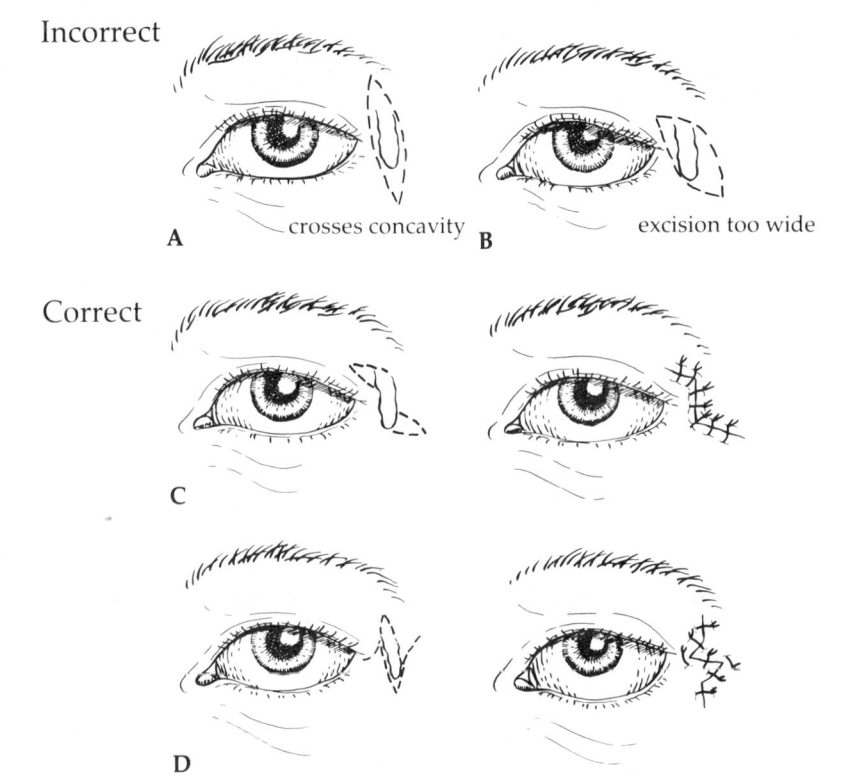

   b. Flaps in concavities or convexities (Fig. 4-25). In concave or convex areas some advantage can be gained by curving the ends of the excision as an S or T.
8. Curvilinear S flaps. Although there is no easy formula for designing a curvilinear S excision, the following guidelines are helpful:
   a. Design the standard 3:1 ellipse. This will tell you how long the limbs of the S will be.
   b. Identify the natural creases or skin lines.
   c. Draw curvilinear lines the same length as the 3:1 ellipse, curving the lines into natural lines or skin creases.
9. T-excision. This method is used when the flap is adjacent to a natural crease.

Large Oblique C Flap

Most large undercut C flaps are caused by impact with standard (non–safety) glass of older automobile windshields and household glass. The glass enters the skin obliquely, creating a large undercut flap. This presents a problem similar to that of the small U flap.

THE PROBLEM—ELEVATED SKIN AND SHADOWS
Large oblique skin flaps tend to form elevated central tissue with depressed scars (Fig. 4-26). Lighting from overhead casts a shadow into the depression. Because these flaps usually are large, excision of the entire flap would cause unacceptable distortion or a wound that cannot be closed.

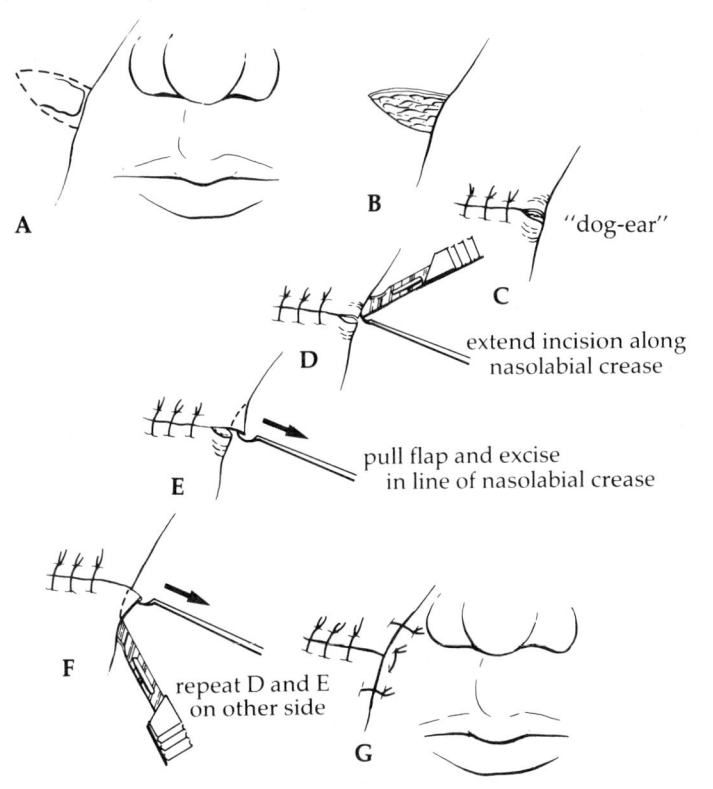

Figure 4-25. Flaps in concavities or convexities.
A. Use the "T-excision" to avoid crossing a natural border with an elliptic excision.
B. Excise the flap up to the nasolabial concavity.
C. Close the wound, leaving a dog-ear.
D. Make an incision in the nasolabial crease.
E. Elevate the resultant flap.
F. Excise the flap, and carry out a similar maneuver on the other bunched side.
G. The resultant closure is T-shaped and does not cross the concavity.

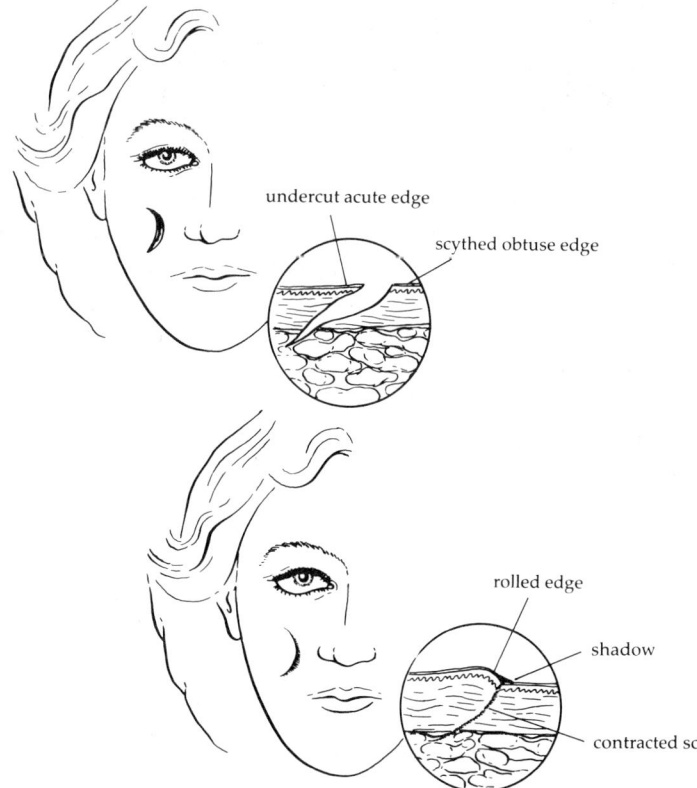

Figure 4-26. The effect of healing with the elevated flap and its shadow. When the acutely undercut edge is simply closed, the resulting scar contracture causes inversion of the scar and rolling up of the acute edge, elevating it above the level of the opposite side. This unevenness causes noticeable shadow calling attention to the scar.

Figure 4-27. Treatment of larger oblique skin flaps.
A. Excise the thin margin of the tip of the flap, creating a perpendicular wound margin. Usually the entire flap cannot be excised, but as much tissue as can be excised and still allow relatively tensionless closure should be debrided. Similarly, excise the oblique margin as illustrated, creating a perpendicular margin of a depth equal to the opposite side.
B. Undermine the margins at a subdermal level. The extent of undermining varies and can be judged by frequently testing the mobility of the margins as demonstrated in Fig. 4-20.

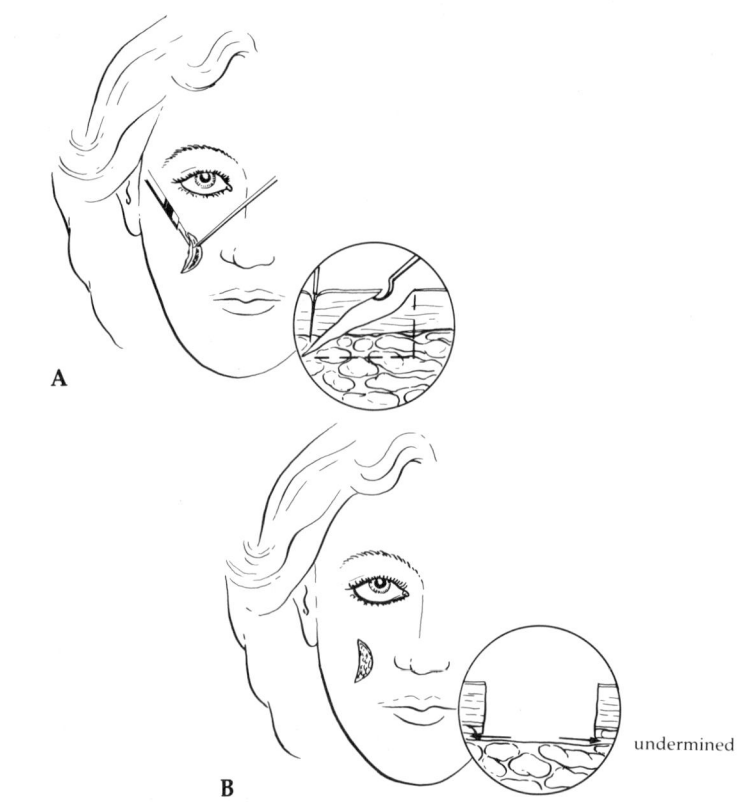

TREATMENT—PERPENDICULAR TRIMMING OF EDGES
1. Slight undercut with minimal flap. Using skin hooks and knife blade the oblique skin edges are trimmed (Fig. 4-27). The anatomic location determines the depth of wound trimming and thus the appropriate level for undermining and advancement.
2. Extreme undercut and flap. If the undercut is extreme or the flap has a tight arc (like a large *U*-shaped flap), a unique iatrogenic problem can be caused by excision. Extensive surgical trimming causes the length of the two sides of the wound to be unequal. *The inner (acute angle) undercut is shortened and the outer (obtuse angle) scythe is lengthened* (Fig. 4-28). This problem is caused by debriding too widely and deeply and attempting to excise the entire undercut. The problem can be minimized by debriding only the dermal undercut but not the undercut of the fat.

Unequal Lengths

Although unequal lengths of the arcs is usually an unnecessary iatrogenic problem created by excessive debridement, some flaps are severely devascularized and must be debrided (Fig. 4-29).

THE PROBLEM
If unequal lengths are sutured, there may be dog-ears because of a relative excess of skin on the longer side.

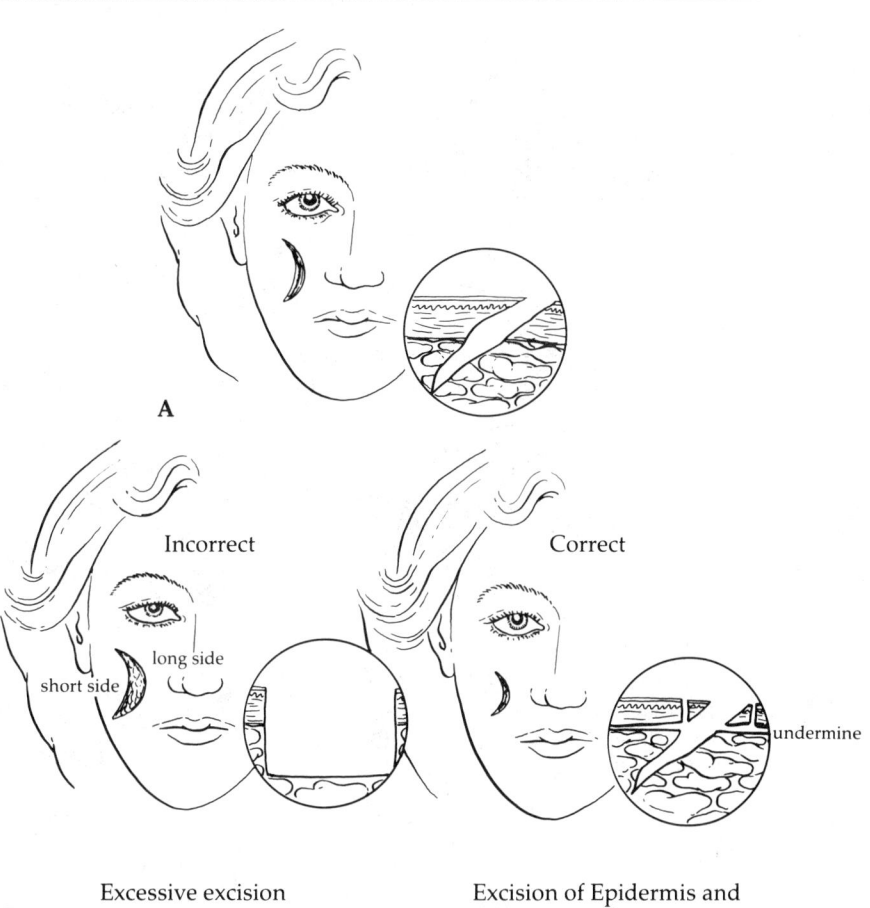

Figure 4-28. Extreme undercut flap.
A. The deep undercut flap and the subcutaneous tissue (if excised) cause the wound edges to be of unequal lengths.
B. If excised in the wound base, the inner edge is shortened and the outer edge lengthened.
C. This can be avoided by excising only the dermis.

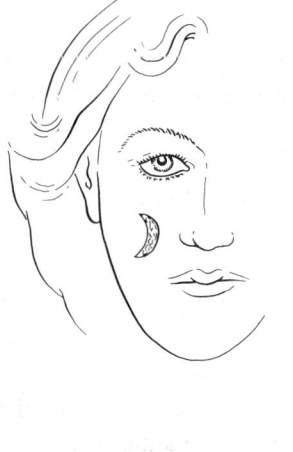
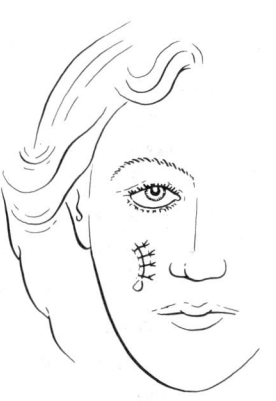

Figure 4-29. Dog-ear. If a wound with sides of unequal length is closed, a dog-ear results at the end of the wound, on the side with the longer arc.

Figure 4-30. Cheating with unequal bites. A minimal (10%) discrepancy in length of the opposite edges can be "cheated" by covering a wider distance on the longer side with each stitch.

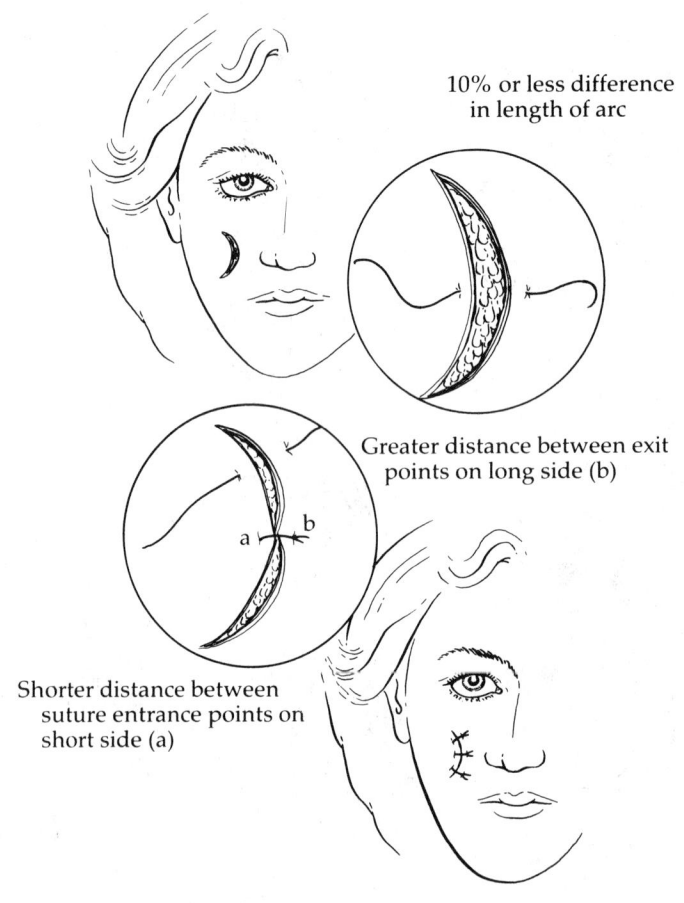

TREATMENT

Alternative treatments include cheating with unequal bites, leaving a dog-ear at one end, shortening the long side, lengthening the short side, or using a ½ Z-plasty.

1. Cheating with unequal bites (Fig. 4-30). This method can be used when:
   a. There is a *minimal length discrepancy* (approximately 10%) between the two sides
   b. The *tissue is flexible* (face, but not forehead)
2. Leaving a dog-ear at one end. This method should be used if the surgeon lacks experience with techniques of plastic surgery.

   It is better to leave a dog-ear at the end of the wound (to be revised later) than to make a mistake in judgment that creates additional scars or to try cheating a wound with unequal bites that create excessive bunching the entire length of the laceration.

   Begin closure at one end of the wound and close with slightly unequal bites as you work toward the other end. If the cheating does not compensate adequately, there will be a dog-ear at the terminal end. This dog-ear can be revised as a final step in the surgery or it can be left for later secondary revision.
3. Shortening the long side. This method—actually the same method used for the ends of the S-plasty or T-excision—can be the next step in lacera-

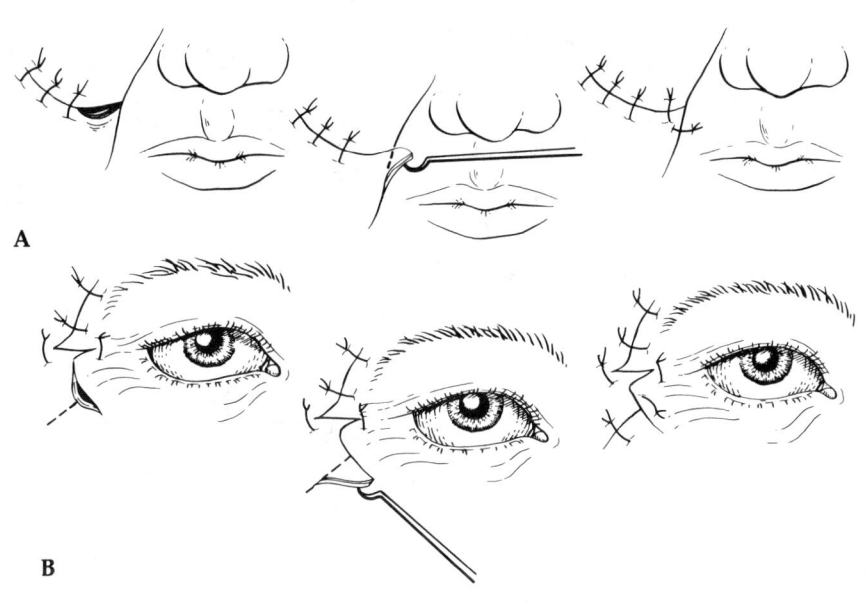

Figure 4-31. Treatment of dog-ear by excision in a natural crease.
A. The method of removing a dog-ear in the nasolabial crease.
B. The skin excess on the cheek is removed in the "crow's-foot" line.

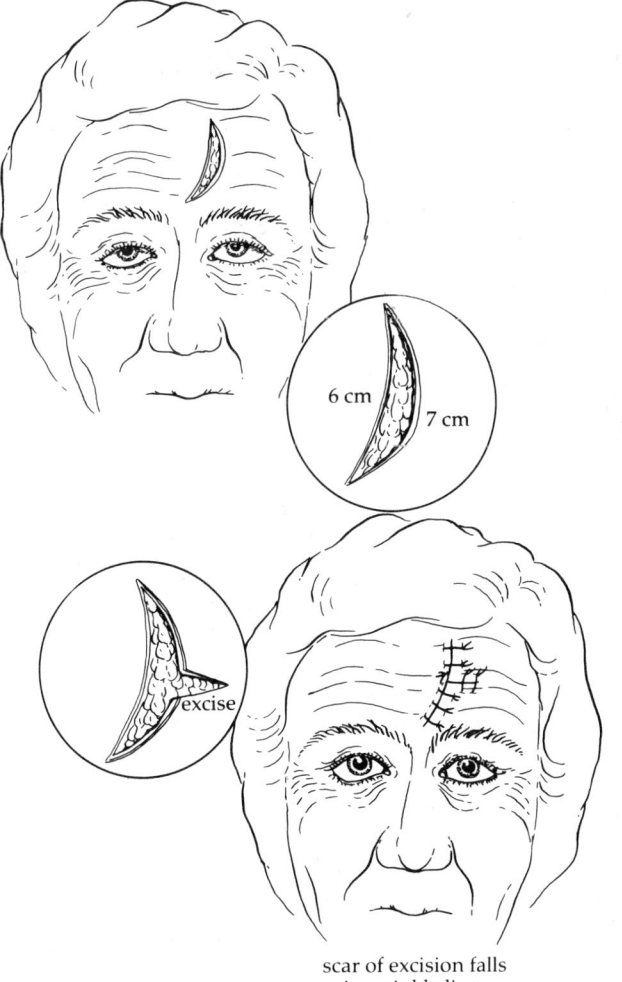

scar of excision falls in wrinkle line

Figure 4-32. Treatment of dog-ear by T-excision. The skin excess after debridement is removed by T-excision in the forehead crease. The excess length of 1 cm is removed so that the additional scar falls into a natural wrinkle line.

Figure 4-33. Treatment of dog-ear if wound is parallel to normal skin crease. The short side is lengthened by an arc extension.

A. Additional incisions extend the wound. These are directed toward or fall within skin wrinkle lines. The total length of the incisions approximates the difference between the long and short sides.

B. The short side is now lengthened by a curving excision (dotted lines) of additional tissue. The wound is then closed by the "halving" method or by "cheating" as illustrated in Fig. 4-30.

This maintains a linear scar parallel to the natural forehead wrinkle. An alternative in this case would be a vertical T-excision in the glabellar crease.

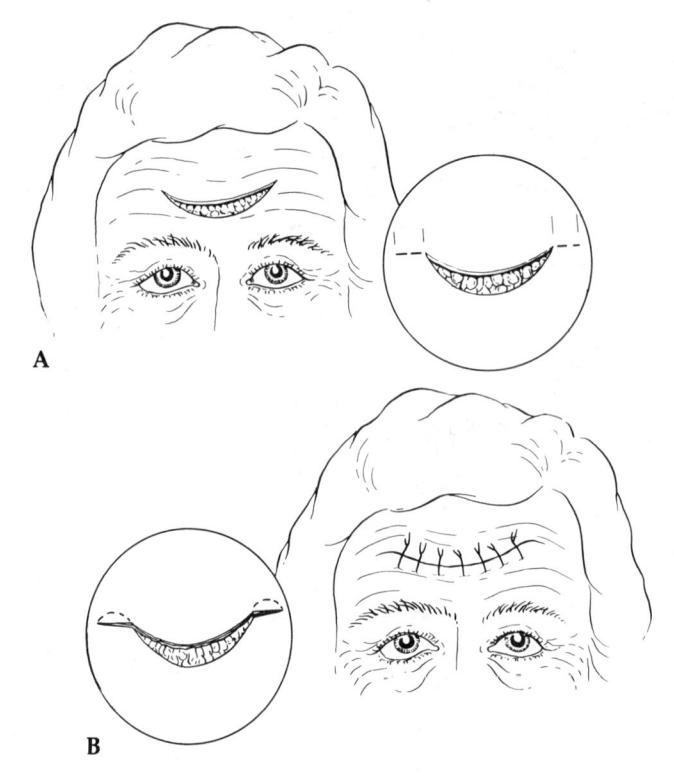

Figure 4-34. Treatment of dog-ear by ½ Z-plasty. The wound crosses several perpendicular skin wrinkles and if closed directly would be noticeable. On the long side, small flaps are created as described in Figure 4-15. The angle of these flaps can vary from 30–60°, depending on the position along the wound margin. Small triangular areas of skin along the shorter side are excised after testing the flap placement by rotating the flap to the most natural position along the opposite margin. With the interdigitation to the flaps, the long scar is "broken-up." This irregular scar is less noticeable than a long straight scar because some portions of the scar now fall into skin creases and are disguised.

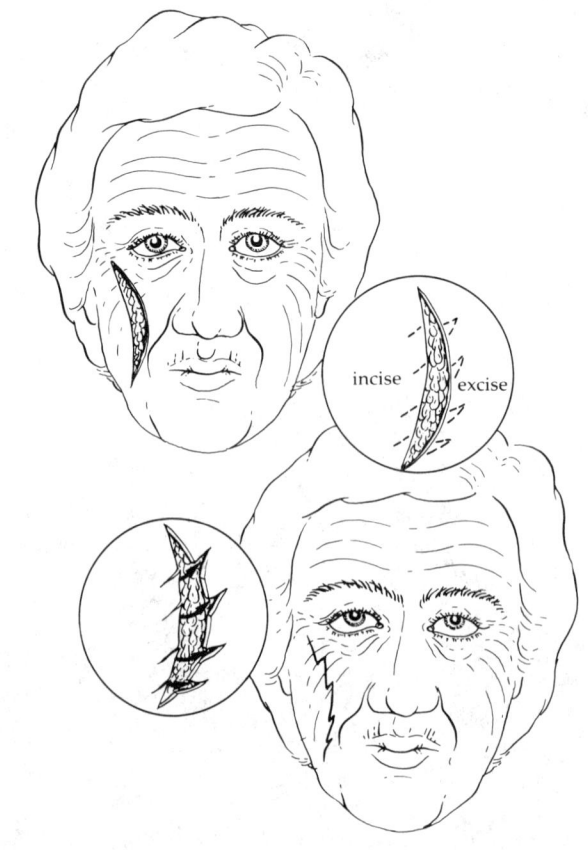

tion closure after creation of a dog-ear. The S-plasty is usually used in the lower face (Fig. 4-31) and T-excision in the forehead (Fig. 4-32).
4. Lengthening the short side (Fig. 4-33). This method is generally not used because it tends to create a longer scar and is technically difficult. The method should be considered if *the wound is parallel to a normal skin crease* and therefore a T-excision would create a new scar that is not in a natural crease. This method may be used for a horizontal forehead laceration.
5. Lengthening the short side and shortening the long side with ½ Z-plasty (Fig. 4-34). This technically difficult method should not be used unless the surgeon is relatively experienced with the principles of plastic surgery. It involves transposition of a flap of tissue from the long side to the short side, and has been termed a *½ Z-plasty*.

   Indications for this method include:
   a. Lacerations situated at or almost perpendicular to a natural skin crease
   b. Very long lacerations that are better interrupted by a Z-plasty to reduce contraction. Plan one or more Z-plasties, depending on the situation. It is generally preferable to place the Z at the straightest part and near the central region of the laceration.

5. AMPUTATIONS AND SKIN LOSS

GENERAL PRINCIPLES

An injury can result in the partial loss of skin and underlying supportive structures, vessels, and nerves, or complete amputation of the entire peripheral projection of an extremity, facial part, or genital organ.

Nose and ear amputations were used as punishment for crimes or adultery for many centuries, and during the early 1800s such amputated parts were often replanted. Hofacker, a Heidelberg physician, picked up amputated parts at the sites of dueling matches, washed them, placed the tissue back in its original position to stop the bleeding, and taped the tissue in place. He said that 50 percent of these replants survived.

Although replantation of amputated parts occasionally has a successful outcome, it is more common for the replanted part to fail to revascularize. The amputated skin or part usually is too severely damaged, is contaminated, or cannot be retrieved. This chapter discusses the indications for replantation of amputated parts and the methods and biology of skin grafts for resurfacing of the amputation site when replacement is impossible or unwarranted. The great majority of amputations require a simple dressing or skin graft. Occasionally, microvascular replantation or a skin flap is indicated.

Fate of the Amputated Part

PARTIAL AMPUTATION

1. Repositioning (Fig. 5-1). Even before a definitive decision is made regarding replantation, the part should be repositioned. The part may be partially attached by a small pedicle of tissue, which may provide adequate vascularity to allow survival of that part. Therefore, *it is of the utmost importance that the part be repositioned as carefully and as soon as possible so that there is no kinking or tension on a bridge of intact tissue.* A very light immobilizing dressing usually suffices to protect the amputation site. Moreover, the amputation should be placed in an elevated position to avoid venous congestion and bleeding.
2. Replantation versus completion of the amputation. When there is a small tissue pedicle, either the flap should be sutured into place or the remaining pedicle severed, thus completing the amputation. This decision is best made by the surgeon after careful evaluation of social and clinical factors and diagnostic testing with fluorescein. When in doubt, it is usually better to attempt replantation because little is lost by the attempt (except time). When early return to work is essential, it may be best to complete the amputation to avoid delay, potential infection, and excessive fibrosis.
    a. Clinical criteria for decision making.
        (1) Size of pedicle and flap. The ratio of pedicle size to flap size and length is the critical variable. A long thin flap is at risk of necrosis at its distal end. A short wide flap has much better potential for vascular flow. Absolute numerical ratios are of minimal clinical value because of the differences in vascularity of various parts of

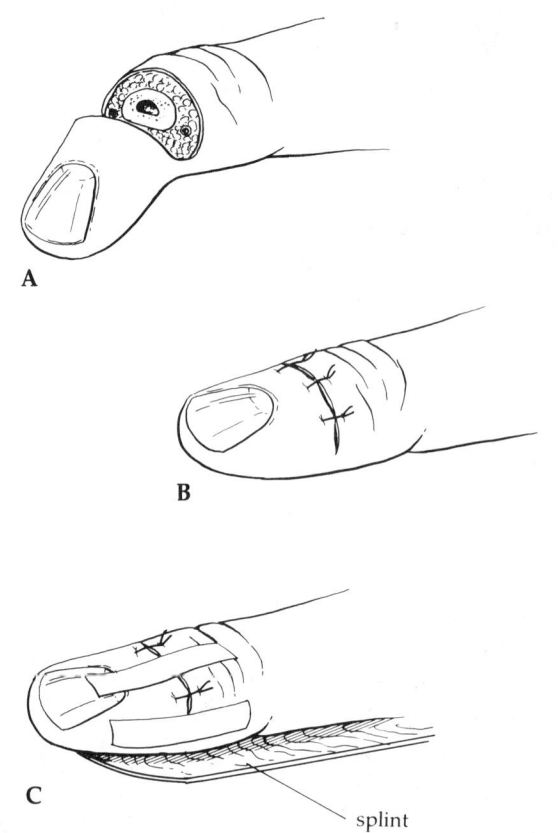

Figure 5-1. Reapproximating a soft tissue pedicle. An incomplete amputation with a residual tissue pedicle of reasonable size at a critical anatomic site should be reapproximated.

A soft tissue pedicle of a marginal size is illustrated.
A. Handle the tissue pedicle carefully, without twisting, kinking, or tension.
B. Reposition with extreme accuracy and use a minimal number of sutures to achieve dermal contact.
C. Immobilize the part with splints or internal wire, and then position at heart level. Do not allow dependency.

the body. Blood flow of the facial structures is better than blood flow to the extremities. A flap that is twice as long as its pedicle width may survive on the face but probably will necrose on the lower extremity. Furthermore, the actual length of the pedicle may be more important than the ratio of length to width. For example, a 10-cm long, 5-cm wide flap (2:1 ratio) on the face may necrose at its distal end, but a 2-cm long, 1-cm wide flap has a better potential for survival. As a general rule, flaps that are longer than they are wide tend to necrose on sites other than the face. Ultimately, clinical judgment and assessment of the specific circumstance are required.

(2) Part of body (blood supply). The part of the body is an important consideration because of differences in inherent vascularity and importance to the patient of function and appearance. The extremes of this concept are exemplified in the following case examples.

A partially amputated small toe of an elderly working man is of little importance functionally and has poor blood supply. Failure of survival after reattachment is likely, and the attempt at replantation would cause considerable delay in healing and increased risks.

An incompletely amputated nose on a young person is of great importance, and the blood supply is excellent. Thus repositioning should be attempted. As a general rule, the face and hand are good sites for replantation because of more satisfactory perfusion and because of their cosmetic and functional importance. The trunk and lower extremities are poor sites for replantation.

- (3) Condition of wound. A tidy, sharp, clean amputation has a better prognosis than a severely contused, contaminated, crushing injury.
- (4) Age of patient. The younger the patient, the higher the probability of a successful repositioning of a partial amputation. Infants under 2 years are excellent candidates; children from 2 to 12 are good candidates; teenagers and young adults are less satisfactory candidates.
- (5) Difficulty of reconstruction. It is extremely difficult or impossible to reconstruct satisfactorily an amputated eyelid or an entire hand, but reconstruction of a nose or ear is possible. Thus greater risks should be taken to retain an eyelid or multiple digits.
- (6) Patient health and other injuries. The patient with fewer minor injuries and good general health is a better candidate for replantation than the patient with severe injury or underlying disease that affects circulation.

b. Fluorescein test—assessment of viability. This test is an adjunct to the clinical decision-making process and cannot be accepted as an isolated test. It is sometimes difficult to assess the viability of the partially amputated part. Abrasions, pigmentation, or ecchymosis may obscure tissue color and blood flow.

One gram of fluorescein dye given intravenously (1 ampule = 500 mg) will, after a 10-minute waiting period, stain most tissues that are adequately vascularized. The Wood's ultraviolet light helps identify the dye distribution and density, particularly in dark-skinned persons.

A stippled yellow appearance of the dye indicates satisfactory flow. Survival following suturing the flap in place is usually assumed. However, absence of fluorescence does not correlate 100 percent with tissue nonviability. Vascular spasm, shock, and other factors can give a false negative result. Ultimately, a clinical judgment must be superimposed on this adjunctive test.

3. Method of replantation (simple suture or microvascular anastomosis). The replanted part can be simply sutured into its correct anatomic position, or additional blood supply can be added by microvascular anastomosis of flap vessels to recipient vessels. This decision is determined by the size and condition of the vessel of the partially amputated part and of the "stump." *Microvascular repair should be used whenever possible for critical structures such as a digit and/or when viability is clearly marginal.* This is a specialized technique that should be performed by trained microvascular surgeons only.

The details of simple suturing are discussed in the following section on composite graft replants of complete amputations. In short, the essence of the technique is:

a. Accurate coaptation of all anatomic layers
b. Minimal number of sutures
c. Careful immobilization

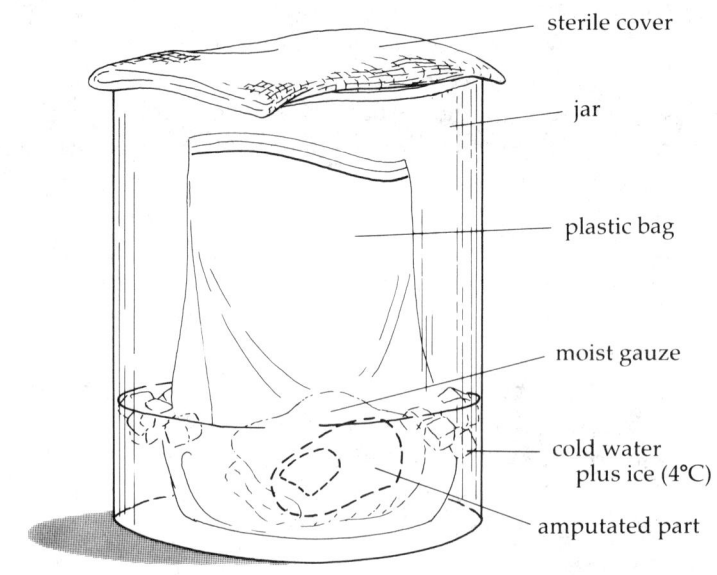

Figure 5-2. Transportation and short-term preservation of an amputated part. The part requires cleansing, humidity (not soaking), and cooling to 4°C (not freezing).

COMPLETE AMPUTATION

1. Transportation of the completely amputated part (Fig. 5-2). We advise that the amputated part be brought to the emergency department wrapped in a moist clean cloth or bandage. Direct immersion in iced solutions or into tap water or other nonisotonic salt solution can be detrimental.
   a. Clean the tissue of as much dirt and foreign material as possible with saline solution irrigations. Do not sharply debride any tissue or debris.
   b. Wrap in clean cloth or gauze dampened with normal saline.
   c. Place in a sealed plastic bag, and immerse the bag in an ice-water mixture. The decision regarding replantation or other use of the part should be deferred until the patient is seen in the emergency department and a complete assessment is made.
2. Preservation. When an amputated part cannot be used immediately, it may be desirable to salvage a specific tissue component or the entire part for subsequent replantation. The part must be preserved by refrigeration. The ability to store the part for prolonged periods until transfer to another facility or until consultation is obtained depends on the type of tissue. The maximum safe interval until replantation depends on the most vulnerable tissue in the amputated part.
   a. Skin. Refrigeration at 4°C can preserve skin for up to 3 weeks. Estimations of survival are 75 to 95 percent at 1 week, 25 to 75 percent at 2 weeks, and 0 to 25 percent at 3 weeks. After 3 weeks, survival is possible but unlikely.
   b. Bone, tendon, and cartilage. Bone and cartilage can be preserved for a considerably longer period than skin—approximately 2 to 3 months. Bone graft replants act as a scaffold for ingrowth and replacement and do not have to have viable cells. Cartilage can survive for extended periods because of its capacity for anaerobic metabolism.

AMPUTATIONS AND SKIN LOSS

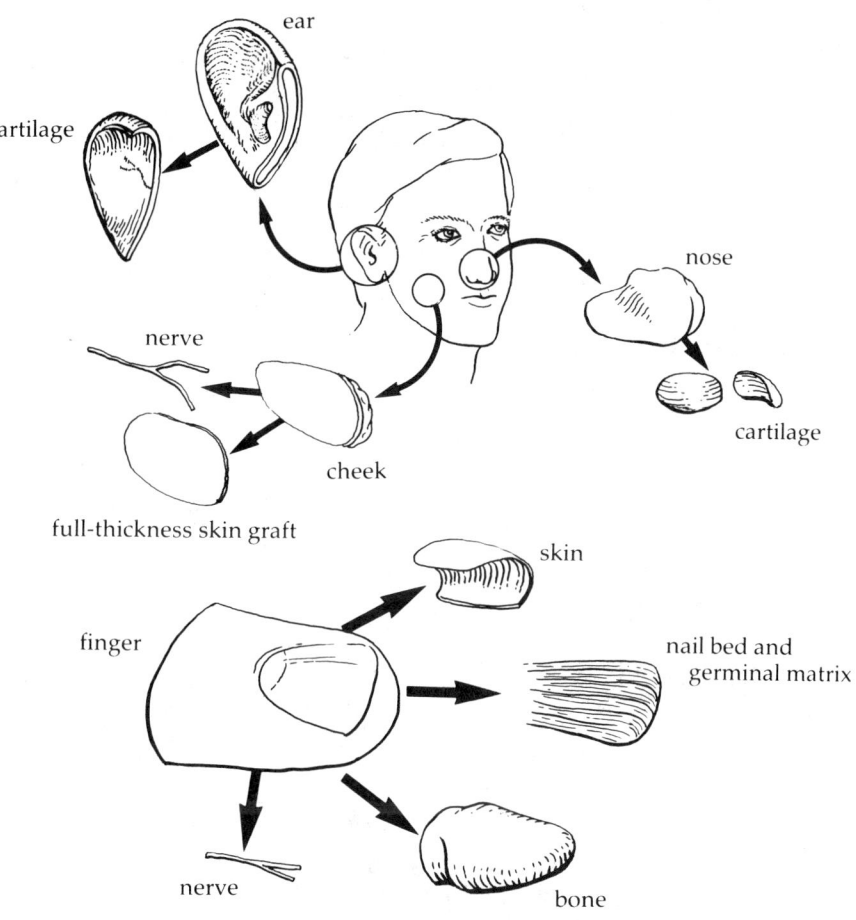

Figure 5-3. The parts most commonly salvaged from amputations: skin, nerve, cartilage, and bone.

  c. **Muscle and fat.** Muscle and fat can withstand only a few hours of devascularization and storage before irreversible damage occurs. There is no reported evidence that intravascular perfusion with saline, heparin, or any other solution prolongs survival. In fact, small-vessel damage may result.
3. **Use of amputated part.** The three alternatives regarding the use of the amputated part include (1) discarding it, (2) salvaging usable components, and (3) replantation (composite or microvascular).
  a. **Discarding the part.** The decision to discard the part is based on criteria similar to those used for partial amputation. The criteria include importance of the part, condition of tissue, age of patient, difficulty of reconstruction, patient health, and other injuries.

  Additional factors regarding completely amputated parts are the time elapsed since the injury and the method and temperature of storage. Any tissue amputated less than 2 hours before can be replanted. After that interval other factors, including tissue size, tissue type, temperature of storage, and contamination, must be considered. With favorable conditions, successful replants have been achieved after 3 days, and the potential exists for success after a longer interval.
  b. **Salvaging usable components (Fig. 5-3).** Once a decision has been made that the entire amputated part cannot be used for replantation

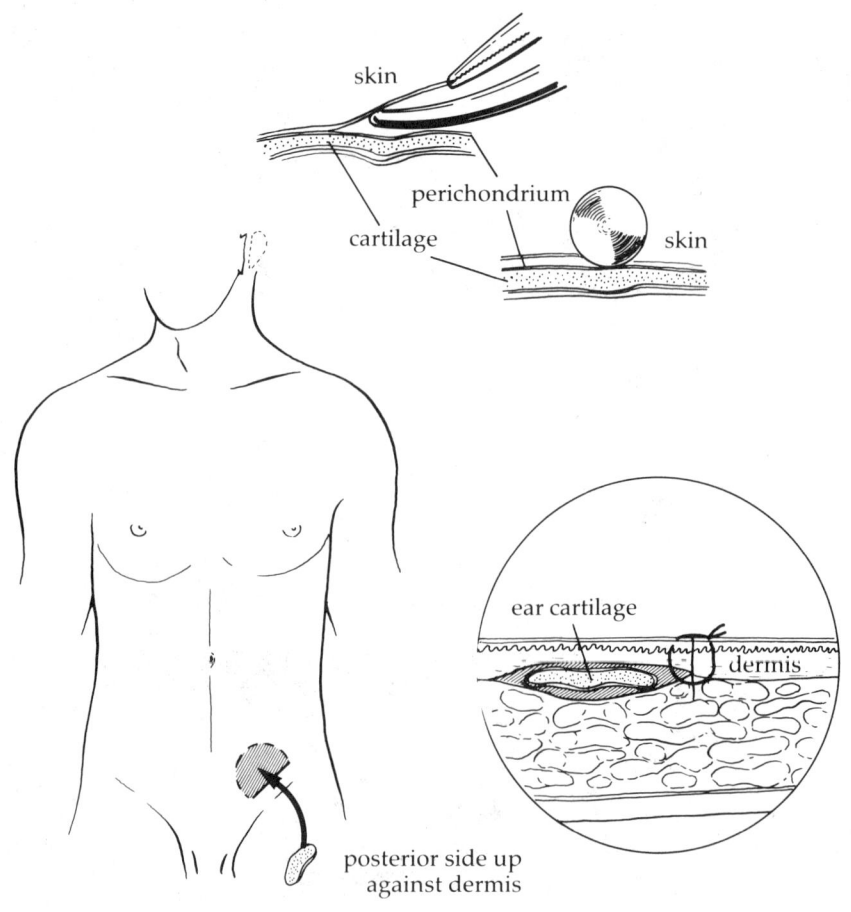

Figure 5-4. Salvage and banking of usable parts. Ear cartilage can be salvaged by removal of traumatized skin and fat, leaving perichondrium on the posterior surface. The anterior skin can be excised, or, if it is in healthy condition, the epidermis can be removed with a dermabrader. This is helpful for later reconstruction because the cartilage retains a more normal delicate architecture. The cartilage is implanted in a subdermal pocket or fascial plane (not in fat). The subdermal placement is used when the cartilage is banked in the mastoid skin. This should only be done by the surgeon responsible for long-term reconstruction.

and must be discarded, consider the possibility of salvaging usable parts. These parts can be either stored in the refrigerator or "banked" in the patient (Fig. 5-4).

Most commonly the skin can be removed and used as a graft, or cartilage from the ear can be removed for subsequent reconstruction. Nail-bed germinal matrix, bone, or nerves may be useful for extremity reconstruction.

The salvaged part should be free from noticeable trauma or contamination. The traumatized portions are discarded.

(1) Skin. If the skin is not severely contused, it can be used as either a split-thickness skin graft or a full-thickness skin graft, depending on the specific requirements of the injured site.

For a split-thickness skin graft, the amputated tissue is pinned to a sterilized wood cutting board or the periphery of the graft is immobilized with towel clips so that a split-thickness skin graft can be harvested. Any of the available dermatomes can be used, but drum dermatomes are less successful for this purpose.

(2) Nail matrix. If an amputated finger is not going to be replanted, but a secondary reconstruction is planned, the nail matrix can be salvaged by careful sharp dissection from the amputated finger and transplanted into the usable stump or to a distant site until needed for definitive reconstruction. The abdomen and thigh are

common sites for in vivo "banking." However, the replanted nail matrix does poorly and may have considerable irregularity and many spicules. False nails are usually a better solution.

   (3) Bone. Bone from the digits, face, or skull can be saved by refrigeration or implantation in the subcutaneous tissues of the abdomen. Revascularization and survival of an entire bone depend on an intact periosteum, which can survive only for a few days with refrigeration. Therefore, in vivo banking is preferred. Because cortical bone is not a good surface for revascularization, it is necessary to split the bone to expose the medullary surface. Furthermore, bone without its periosteum has little potential for survival, but it undergoes slow resorption unless there is direct contact with bone from the recipient site. If there is direct bone contact, the bone is replaced by "creeping substitution." Therefore, refrigeration is satisfactory for partial bone amputation with medullary bone contact.
   (4) Cartilage (Fig. 5-4). Cartilage survives transplantation extremely well and can be "banked" either in the abdomen or adjacent to the amputation site, such as in the submastoid skin following amputation of the ear. The cartilage should be transplanted with intact perichondrium because of better blood supply and potential for new cartilage formation. Cartilage should not be incised to expose its inner surfaces. Severe warping can occur if incisions are made into the cartilage.
   (5) Nerves. There are numerous circumstances in which nerve grafts may be required following limb amputation and, occasionally, following severe facial skin losses that involve the facial nerve. These nerves can be used for subsequent nerve grafts or, in certain circumstances, during a primary reconstruction.

   Clearly, the decision regarding salvage of useful parts depends on definition by the physician of long-term needs for reconstruction. These decisions are most appropriately deferred to the reconstructive surgeons who are responsible for the long-term care of the patient.

c. Replantation. The three forms of replantation are free composite graft, microvascular anastomosis, and added flap blood supply. Choosing among these requires considerable judgment and skill. General guidelines follow:
   (1) Composite graft. Fig. 5-5 illustrates the mechanisms of revascularization. Amputation usually results in composite tissue loss (in addition to epidermis and dermis). A composite tissue includes skin (epidermis, dermis, and fat) and additional contiguous tissues such as areolar connective tissues, cartilage, bone, muscle, and the associated nerves and arteries. Composite tissue replants have limited potential to survive because there is minimal surface area of contact of the vascular surface of the replanted composite tissue (relative to the tissue volume and the distance into the tissue that must be revascularized). A composite graft is revascularized at the dermis along the peripheral margins because blood vessel cannot effectively invade the graft through the fat, muscle, and other tissues. In contrast, a skin

Figure 5-5. Revascularization of grafts.
A. Split- and full-thickness grafts revascularize from the base, and tissue volume is minimal; thus, size of the graft is "unlimited."
B. Composite grafts revascularize from the peripheral dermal margin and areolar fascia but not the base of fat, muscle, or cartilage. Tissue volume is large relative to vascular surface.
C. Example of a nose tip. Amputation and replantation may be limited by its size. The composite tissue should be no more than 1½ cm from the vascularizing surface.

Split- and full-thickness skin graft

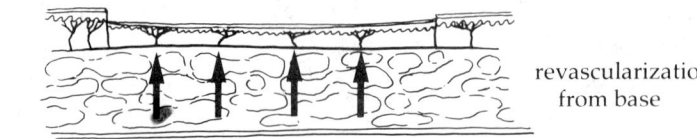

revascularization from base

Composite graft

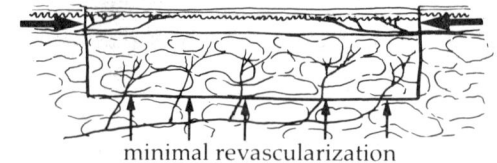

revascularization from periphery (dermis)

minimal revascularization

Composite tissues

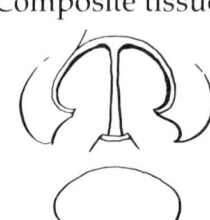

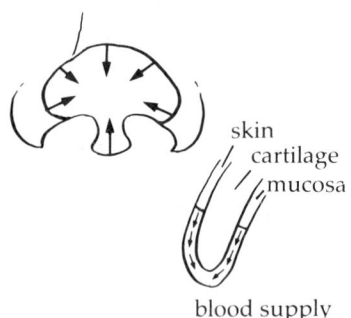

skin
cartilage
mucosa

blood supply from dermis

---

graft is revascularized by ingrowth of vessels from the broad wound base into the thin dermis on the underside of the graft. Thus, a split skin graft has its entire dermal undersurface in contact with the wound for vascularization, whereas a composite graft has a limited dermal contact area around the periphery. Furthermore, there is a much greater tissue volume that must be nourished in a composite graft. *As a general rule, therefore, the maximum amputation that can be replanted successfully as a free composite graft is 2 to 3 cm, so that no part of the composite tissue is more than 1 cm from a vascular source.*

(a) Technique
  (i) Tidy amputation. Debridement should not be performed. Survival of the replant is achieved by exact repositioning in the original bed so that vascular realignment in the dermis is most likely to occur. This process of vessel-to-vessel contact and revascularization is termed *inosculation*.

  The strength and stability of the repair should come from the fixation of bone, cartilage, fat, and fascia—not from the dermis.

  Use a minimal number of "flap" sutures in the dermis. The tissue can be aligned with a few sutures and tapes. Excessive suturing destroys vascularity and predisposes to infection.

(ii) Untidy amputation. With ragged amputations or contaminated wounds, such as bites, the edges must be debrided to reduce the risk of infection and tissue necrosis. This should be done in the manner described for lacerations.

   A very small number of subcutaneous and subdermal sutures are used in a layered closure to obliterate dead spaces and approximate dermis.

   A minimal number of "flap" sutures should be used in the skin.

(b) Postoperative care
   (i) Splinting and immobilization. A firm dressing and splints immobilize the surgical site.
   (ii) Elevation. Elevation for 1 week is perhaps the most important factor in postoperative management.
   (iii) Dressing. It has been suggested that ice packs be applied to the replantation site to reduce the metabolic requirements. There is, however, no confirmation that ice is beneficial, and we do not use postoperative ice packs. A simple, light gauze pad or wrap is sufficient.
   (iv) Dressing change. The graft should be left undisturbed for 5 to 7 days. The initial graft pallor turns to a deep cyanosis within a day or 2, and that cyanotic color is maintained without evidence of revascularization until 3 to 5 days postreplantation. A pink color returns if revascularization occurs.
   (v) Graft care. If incomplete survival has occurred, the outer layer of skin may form a dark eschar with loss of the most superficial dermis and epidermis. However, a layer of dermis and epithelium remnants survives underneath. After 2 to 3 weeks and removal of the eschar, reepithelialization occurs from the remnants. Be careful not to remove the entire composite graft. This process is promoted with an occlusive dressing using topical antibiotic ointments.

(2) Microvascular anastomosis. The technique of microvascular surgery involves the suturing of small blood vessels of 1 to 3 mm in diameter using special instrumentation and magnification. The technique requires considerable experience and should be undertaken only by practiced surgeons. The most common application of microvascular anastomosis is in digit and limb replantation, but scalp and other tissue replantations also have been successful. The methods are not detailed here, but the indications for replantation are discussed in the section on specific anatomic sites later in this chapter.

(3) Added flap blood supply. Large (2–3 cm) pieces of amputated tissue may be too large to replant as a composite graft and may not have identifiable blood vessels for microvascular anastomosis. The tissue can be replanted by adding blood supply by dermabrasion of epithelium and burying in a pocket or by removing an epithelial surface and lining with a skin flap. Examples of this

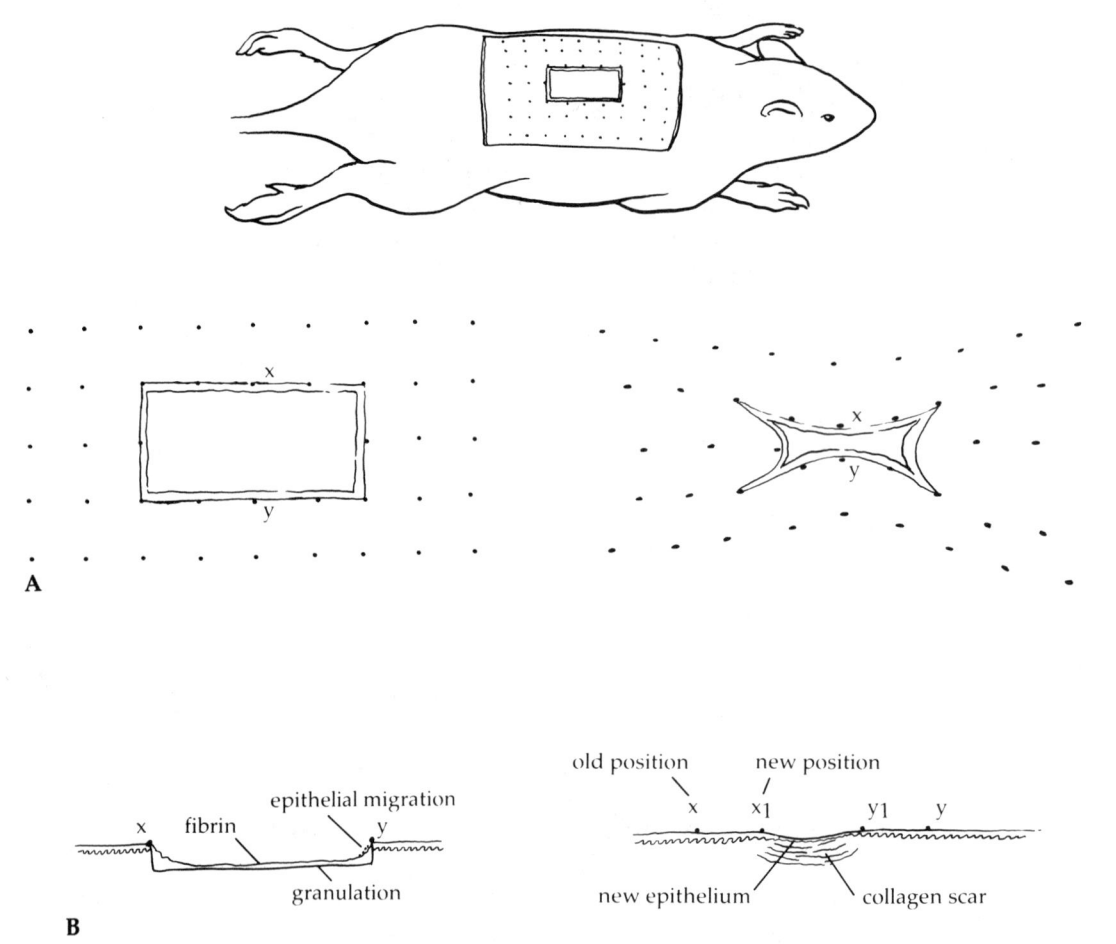

Figure 5-6. Experimental model of a rat's back.
A. The tissue deficit is spontaneously closed by the inward migration of the entire skin border with the epithelium growing across the most central portion. Contraction is achieved by stretching of the surrounding supple skin.
B. Diagrammatic cross section, showing that this is achieved by myofibroblasts pulling the edges centrally. In addition, epithelium migrates across the surface.

principle are presented in the section on specific anatomic sites later in this chapter.

Management of the Wound (Stump)

What should be done with the open wound when the amputated part cannot be replanted? The alternatives include (1) leaving an open wound (with dressing) and allowing it to heal by wound contraction and epithelialization, (2) applying a skin graft, and (3) performing an immediate flap reconstruction or tissue advancement.

We describe here the biologic basis for each of these alternatives and the methods available. In general, a dressing or a thin split graft is the best alternative in the emergency department.

OPEN WOUND—CONTRACTION AND REEPITHELIALIZATION
Some small wounds do not require surgical addition of tissue as a graft or flap. An open wound can close spontaneously through a combination of contraction of the wound size by pulling in of surrounding skin and growth of new epithelium across the granulated wound base (Fig. 5-6).

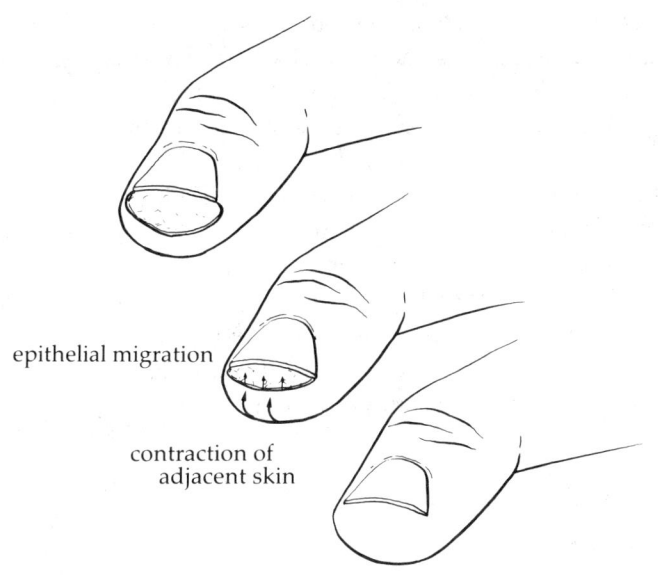

Figure 5-7. Small fingertip wound provides an example of using wound contraction for clinical advantage and simplicity.

1. Indications and contraindications. Management of an open wound by contraction and epithelialization is indicated for some small wounds that have sufficient adjacent tissue that will not be distorted by wound contraction. If a large wound is allowed to contract and reepithelialize, the distortion and tissue redistribution can be unacceptable cosmetically and functionally.

    This method is indicated primarily for wounds of the proximal extremity and trunk, but it can be used on the fingertip and parts of the face (Fig. 5-7). In particular, secondary healing by the processes of wound contraction and epithelialization is indicated for:
    a. Severely contaminated wounds with ground-in dirt, oil, grass, or other foreign material
    b. Clinical infection
    c. Human or animal bites (particularly of the hand) that require extensive debridement
    d. Contaminated wounds older than 6 to 12 hours
    e. Situations in which viability of tissue is improbable. It is sometimes difficult to predict the viability of tissues accurately. In critical, functional, or cosmetic areas, a period of watchful waiting is indicated to avoid unnecessarily debriding healthy tissue or unnecessarily grafting the wound.

    The wound should be packed with a weakly antiseptic, nondesiccating dressing, and the dressing should be changed frequently. Povidone-iodine (Betadine), gentamicin, Neosporin, and saline are examples of useful agents. The wound is then covered with 4 × 4 gauze pads, held in place with adhesive tape or an elastic gauze wrap.
2. Skin flaps. These are used for (1) joints (particularly flexion surface or when the joint space is exposed), (2) some weight or pressure sites (soles, ischium), and (3) underlying tissue that must be protected (nerves, vessels).

When the decision is made to cover a wound, the safest, simplest, and usually most effective method is to apply a skin graft, although there are definite circumstances under which flap coverage is preferable.

Flap surgery is more complex than skin grafting and can cause additional problems. We discuss here the indications for a flap but do not describe techniques. If a flap is required, a plastic surgeon should be consulted. When in doubt, a skin graft should be used.

The criteria for choosing between a graft and a flap are based primarily on three considerations: anatomic site, wound condition, and surgical expertise. These have been discussed, in part, in relation to wound contraction. The indications for a flap are usually related to anatomic sites that have exposed tissues of functional importance:

- a. Exposed tendons (without paratenon)
- b. Exposed nerves
- c. Open joints
- d. Cortical bone (without periosteum)
- e. Cartilage (without perichondrium)
- f. Cosmetic defects of the face
- g. Some weight or pressure sites (soles, ischium)

3. Skin graft. For almost all other open wounds with acceptable wound conditions and unexposed deep tissue, a skin graft is the preferred treatment. A thin skin graft is a simple technique that all physicians should be able to perform. For this reason, the indications and techniques of skin grafting are discussed in detail below.

Great benefits with minimal danger of causing harm can be anticipated from a thin graft. *When in doubt, thin graft is the treatment of choice!*

SKIN GRAFTS

Reverdin in 1869 first treated a large granulating wound of the arm of a 35-year-old man with a skin graft from the abdomen. He removed two small slivers of epidermis with the point of a lancet and placed them in the middle of the wound, their deep surface in contact with the granulation. He observed that the islands enlarged.

The following section discusses skin grafting, including:

Classification of graft types
Physical characteristics of graft types
Choosing a donor site
Method of obtaining grafts
Dressing the donor site and postoperative care of the donor site
Method of graft application
Biology of graft healing
Graft dressings and postoperative care
Failures of graft take

Classification of Skin Grafts

A skin graft is a segment of skin composed of epidermis and varying amounts of dermis that has been completely separated from its blood sup-

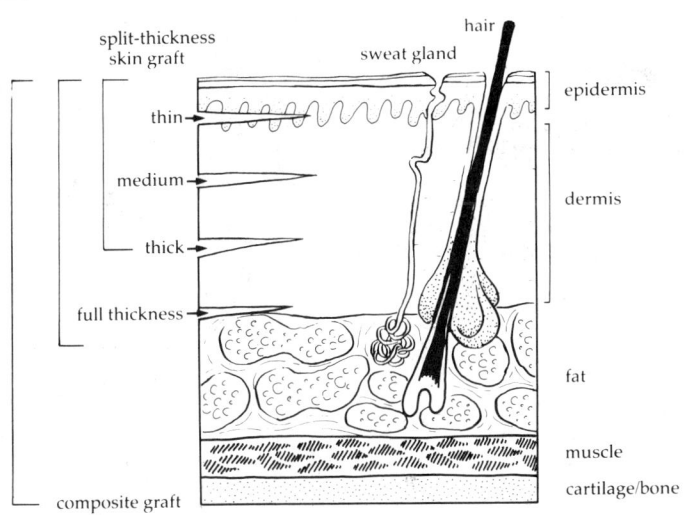

Figure 5-8. Thickness of a skin graft, measured in thousandths of an inch, is correlated with the anatomy of the skin. Split grafts are within the dermis, full-thickness grafts are all dermis, and composite grafts contain fat and other deep tissue.

ply (the donor site) and transplanted to another area of the body (the recipient site) that is devoid of epithelium. Ultimately, the skin graft must be revascularized to survive.

Skin grafts can be classified according to various criteria, including thickness, donor source, and physical characteristics.

THICKNESS OF GRAFT

Fig. 5-8 shows the tissue contained within grafts of different thicknesses.

1. *Split-thickness skin grafts (STSG)* are split within the dermis by a dermatome or knife. The skin graft contains all of the epidermis and the superficial portion of the dermis and skin appendages. The donor site retains the deeper component of the dermis with the remaining epidermal skin appendages. In some instances of very thin skin grafts, portions of the downward projections of the epidermis itself (the rete pegs) can also be left as part of the donor bed.

   A split-thickness skin graft can be additionally described as thin, medium, or thick, according to the amount of dermis on the graft.
   a. A thin graft is generally considered to be between six- and ten-thousandths (0.006–0.010) of an inch.
   b. A medium graft is between ten- and eighteen-thousandths of an inch.
   c. A thick graft is eighteen-thousandths of an inch or more.
2. *Full-thickness grafts* contain all of the dermis but little or no fat. They are usually obtained by free-hand excision of an ellipse of skin. Any fat on the undersurface is removed with a pair of curved scissors. The donor site is closed with sutures.
3. *Composite grafts* contain the entire thickness of epidermis and dermis and some additional fat, cartilage, or muscle.

BIOLOGIC SOURCE

Grafts also can be classified according to the source (Fig. 5-9).

1. *Autografts* are grafts taken from one site and transferred to another site on the same person.

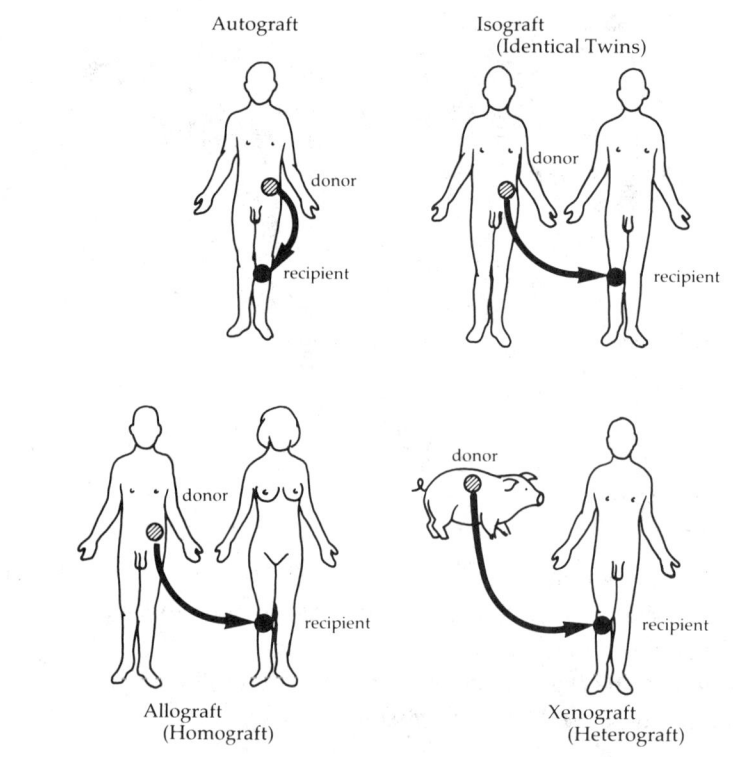

Figure 5-9. Types of skin grafts classified according to donor. Only autografts and isografts can be used as permanent replacement. In the emergency situation, an allograft or xenograft, such as commercially available porcine skin, can be used as a temporary dressing if removed within a few days.

2. *Isografts* are grafts between *genetically identical people* (twins, triplets) or between members of an inbred strain of animals.
3. *Allografts (homografts)* are taken from one person and transferred to another person of different genetic makeup of the same species.
4. *Xenografts (heterografts)* are taken from an animal of one species and transferred to an animal of another species.

Only the autograft and isograft can serve as a permanent skin replacement. The allograft and xenograft may be revascularized (take) but will be immunologically rejected because of the body's ability to recognize foreign antigens. *For emergency room use, the autograft is to be considered the prime method.*

PHYSICAL CHARACTERISTICS

A graft can be described according to its physical appearance, which is an indication of the manner in which the graft was obtained (Fig. 5-10).

1. *Sheetgrafts* are single sheets of skin that are usually obtained with specialized knife blades or dermatomes. The Goulian-Weck blade, Humby knife, Silver dermatome, Brown dermatome, Reese dermatome, Davol dermatome, and Padgett dermatome are some of the more common instruments for obtaining sheet grafts.

   Sheetgrafts are usually of relatively large size, varying from a few to several hundred square centimeters.
2. *Pinch grafts* are small mounds of skin with a saucer-like shape that are obtained by grasping the skin with a hook or forceps and snipping it with a pair of scissors or small scalpel blade.

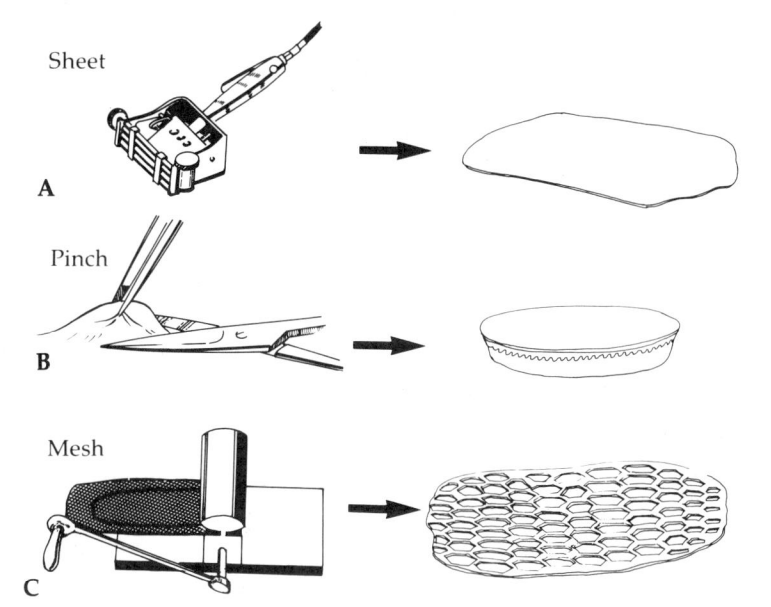

Figure 5-10. Types of graft configuration.
A. Sheet grafts of split thickness skin are used for most emergency situations.
B. Pinch grafts, almost never used, are mainly of historical interest as the first method developed.
C. Mesh grafts are used for contaminated or draining (blood serum) wounds to allow passage of drainage materials through the interstices.
   The open areas between grafts heal by epithelialization.

3. *Mesh grafts* are sheet grafts that are subsequently passed through a special instrument that makes numerous cuts through its thickness, allowing it to expand in an accordion or meshlike pattern.

Characteristics of Grafts

CONTRACTION

A raw open wound heals by the process of wound contraction. This process of contraction is modified by the presence of skin grafts and flaps. In general, the thicker the graft or flap, the less wound contraction occurs. The actual percentage of wound contraction correlates not only with the thickness of the grafted tissue, but also with the length of time the wound was left open before grafting and with the region of the body. The longer the wound was open and therefore the more granulation tissue with myofibroblasts, the greater the contraction. Open wounds about natural concavities and flexion creases tend to contract more than comparable wounds on extensor surfaces or areas in which there is a rigid underlying structure, such as cartilage or bone.

The range of wound contraction that might occur even with a skin graft is indicated below. The lower percentage represents contraction under ideal circumstances, and the higher figure represents contraction under adverse circumstances.

Thin grafts—50 to 90 percent
Medium grafts—40 to 75 percent
Thick grafts (full thickness)—5 to 50 percent
Flaps—0 to 25 percent

SENSIBILITY

The return of sensation to a skin graft or skin flap is primarily related to the following factors:

1. Number of nerve endings at that recipient site. For example, skin of the hand or face has more recipient sensory end-organs than skin of the back or trunk. The two-point discrimination of a thigh graft placed on the finger would be better than a thigh graft placed on the back.
2. Number and type of sensory receptors of the donor skin. Although this factor provides less variation, a donor graft of the hand or face has more end-organs than a graft taken from the trunk or proximal extremities.
3. Thickness of the graft. Paresthesias or other uncomfortable dysesthesias are more common with thin skin grafts than with thick grafts or with flaps; in general, thick grafts provide better two-point discrimination.

DURABILITY

The thicker the graft, the greater the durability. There is a correlation between the amount of dermis and subcutaneous tissue in the donor graft and its ability to resist trauma. The additional dermis and subcutaneous tissue provides a cushion and contains additional epidermal elements necessary to heal an abrasion of the previously grafted tissue. In particular, any fat in the graft, flap, or recipient bed allows a side-to-side mobility that protects against shearing forces. In contrast, a thin skin graft on a nonyielding surface such as a bone is highly susceptible to reinjury.

"TAKE" (REVASCULARIZATION)

1. Healthy wounds. A thin graft is more likely to "take" on a normal, healthy wound than is a thick graft. This is partly because of the diminished volume of tissue in the graft and therefore lower metabolic demand. Most important, there are more blood vessels within the upper dermis (the base of a thin graft) than there are in the lower dermis (the base of a thick graft). The increased number and smaller size of vessels at the base of a thin graft make vascularization more likely. The full-thickness graft or composite graft with fat at the undersurface has fewer blood vessels at the base, but revascularization can occur around the margins of the dermis (Fig. 5-5).
2. Avascular tissues. Thin- or medium-thickness STSGs do not survive, or "take," over an avascular bed. In contrast, a very thick skin graft, or full-thickness graft, can survive on an avascular wound (cortical bone, cartilage without perichondrium, tendon without paratenon, or irradiated tissue) because of the "bridging phenomenon." However, the margins of the wound surrounding the avascular area must have a good blood supply, and the wound must be no greater than 2 to 3 cm across. The thick or composite graft picks up its blood supply from the vascular margin and bridges across the avascular defect. In essence, the graft derives its blood from the periphery rather than the base.

COLOR AND TEXTURE

In general, skin flaps have a more natural appearance than thick grafts, and thick grafts have a more natural appearance than thin grafts. *The best color and texture match is achieved by taking a donor graft at an anatomic site close to the recipient site.*

Donor Sites

Fig. 5-11 shows the most frequently used donor sites.

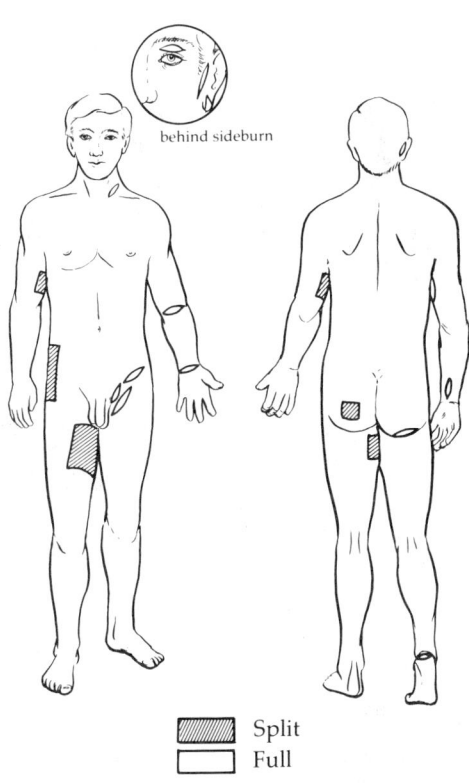

Figure 5-11. The most common donor sites. The split graft sites are indicated by the shaded marking and the full-thickness sites are simply outlined.

SPLIT-THICKNESS SKIN GRAFTS

In theory, any cutaneous site on the body could be used for a split-thickness skin graft, but various practical considerations limit the favorable sites. Skin grafts should not be taken from an important functional area, and the donor site should be hidden so that if scarring occurs, there is not an obvious cosmetic deformity. The preferred sites for split-thickness skin grafts for achieving wound healing (temporary biologic dressings) on the face or for permanent cover in any other area of the body are the:

Lateral buttock in the "panty area"
Posterior buttock (this has the disadvantage that the patient can't sit comfortably while the donor site is healing)
Medial thigh (this is a relatively hidden area but has the disadvantage that the site can be seen when the patient is wearing a bathing suit or shorts)
Medial aspect of the upper arm

Although the volar surface of the forearm and the anterior surface of the thigh have been suggested as useful donor sites because of their easy accessibility, these sites can develop unwarranted difficulties. A tender and very noticeable hypertrophic scar can occur if there is delayed healing, if there is an inadvertent full-thickness graft, or if infection intervenes (infection can convert a split-thickness donor site into a full thickness loss). Therefore, we discourage the use of these visible sites if cosmesis is of concern to the patient.

1. Healing potential. The most essential quality of a split-thickness donor site is the capability of healing. As we discuss later, the healing occurs

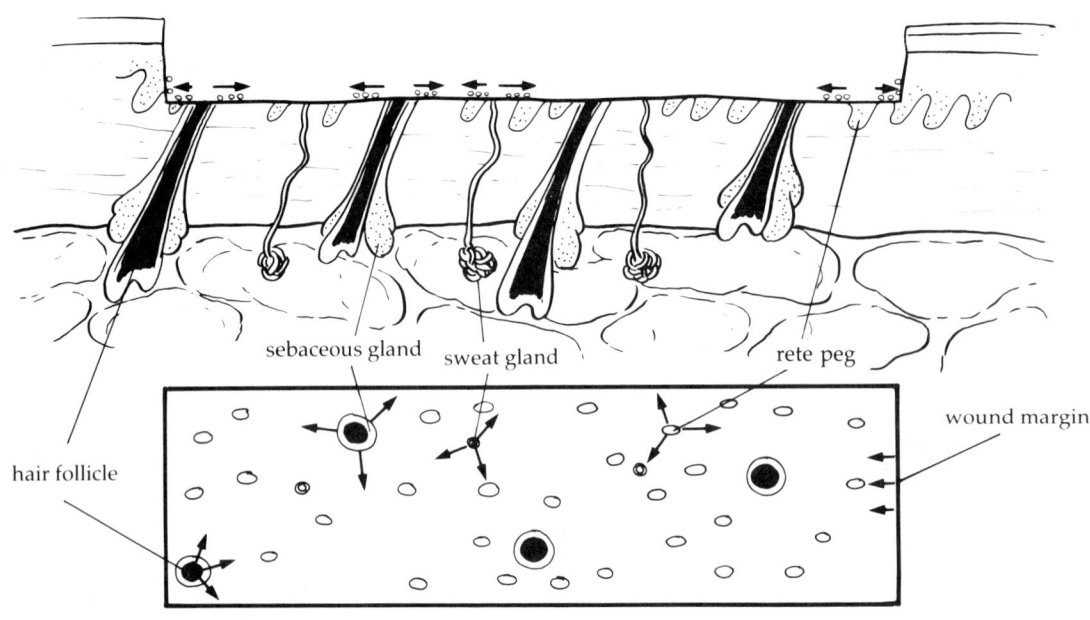

Figure 5-12. The healing of a split graft donor site occurs from epithelial appendices (hair follicles and sebaceous and sweat glands).

from preexisting skin appendages. Therefore, choose a site with adequate thickness of skin and skin appendages, and without burns or other scars.

2. Cosmesis. Although it is preferable to choose a site with the best possible color and texture match, the donor site should be hidden. Therefore, the buttock and lateral thigh are preferred sites.

3. Mechanism of healing (Fig. 5-12). The donor site of a split-thickness skin graft normally heals by reepithelialization. Epithelial cells from the margins of the wound, sweat glands, sebaceous glands, hair follicles, and rete pegs are potential sources for new epithelium.

The rate of healing is affected by the thickness of the split graft. The thin graft leaves considerably more epithelial appendages and less exposed dermis. With an extremely thick split graft, there are no rete pegs, sebaceous glands, or epithelial cells, leaving only the very base of the deepest hair follicles as a source for epithelialization. In fact a thick split graft donor site can be so deep that there is inadequate epithelium within the donor site and healing may be extremely delayed. Healing eventually occurs from wound contraction and reepithelialization from the margin. A dense hypertrophic scar usually results.

Healing of the donor site also can be affected by the type of dressing. Epithelialization occurs more rapidly on a moist occluded surface than it does on a dry open surface. Although using a wet dressing technique for healing of a donor site would seem preferable, this advantage of rapid healing is counterbalanced by a considerably greater risk of wound infection and resultant destruction of epithelial remnants.

Considering all factors, an extreme variation in healing time is possible. A very thin graft treated with wet dressings heals in 3 to 4 days, and a very thick graft treated as a dry open wound heals in 3 to 4 weeks.

Table 5-1. Facial grafts

	Retroauricular	Preauricular	Upper eyelid	Supraclavicular	Earlobe
Texture and color	Relatively red and smooth	Somewhat less red than preauricular and a slightly more irregular texture	Slightly more pale and tan, with an extremely smooth surface	Darker tan and somewhat less smooth	Paler tan, red, smooth
Size	1.5 × 4.0 cm safe size, to 2.5 × 6.0 cm maximum	1.0 × 4.0 cm safe size, to 2.0 × 6.0 cm maximum in aged adults with excess skin. Skin is thicker than retroauricular skin	1.0 × 3.0 cm, very thin and flexible	2.0 × 6.0 cm safe size, to 3.0 × 9.0 cm	1.0 × 3.0 cm and thicker dermis than other skin
Problems and clinical considerations	Ears are "pinned back" very slightly. Choose the more prominent ear	Gives a slight "face lift" effect on one side, and asymmetry is created. Can be used only in adults with excess skin. In men, pulls the sideburns against the ear tragus and makes shaving difficult. Beard may grow from transplanted graft	Should be used only on adults with excess eyelid skin. Creates a unilateral blepharoplasty and asymmetric eye appearance. Excess skin removal may prevent closure of the upper eyelid	Donor site scar can be quite noticeable, even with minimal skin excision because of tension associated with neck movements. The scar tends to be very wide and atrophic	Earlobe size asymmetry occurs but is usually not noticeable. There may be hair growing from earlobe skin
Primary use	Cheeks and eyelids	Nose, cheeks	Lower eyelid	Lower face	Nasal-dorsum and glabella

FULL-THICKNESS SKIN GRAFTS

A full-thickness skin graft is taken with a scalpel, and skin margins of the donor site are advanced and sutured. There are no special dermatomes used for full-thickness skin grafts.

In general, the best donor sites are in areas of relative tissue excess so that when an ellipse of skin is excised, the donor site can be closed by advancement of the skin edges and suturing. The area of the donor skin is limited by the necessity of closing the wound. If a very large full-thickness graft is required, the donor site can be covered by a split-thickness skin graft from another area. This technique, however, is not used in emergency situations.

The preferred sites for full-thickness grafts are not the same as those for split-thickness grafts. In general, full-thickness grafts are used for permanent cover to provide better cosmetic or functional skin.

Most full-thickness graft donor sites are in natural concavities (retroauricular, supraclavicular, upper eyelid), parallel to and/or within a flexion crease (groin, medial thigh, buttock, elbow, wrist), or in areas of relative tissue excess (e.g., hypothenar, preauricular, medial upper arm).

The choice of donor site depends on various factors, including the nature of the injury, anatomic location, size of the defect, and functional requirements (Tables 5-1 and 5-2).

Decide on a donor site to match the size and clinical needs of the recipi-

Table 5-2. Extremity grafts

	Medial upper arm	Antecubital crease	Wrist crease	Hypothenar crease	Groin	Buttock crease	Sole
Texture and color	Slightly tan, smooth, hairless	Darker pigment, rougher texture, and hairless	Darker tan, rough, hairless	Very pale, slight ridging from "palmprint" creases, hairless	Darker tan, yellow, slightly irregular texture, some hair	Pale, tan, much yellower, cobblestone surface	Very pale, rough, hairless
Size	Up to 4.0 × 12.0 cm, very thin	1.5 × 1.5 cm	1.0 × 3.0 cm	1.0 × 3.0 cm, very thick dermis and stratum corneum	3.0 × 9.0 cm, relatively thick	3.0 × 9.0 cm, thick dermis	1.0 × 3.0 cm, very thick stratum corneum and dermis
Problems and clinical applications	Donor scar may be visible. Excess skin removal may cause a tourniquetlike constriction around the upper arm. Numbness may occur in the region of the medial branchial cutaneous nerve	Scar tends to become quite wide and atrophic. If excess skin is removed, there may be limitation of elbow extension and permanent periarticular stiffness	May limit wrist extension. Injury to midpalmar branch of median nerve can cause paresthesia or anesthesia	May cause a tender scar from bumping or rubbing against the hypothenar eminence	May grow pubic hair if donor site is too close to perineum. Scar may mimic an appendix or hernia scar and cause confusion in surgical diagnosis (choose the left groin whenever possible)	Can change buttock configuration; may cause a tender scar, and sitting can be uncomfortable	May cause tender scar, which can impair walking and running
Primary use	Face or hand	Palm or volar finger	Palm or volar finger	Volar finger	Dorsal hand	Dorsal hand	Hand

ent area, remembering to avoid donor sites that are more likely to result in complications.

Technique

The technique for obtaining a skin graft is different for split- and full-thickness grafts. Full-thickness grafts are usually quite small and are precisely shaped to fit the defect, whereas split grafts are usually larger and do not have to fit precisely. Full-thickness grafts are taken with a scalpel blade, and split grafts with a scalpel or, more frequently, a dermatome.

TAKING A FULL-THICKNESS GRAFT
1. Determine the size and shape of the graft with a pattern (Fig. 5-13). In most circumstances, the recipient defect appears to be larger than it

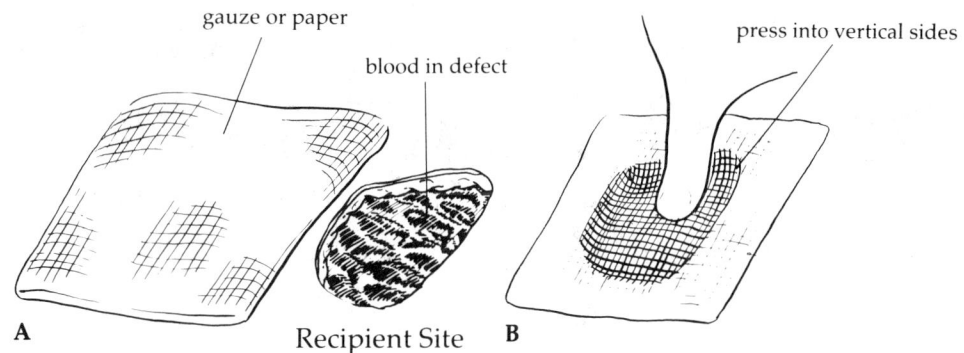

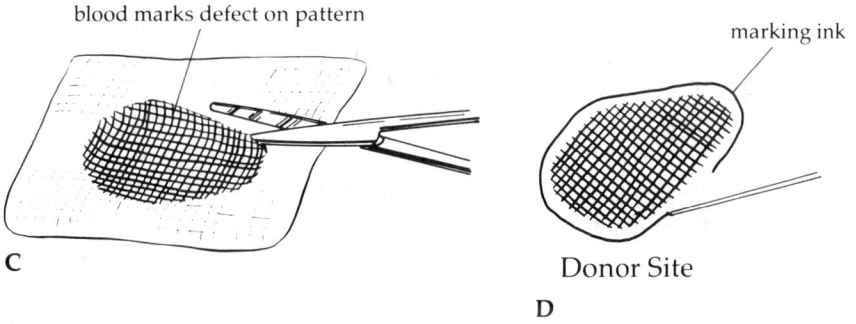

Figure 5-13. Determining size and shape of graft.
A and B. Take the pattern, including the vertical wall, with paper wrapping.
C and D. Cut out the pattern and transfer it to the donor site to use as an outline for methylene blue marker.

actually is because of the retraction of skin margins caused by internal elasticity. The actual defect size can be estimated by pushing in or suturing the wound margin. Nonetheless, as a general rule it is best to take a pattern to fit the measured size of the defect.

Take a pattern using an absorbable elastic material, such as cotton gauze or glove paper wrappings. The material should be such that blood absorbs into the pattern. Remember when pressing the gauze into the defect that the vertical wall of the defect also must be included.

Cut out the pattern and transfer it to the proposed donor site. Place the long axis of the pattern parallel to the most natural axis of the donor site that facilitates closure of the donor site. Be sure to keep the pattern "right-side-up."

Use a marking pen or some ink material (e.g., methylene blue, gentian violet, Bonney blue) on a cotton-tipped applicator to trace the pattern onto the skin.

2. Excise the graft. Incise the lateral margins through the dermis to the level of the subcutaneous tissue. Place a skin hook (or a clamp if the tip of the graft is to be discarded) into the end of the skin graft. With a scalpel blade, begin to sweep the blade from side to side carefully to separate the dermis of the skin from the subcutaneous tissue, and remove the graft.

3. Defat the graft (Fig. 5-14). Roll the edge of the skin graft over your long finger and stabilize with the adjacent fingers and thumb. A stable surface for cutting is achieved, and also there is a better "feel" for the

Figure 5-14. Removing the excess fat on the deep surface from the graft.

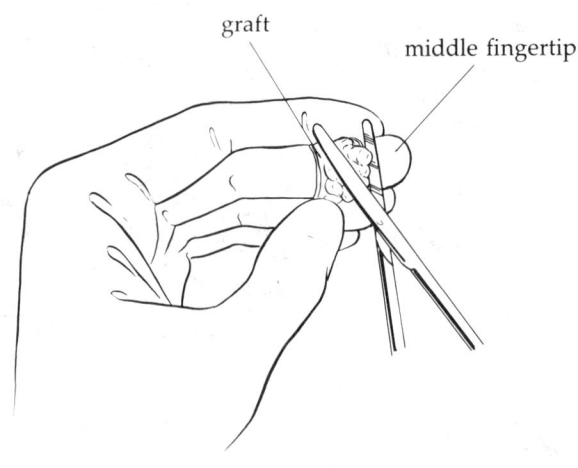

proper depth of excision by scissors of unwelcome subcutaneous fat of the dermis.

Examine the underside of the skin graft as you proceed. You should note small flecks of fat adherent to the underside of the dermis, giving it a more yellow appearance. Care must be taken that a hole is not made through the dermis.

TAKING A SPLIT SKIN GRAFT

The various means of obtaining a split-thickness skin graft all require some type of knife blade that is capable of splitting the skin through an intradermal plane to obtain a sheet of split-thickness skin.

1. Choice of knives and dermatomes. The instruments used for obtaining a skin graft vary in size and mechanical principles. For emergency department use, however, some of the smaller and relatively simple instruments are suitable for thin, small, split skin grafts.

   The two general types of instruments are knife blades and dermatomes.

   a. Free-hand knife blades (Fig. 5-15)
      (1) Scalpel (#20) with handle
      (2) Razor blade
      (3) Weck blade
   b. Dermatomes (small, calibrated) (Fig. 5-16)
      (1) Silver dermatome
      (2) Humby knife
      (3) Davol dermatome
   c. Dermatomes (large, calibrated)
      (1) Brown dermatome
      (2) Padgett dermatome
      (3) Reese dermatome

      Free-hand skin grafts using scalpel, razor, or Weck blade are usually not as uniform or predictable in their thickness and margins as those obtained with dermatome blades. However, many emergency departments do not have calibrated dermatomes available.

      The Silver, Weck, and Davol dermatomes are quite simple to use,

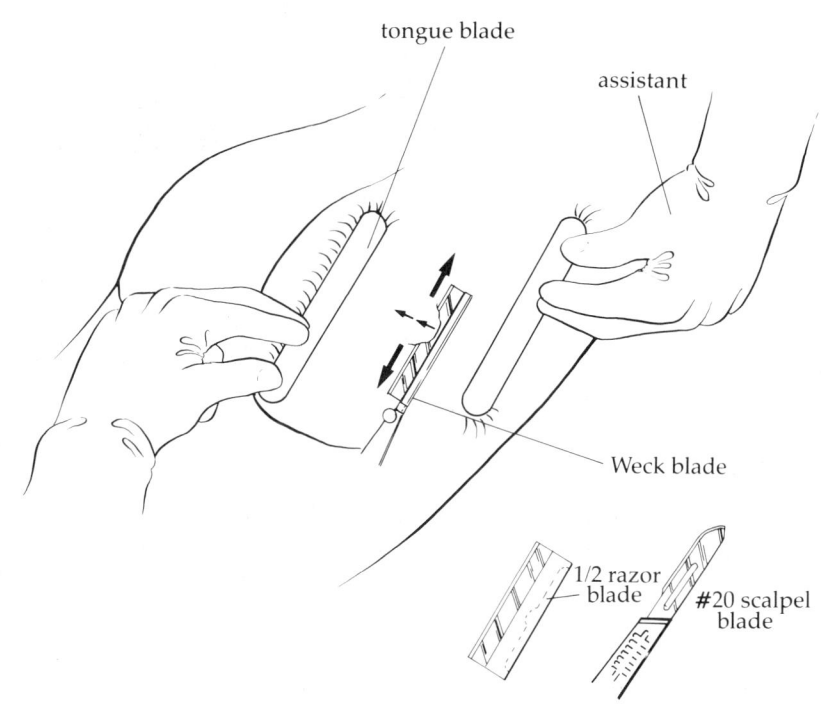

Figure 5-15. Blades with which free-hand skin grafts can be taken. These grafts should be taken as thinly as possible, using a back-and-forth slicing motion on a lubricated flat surface. Countertraction should be used to keep the skin under tension.

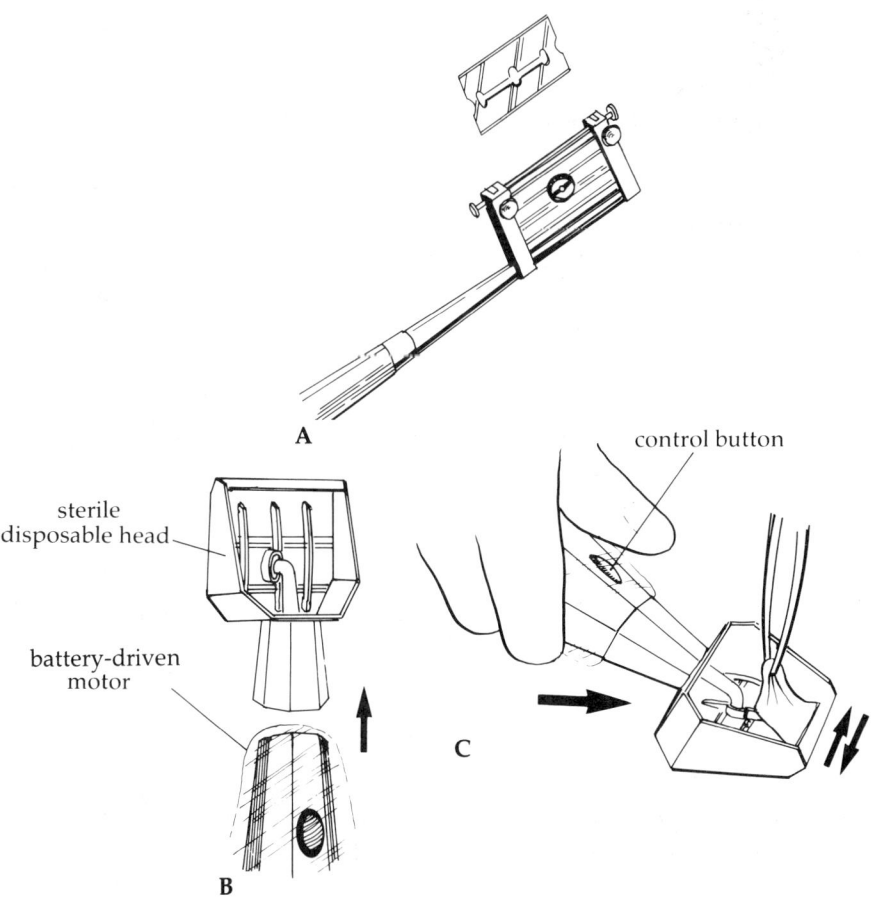

Figure 5-16. Calibrated dermatomes for small grafts taken in the emergency department.
    A. Silver dermatome.
B and C. Davol dermatome, demonstrating mode of action.

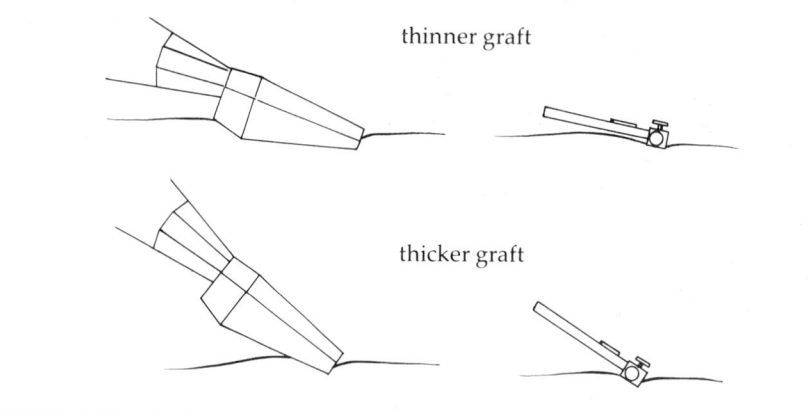

Figure 5-17. The thickness of the graft can be increased by increasing the angle of the blade.

and a very uniform graft can be obtained with minimal practice. Every emergency room should have at least one, if not all of these, available.

The Silver dermatome has an adjustable calibration for determining the thickness of the skin graft such that a graft of any size from 4/1000 to 24/1000 of an inch can be obtained. The cutting edge for the Silver dermatome is a standard double-edged razor blade, and the width of the graft is limited, therefore, to 2.5 cm. This dermatome is probably the most useful for standard emergency department situations because of its simplicity and the ready access to standard shaving blades.

The Davol dermatome is a battery-powered unit kept in a rechargeable holder when not in use. Special disposable dermatome blades for this unit are available. The Davol dermatome is probably the simplest of all the units available but has the drawback that only a medium-thickness graft of about 14/1000 of an inch can be obtained. There is no adjustable setting for thinner or thicker grafts, although by changing the angle of the blade, as is illustrated in Fig. 5-17, some variation in thickness can occur.

Other dermatomes, such as the Humby, Brown, Padgett, and Reese dermatomes, obtain large grafts for major resurfacing and are not for emergency department use. If larger skin grafts are required than can be obtained by the smaller dermatome, the patient should be taken care of in an operating room by surgeons experienced in managing major tissue losses.

2. Method of cutting the graft (Fig. 5-15)
    a. Positioning. All the aforementioned instruments for obtaining split-thickness skin grafts require the following procedure:
        (1) *Choose a flat surface* that is unobstructed by clothing, drapes, or table.
        (2) *Lubricate the skin* with a sterile mineral oil, antibiotic solution, or water.
        (3) *Stabilize the skin with traction.* Traction over a broad surface can be effected with the use of tongue blades, a block of wood, or any other flat, broad-surfaced object.

One tongue blade places traction in front of and in a direction away

AMPUTATIONS AND SKIN LOSS

from the intended direction of the dermatome. An assistant should place traction behind the dermatome.

The instrument is positioned in preparation for cutting.

b. Angle of blade (Fig. 5-17). The steeper (i.e., more obtuse) the angle between the plane of the skin and the plane of the dermatome, the deeper these blades cut into the skin regardless of dermatome setting. Most dermatomes are designed so that the base of the dermatome is flush with the skin, and the actual angle of the blade with the skin is about 10° or 15°. This angle usually cuts a graft of the proper thickness.

If the handle of the dermatome is dropped toward the skin, the angle of the blade at the anterior surface is more acute (0°–10°), and therefore a thinner graft may be obtained than desired.

If the handle of the dermatome is elevated, the blade angle increases to 20° to 30°, and a thicker graft is obtained.

c. Pressure. There is an optimal pressure for taking skin grafts of precise and even thickness. Success follows learning the "feel" of the instrument. A guideline to the correct amount of pressure can be developed by examining the contact point of the dermatome with the skin.

There usually is a slight depression of the skin at the site of contact. If the knife is deeply indented into the skin, there is probably too much pressure and a thicker graft is obtained. If there is no indentation on the skin, however, and therefore not enough pressure, a thinner graft is obtained.

d. Cutting motion. With the Silver dermatome or a free-hand knife, there are two component movements occurring simultaneously:
   (1) A rapid, short, side-to-side movement of the knife handle, which varies from 1 to 3 strokes per second
   (2) A slow, forward advancement such that it usually takes between 10 and 20 seconds to advance the dermatome 2 to 3 cm

   With the Davol dermatome, there is only a forward motion because the motorized blade has its own side-to-side component. The rate of forward movement is somewhat more rapid than that of the Silver dermatome.

e. Check of thickness of graft. From the very first cutting of the graft, a simultaneous check should be made that the proper thickness is being obtained. This can be done in several ways:
   (1) An assistant, if available, can grasp the skin graft with forceps or a clamp and keep it under slight traction so that the thickness of the graft can be observed.
   (2) Look at the donor site. In particular, the margins of the graft site should be checked to make sure the blade has not inadvertently dug deeply into the skin, taking out a large divot of full-thickness skin graft. This can occur easily if pressure on the dermatome is not uniform throughout the surface and there is a tilting of the blade in one direction or the other.
   (3) If an improper thickness or a divot of full-thickness skin is being obtained, the cutting should be stopped and the blade readjusted. If this cannot be done, a new donor site should be picked.

f. Final separation of graft from bed. To separate the graft from the bed, the dermatome or blade should be tilted upward away from the

plane of the skin so that it will cut through the base of the skin graft. As an alternative, the cutting motion can be stopped and a separate knife blade used to cut the graft from the bed.
3. Hemostasis. Immediately after a skin graft is taken, the donor site may bleed profusely. Application of a cool moist gauze pad facilitates hemostasis and absorbs most of the blood. A light pressure wrap also may be of benefit. After 5 to 15 minutes, most of the gauze can be removed, and if there is no active bleeding, the final dressing can be applied.

Dressing the Donor Site

The split-thickness donor site is comparable to an abrasion in which the epidermis and a portion of the dermis are removed, but epithelial remnants including the rete pegs and skin appendages remain in the deep dermis for reepithelialization. The principle of healing of the donor site has been reviewed. The choice between using an occlusive, closed antibiotic dressing or a dry open technique depends on the clinical conditions. The closed dressing (Opsite, Biobrane, N-terface) is simple and more comfortable for the patient but increases the risk of infection; therefore, it is preferred for most donor graft sites except in the patient with severe cutaneous infection. The open technique or closed antibiotic dressing are used for contaminated wounds. Also see Chapter 8.

CIRCUMSTANCES FAVORING AN OPEN TECHNIQUE
1. Predisposition to infection:
   a. Patients with other, nearby cutaneous infections
   b. Patients treated as outpatients in whom adequate follow-up is difficult
   c. Donor sites around the thigh, buttock, and perineum, in which contamination is probable in spite of a closed dressing.
2. Areas in which it is difficult to apply a dressing because of movement, contour, or hair:
   a. For a dry open technique to be used, the patient must not be wearing clothing in the donor area.
   b. A fan or heat lamp is used to facilitate drying.
   c. After 24 to 36 hours, a dry crust is formed.
   d. This is kept dry, and exposed for 7 to 10 days until the crust begins to separate spontaneously.

CIRCUMSTANCES FAVORING A CLOSED ANTIBIOTIC DRESSING
A *very thick skin graft* removes most sources of epithelial regrowth; therefore, desiccation of the dermal appendages may convert the donor site to a full-thickness wound that may itself require skin grafting. Ideally, the donor site should be completely occluded, but if there is local infection, it should be treated with a closed antibiotic dressing changed frequently. The method of applying a closed antibiotic dressing follows:

1. Apply an antibiotic cream (Neosporin, gentamicin, silver sulfadiazine [Silvadene]). The antibiotic ointment reduces the possibility of infection and at the same time provides some degree of occlusion and protection against desiccation.

2. Apply wide-mesh gauze (Adaptic, N-terface). This layer serves as an interface that allows drainage to pass through the gauze.
3. Apply a layer of absorbent cotton gauze (4 × 4, Surgipad, Fluffs). This layer absorbs any hemorrhage or serous drainage that may occur.
4. Fix in place. A wrap (Ace bandage, Kling, Kerlix, bias-cut stockinette, tube gauze) or tape will hold these in place.
5. Change the outer two layers daily or twice a day.

CIRCUMSTANCES FAVORING A CLOSED OCCLUSIVE DRESSING
For most wounds with uncontaminated, clean, hairless, smooth contours, a synthetic membrane (Opsite, Biobrane, N-terface) is used. This allows rapid, relatively painless healing, with a minimum of intervention by patient and physician. The method follows:

1. Hemostasis is obtained.
   a. The skin surrounding the donor site is dried and the membrane applied.
   b. The membrane is removed when reepithelialization is complete (7 to 24 days).
2. Postoperative course:
   a. The patient should be instructed to:
      (1) Elevate the donor site
      (2) Engage in essential activities only
      (3) Apply no pressure (such as lying down), no shearing, and no rubbing
      (4) Be aware of signs of hemorrhage and infection
   b. The patient should return to the physician on the second or third postoperative day, at which time the entire outer layers of the dressing (except a synthetic occlusive membrane) should be removed as long as they are not adherent to the healing wound. In some instances the second absorbent layer of gauze is incorporated into the crust of the healing wound. If this is so, it should not be removed because the healing epithelium will be torn off with the gauze.
   c. If there is no sign of infection, a light covering of dry gauze should be applied and the patient allowed to resume more normal activities but no bathing is allowed until the seventh postgraft day.
   d. On the seventh day, the inner gauze can be removed. The patient can begin bathing with instruction to peel away the gauze carefully that is adherent to the crust. This is best done in the bathtub when the gauze is wet. If bleeding or disruption of epithelium is occurring, the donor site should be left open to the air until it is dry and an additional 4 or 5 days allowed to pass before another attempt is made at removal of the adherent gauze.
   e. If there is infection at the donor site, the entire gauze should be removed by soaking. This is best done in a bathtub, Jacuzzi, or Hubbard tank.

      After all layers of gauze are removed, the wound can be treated in two ways:
      (1) If the patient cannot be admitted to the hospital or is reliable, the donor site can be treated as an infected open wound by applica-

tion of topical antibiotics, bathing to remove the antibiotic gently, and reapplication of antibiotic dressings. This should be repeated three to four times a day.

(2) An alternative for patients who must be treated on an outpatient basis is to leave the wound open or covered with a gauze to absorb the drainage. In most instances systemic antibiotics are not required, but it is advisable to obtain a culture in case systemic symptoms develop or there is spread of infection with lymphangitis or cellulitis to adjacent areas.

Remember that if the donor site is infected, there is a higher probability that the grafted recipient site is also infected, and it should be closely inspected.

Application of the Graft

The recipient defect must be judged suitable for grafting after evaluation for these characteristics:

1. Adequate vascularity
2. Smooth contours
3. No necrotic debris or foreign material
4. No bleeding

If the wound is not suitable, it should be dressed and a delayed skin graft done several days later, after dressing changes, or after surgical debridement.

METHOD
If the wound is suitable:

1. Apply the graft to the wound, making certain that the raw dermal side is against the wound (Fig. 5-18A). Although this seems simple and obvious, it is sometimes difficult to determine with *very* thin grafts.
2. Distribute the skin graft over the entire recipient surface using the back of the forceps or a cotton-tipped applicator (Fig. 5-18B).
3. Be certain that the graft is evenly contoured against the raw surface. The most common mistake is to arch the graft over the defect because the bed is irregular (Fig. 5-18E) or the graft is too small (Fig. 5-18F).
4. Suture or staple the graft to the skin margin (Fig. 5-18C).
   a. Thin split-thickness skin grafts do not need to be carefully coapted. They can overlap onto the epidermis around the margin. Staples can facilitate application.
   b. Full-thickness skin grafts need careful approximation of the edges in the same manner as lacerations. This is to ensure that a good cosmetic scar is obtained and also to provide additional blood supply to the graft through the margins.
   c. The needle containing suture should pass first through the graft and second into the normal skin. If the needle is passed in the opposite direction, the graft will be lifted off the bed.
   d. The suture is tied and the end cut (cut long if a tie-over stent dressing is to be used).

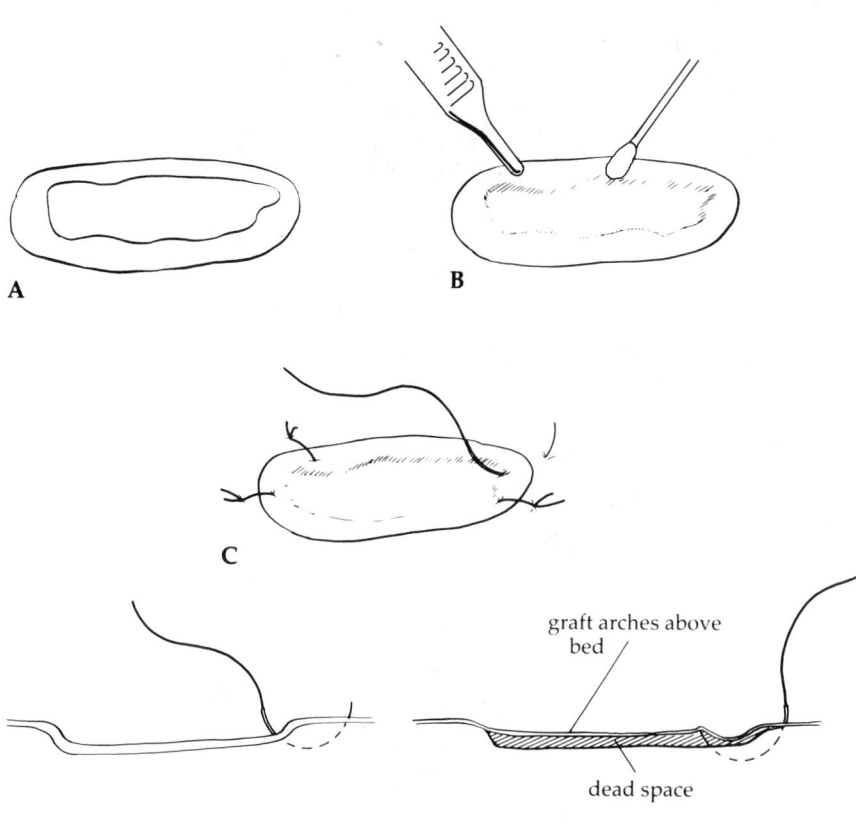

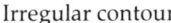

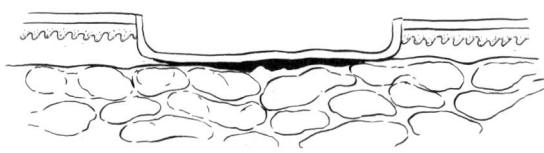

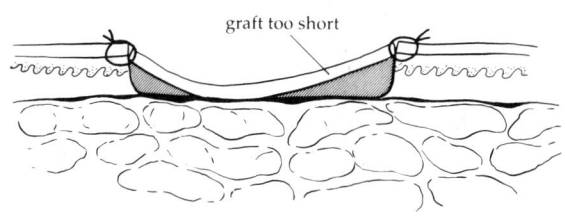

Figure 5-18. Application of graft to wound.
A. Apply graft with raw dermal side against wound.
B. Distribute graft evenly over surface.
C. Suture or staple—the needle passes from graft to skin edge.
D. When the needle is passed in the appropriate direction, the graft remains in good contact to its bed. If passed incorrectly, the graft will be lifted away from its bed. This creates a potential dead space in which blood or serum collects, inhibiting skin graft "take."

Check the graft to ensure that it is in direct contact with the bed and not over an irregular bed (E) or arching above the surface with an underlying dead space (F).

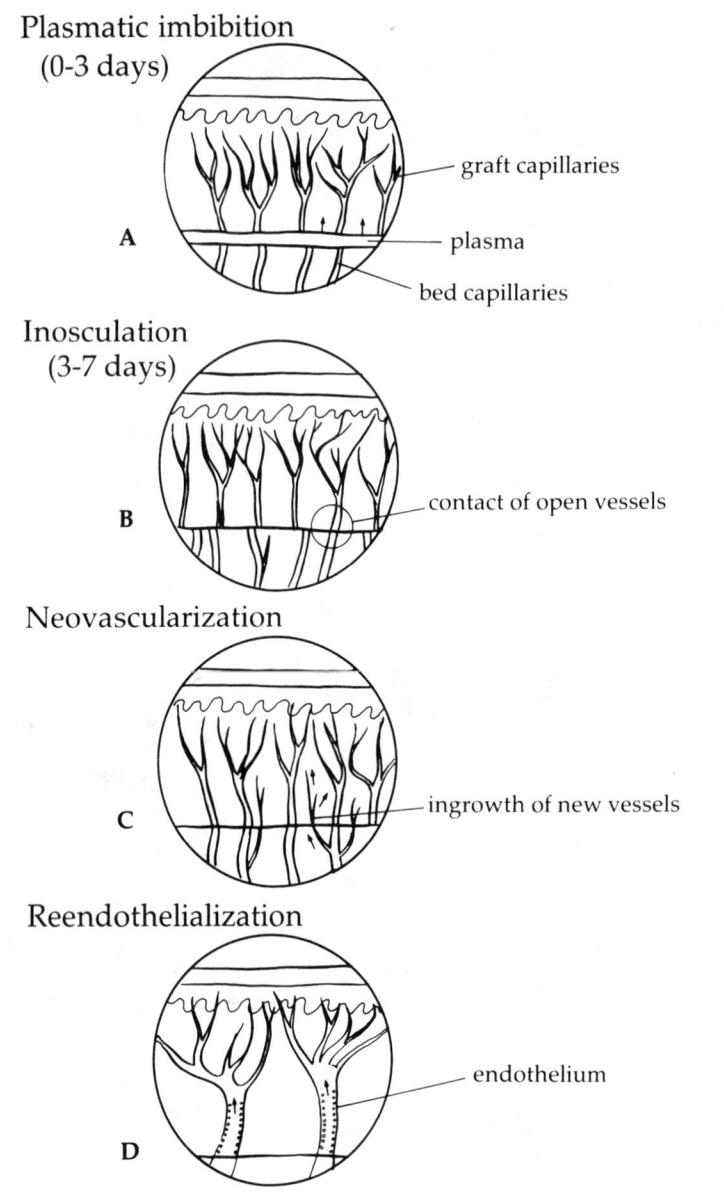

Figure 5-19. Revascularization of graft.
A. For the first 3 days, a skin graft revascularizes by plasmatic imbibition.
B, C, and D. After 3 days, blood vessels grow into the graft primarily by reendothelialization and inosculation.

Graft Healing

The healing of a skin graft can be considered as two separate processes: revascularization and adherence. Revascularization achieves graft viability, and adherence maintains the graft position by scar formation. A graft can be revascularized but not adhere to its bed. This can occur in patients taking steroids or with grafts placed on avascular tissue or over alloplastic foreign materials. However, adherence cannot occur with revascularization.

REVASCULARIZATION—THE BIOLOGY OF GRAFT HEALING

When a skin graft is transplanted to its recipient site, the graft must be revascularized by the ingrowth of blood vessels from the recipient bed into the transplanted skin (Fig. 5-19). If this process of revascularization does not occur, the skin graft will die (nontake). During the interval between placement of the graft and actual revascularization, the graft survives by diffusion of nutrients (plasmatic imbibition). At body temperatures, the period of survival by diffusion is approximately 72 hours.

1. Plasmatic imbibition. For 3 days the graft is nourished by plasmatic imbibition. Plasma passively moves into the existing vasculature of the skin graft. The graft may double or triple in thickness from this fluid intake. There is not a true circulation of plasma. The graft survives primarily by anaerobic metabolism, but there is a small amount of oxygen available by diffusion. The graft cannot survive, however, if there is blood separating the graft from the recipient bed. Apparently, there are toxic products within blood that cause cell necrosis. Furthermore, nutrient materials are not capable of diffusion into the graft because of the clot.

   During these first 3 days, a fibrin clot adheres the graft dermis to the recipient tissue.
2. Capillary ingrowth. For 3 to 7 days, capillaries grow from the bed into the graft. Three distinct processes have been implicated: inosculation, neovascularization, and reendothelialization. Numerous studies have indicated that the original vascular tree maintains its anatomic pattern throughout the period of revascularization. Therefore, a combination of inosculation and reendothelialization seems to be the predominant mechanism.
   a. *Inosculation* involves the random contact of blood vessels in the recipient site with preexisting blood vessels of the graft. The vascular pattern of the graft does not change but is reestablished, and the endothelium within the graft vessels is the original endothelium.
   b. *Neovascularization* is the ingrowth of new capillary endothelial buds into the dermal collagen to form new vascular channels. Neovascularization has not been clearly documented.
   c. *Reendothelialization* is the ingrowth of new endothelial buds directly into the original vascular channels of the graft. This is similar to inosculation because the vascular pattern is maintained, but the new endothelial buds use the old vascular system as a conduit for their ingrowth, and there is replacement of the graft endothelial cells.

GRAFT ADHERENCE

Adherence of a graft involves the same processes as the healing of the opposed margins of a skin laceration.

1. 0–3 days—fibrin clot attaches graft dermis to recipient tissue bed.
2. 3–7 days—vessel ingrowth adds additional strength.
3. 7 days onward—collagen (scar) causes adherence of graft and bed.

Dressing the Recipient Site

The requirements for a skin graft dressing are (1) a nonadherent contact layer, (2) an absorbent middle layer, and (3) an immobilizing pressure outer layer (tie-over stent, circumferential wrap or tape).

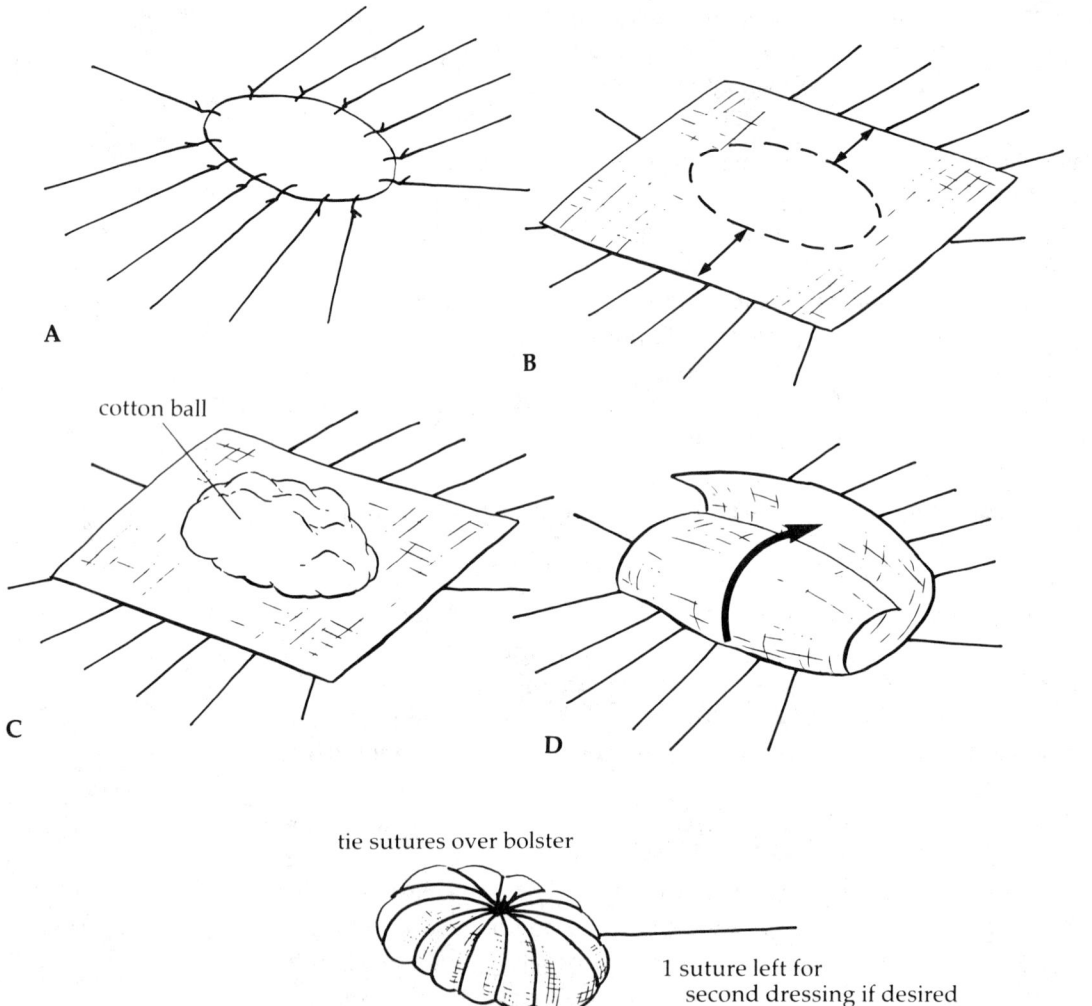

Figure 5-20. Technique for a tie-over dressing.
A. Suture the graft, leaving the ends 5 to 10 cm long.
B. Apply a soft petrolatum gauze.
C. Pack cotton wadding into the wound.
D. Fold the gauze over.
E. Tie the sutures over in pairs.

INNER LAYER

The inner layer can consist of any of the commercial gauzes or a gauze dressing can be made by impregnating a cotton gauze pad with antibiotic cream or ointment.

The gauze should be applied carefully so that there are no ridges.

MIDDLE LAYER

The middle absorbent layer can be of cotton gauze or cotton wadding. It should carefully be made to conform to the wound contour so that when the outer pressure is applied, the pressure is evenly distributed.

The gauze can be dry or moistened with glycerin if better conformity is required. Wetting with saline or water is not done because the water evaporates, leaving a very hard, somewhat smaller gauze that does not conform as well.

Other materials, such as Reston foam or silicone sponge, can be used for distribution of pressure and padding. However, because these materials are nonabsorbent and may lead to maceration of serous or bloody wounds, they are used over a more absorbent layer.

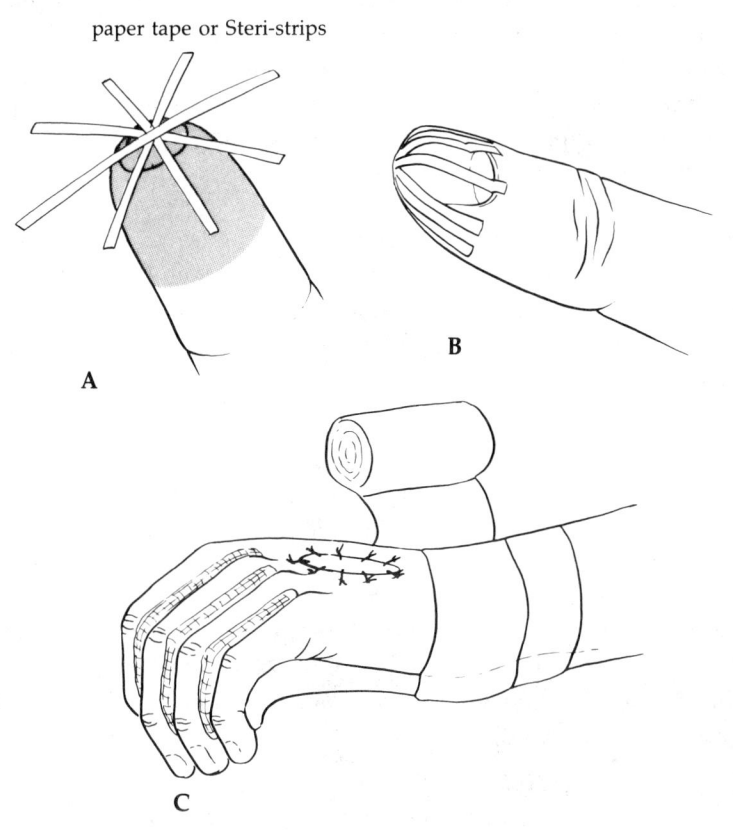

Figure 5-21. Circumferential wraps.
A and B. Sterile paper tape is useful for fingertips and other areas difficult to wrap. This can be combined with tube gauze (not illustrated) for protection and immobilization.
C. Circumferential wraps are effective on the extremities.

OUTER LAYER

The outer layer should apply firm pressure and immobilize the inner and middle layer. There are three alternatives: tie-over stents, circumferential wraps, and tape. The choice depends on the anatomic site:

1. Tie-over stents (Fig. 5-20). This method can be used anywhere but is best for concave or flat surfaces around the mouth, eyelid, fingertip, and hand.

    This very popular and effective method must be properly applied. Otherwise, there is a tendency for the peripheral part of the graft to pull away from the bed and the central graft to have too much pressure.

    It should not be used for very large grafts placed over mobile areas (such as chest wall).

    At 3 to 5 postoperative days, the tie-over is removed without dislodging the skin graft. First, cut the tie-over sutures near the skin surface. Grasp the bolus, and slide a moistened applicator stick between the graft and bolus. Roll the applicator stick between these and gently tease off the bolus with the applicator stick. Do not lift the bolus up because the graft can be elevated. Any seroma or hematoma can be expressed from the edge or through a small slit in the graft.

2. Circumferential wraps (Fig. 5-21). The circumferential wraps (e.g., Ace bandage, bias-cut stockinette, Kerlix gauze) are best used for grafts on convex surfaces, such as the extremities, scalp, and forehead.

    The wrap can also be used in conjunction with a tie-over stent for additional immobilization.

3. Taping (Fig. 5-21). This is an insecure method because the tape can become wet and come off. However, it is sometimes useful for
   a. Children, because of the ease of removal
   b. Large areas, to save time of suturing
   c. Tenuous composite grafts, in which additional trauma from suturing is to be avoided
   d. The fingertip

   The surrounding skin should be thoroughly dried and made sticky with Ace adherent or benzoin. Steri-strips are then taped directly over the graft. The inner and middle gauze layers are not used or are applied over the tape.

Failures of Skin Graft Take

A skin graft may fail to take (revascularize) because of a wide variety of factors. The factors may be intrinsic to the health of the patient, related to the nature of the injury, caused by poor surgical judgment or technique, or resulting from inadequate postoperative care.

We have divided the reasons for failure into four groups: hypovascular bed, hematoma, technical error, and noncontact and infection. Each factor itself or a combination of these factors can contribute to ultimate failure.

HYPOVASCULAR RECIPIENT BED

In this situation, the bed on which the skin graft was placed has inadequate vascularity to support a skin graft. In most instances the surgeon can make this determination by considering the general health of the patient, nature of the injury, and quality of the tissues on which the graft is to be placed.

1. Disease states. The patient may have an underlying disease process such as arteriosclerosis, diabetes, or an autoimmune arthritis. Any of these conditions could preclude the normal availability of capillaries for revascularization. This does not mean that a skin graft should not be attempted if the patient has one of these conditions. Rather, both the surgeon and patient should be aware of the potential for failure and need for a greater period of immobilization.
2. Trauma. The nature of the injury may be a severe crush or associated vascular injury that renders the tissues ischemic. Adequate debridement may create a more suitable vascular bed; in many instances, however, the demarcation between ischemic and nonischemic tissues is not readily apparent, and a waiting period to allow demarcation may be indicated, followed by delayed grafting.
3. Hypovascular normal tissues. Bare bone without its periosteum, cartilage without perichondrium, tendon without its peritenon, and fascia without the overlying areolar tissue are poor vascular beds. The number of capillaries that can grow from these tissues is usually insufficient for sustaining a skin graft. If adjacent tissues have normal vascularity, however, it is possible to put on a thicker skin graft that obtains its vascularization from those tissues and bridges across the small (less than 1 cm) hypovascular tissues.

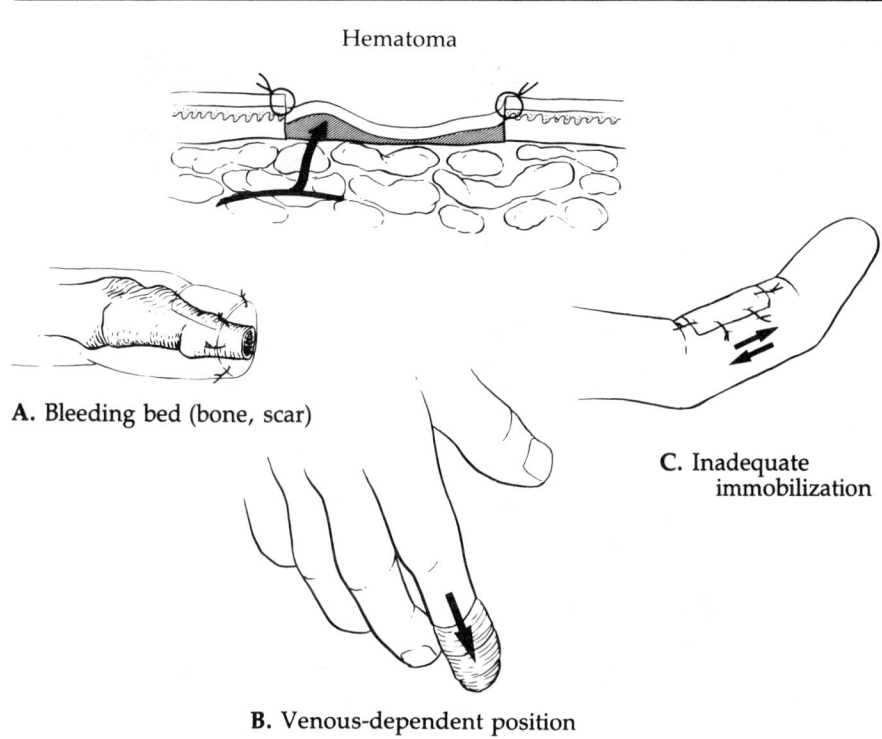

Figure 5-22. Hematoma formation is often caused by bleeding from a bed of bone or scar (A), dependency causing venous hypertension (B), or poor immobilization causing shearing between the graft and bed (C).

HEMATOMAS

A hematoma prevents revascularization for two reasons (Fig. 5-22). The hematoma fills the space between the graft and the bed such that capillaries in the bed cannot grow into the skin graft. That is, the hematoma is a physical obstruction to capillary ingrowth. The second reason is that a hematoma produces metabolic breakdown products, which are toxic to skin. It is well established that a skin graft can survive for extended periods when resting on a seroma, but the graft will die within 12 to 24 hours if it is on top of a hematoma. The reasons for hematoma are:

1. Abnormal vascular bed. Injuries within old scar or on cancellous bone tend to bleed in spite of otherwise adequate surgical efforts to obtain hemostasis. The multiple vessels within fibrous tissue are incapable of vasoconstriction, and therefore normal hemostasis is more difficult to obtain. Bone has open vascular lacunae, which tend to ooze for the same reasons. In these tissues it is often preferable to do delayed skin grafts after a prolonged period of hemostasis.
2. Inadequate postoperative immobilization. Bleeding may occur after the skin graft has been placed on the wound because of inadequate postoperative immobilization. The graft site should be stabilized with dressings or splints so that shearing between the graft and its bed is not possible. If there is inadequate immobilization, the movement of the graft across the recipient bed can disturb ingrowing capillaries and lead to hematoma.
3. Venous oozing from dependency. The other major postoperative problem is venous oozing when the grafted part is in a gravity-dependent

Figure 5-23. Technical errors most commonly causing graft failure are an irregular bed preventing contouring of graft (A), a graft that is too small and bridges across the surface (B), and poorly distributed or excessive pressure (C).

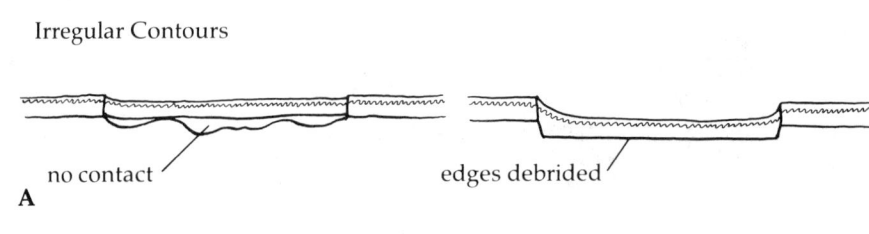

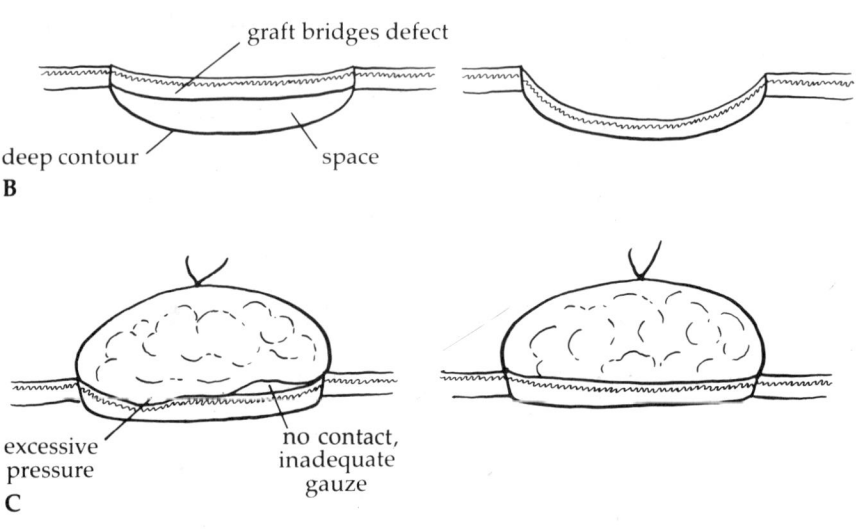

position. It is absolutely essential that a skin graft site be elevated to prevent venous oozing. In particular, skin grafts of the lower extremity require 1 week at a minimum and often 2 weeks of continuous elevation. Otherwise, hemorrhage occurs underneath the graft because of the increased venous pressure accompanying dependency. Facial wounds do not require special elevation other than maintaining a sitting posture or lying in bed with one or two pillows. Injuries of the upper extremity can usually be elevated adequately in a sling.

TECHNICAL ERRORS

Fig. 5-23 shows three of the most common technical errors that cause graft failure.

1. Failure to recognize irregular wound contours caused by the injury. Some injuries produce an irregular contour with alternating depressions and elevations or gouges. Either the graft must be pushed down into the depression, or the surface must be made more regular by debridement or advancement of tissues.
2. Poor design of skin graft. If too small a skin graft is sutured to the wound margins, the tension on the graft causes it to bowstring above the wound surface. This problem is usually caused by the surgeon measuring only the horizontal plane of the wound, forgetting that tissue is required to fill in the vertical walls of the defect. If this does occur, the alternatives are (1) simply to lay the graft down into the concavity of the wound and leave the vertical wall ungrafted, or (2) to take an addi-

tional skin graft either to place around a vertical wall or to seam the two grafts together to make one large graft.
3. Poor dressing. The dressing may be poorly designed and cause the graft to pull away from its bed. Common situations in which this occurs include grafts that have been dressed with a tie-over stent and grafts in a natural concavity or flexion crease. Even though the graft fits the contour perfectly with the joint in flexion, the distance across the flexion crease is greater when the joint is in extension. Therefore, the joint must be splinted in the same position as when the graft was placed on the bed. In fact, it is almost always preferable to place a skin graft across a flexion crease with that joint in maximum extension.

The opposite problem occurs when a skin graft is placed across an extensor joint surface. The graft should be placed with the joint in maximum flexion so that an adequate amount of skin covers the joint.

Tie-over stents may be poorly designed and place too much or too little pressure (Fig. 5-23C).

INFECTION

Infection prevents graft revascularization, and hematomas additionally increase the potential for infection. The most devastating organisms are β streptococcus, *Staphylococcus aureus*, and *Pseudomonas aeruginosa*. They are particularly pathogenic in their effects on skin graft revascularization. Other organisms in relatively lower concentration may be sterilized by a skin graft, but if the concentration of the organism in the tissue exceeds 10^5 organisms per cubic centimeter of tissue, clinical infection may occur and graft loss is quite likely. Thorough irrigation, debridement, and, in some circumstances, antibiotics are required to prevent infection. Systemic antibiotics are required for potentially contaminated wounds.

In summary, the basic requirements for a successful skin graft include an adequate vascular bed, lack of hematoma, adequate measures against infection, good contact between graft and bed, a dressing that immobilizes the grafted area, and postoperative elevation.

SPECIFIC ANATOMIC SITES

We describe here the management of some common, difficult, and dangerous types of tissue loss and amputation. We have subdivided these by the anatomic areas of the head and neck and upper limbs because of the unique function, anatomy, importance, and frequency of injury of these parts. Soft tissue losses over the trunk and lower limbs are far less common and their treatment somewhat simpler than the following tissue losses.

The critical factors for determining appropriate therapy are size and configuration of the defect and tidiness and contamination of the wound. Most of these decisions and procedures are best accomplished by an experienced surgeon; the techniques shown here are not meant to be followed in a "cookbook" fashion, but to be used as a guideline for deciding when to seek consultation.

As a general principle, we suggest replanting healthy amputated tissue as a composite graft or by microvascular surgical means whenever possible. Even if all or part of the replant does not survive, there is no additional loss, and some benefit may be achieved. The second principle is to achieve

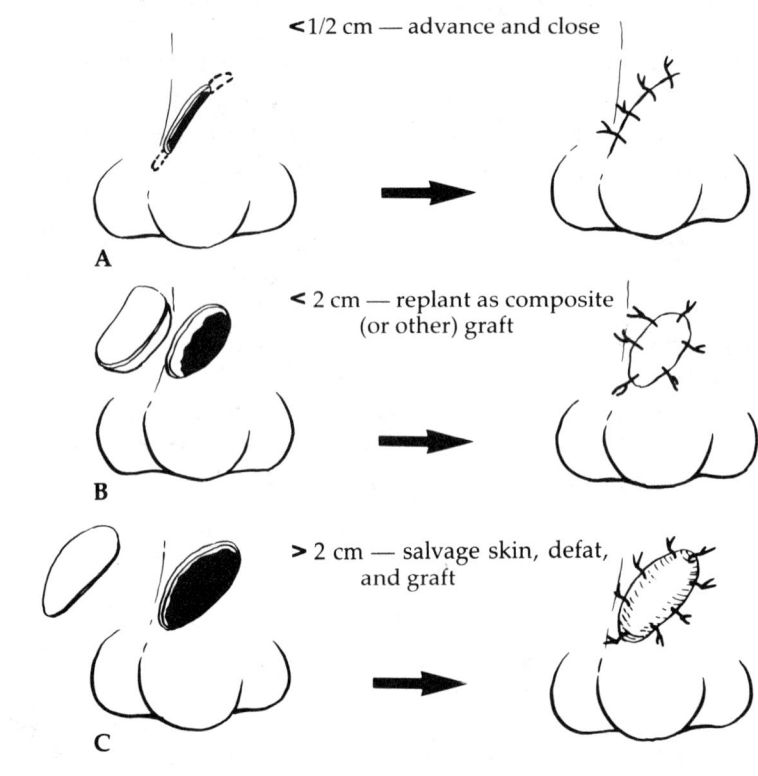

Figure 5-24. Amputation of the skin of the nasal dorsum is repaired by excision and closure (A), composite replantation (B), or defatting as a full-thickness graft or a split graft (C). The method chosen is determined by size of defect and health of tissue.

primary healing with a split-thickness graft. If these methods are not possible, the final alternative is to use full-thickness grafts or flaps for unusual circumstances.

Facial Amputations

AMPUTATIONS OF THE NOSE
1. Amputations of skin only. The size of the amputated part is critical to the choice of therapy (Fig. 5-24).
   a. *Small defects* (less than ½ cm) can be closed primarily by adapting and advancing adjacent tissue. Elliptic excision should extend into natural skin lines if advancing the edges creates "dog-ears."
   b. *Intermediate defects* (2–3 cm). If the tissues are healthy (i.e., a tidy wound), the tissue should be replanted as a composite graft. If the tissues are untidy, the edges can be debrided and replanted. If the tissue is severely contused or contaminated, a temporary biologic split graft is appropriate.
   c. *Larger defects* (greater than 3 cm) can be covered by defatting the amputated skin and replacing it as a full-thickness skin graft. If the skin is severely damaged, a full-thickness skin graft from the preauricular region will give a good definitive result with ideal tidy wounds. A split graft should be used for untidy wounds.
2. Amputations of skin and cartilage (with or without intranasal lining) (Fig. 5-25). This is an unusual type of injury because the mucosa is strongly adherent to the cartilage.

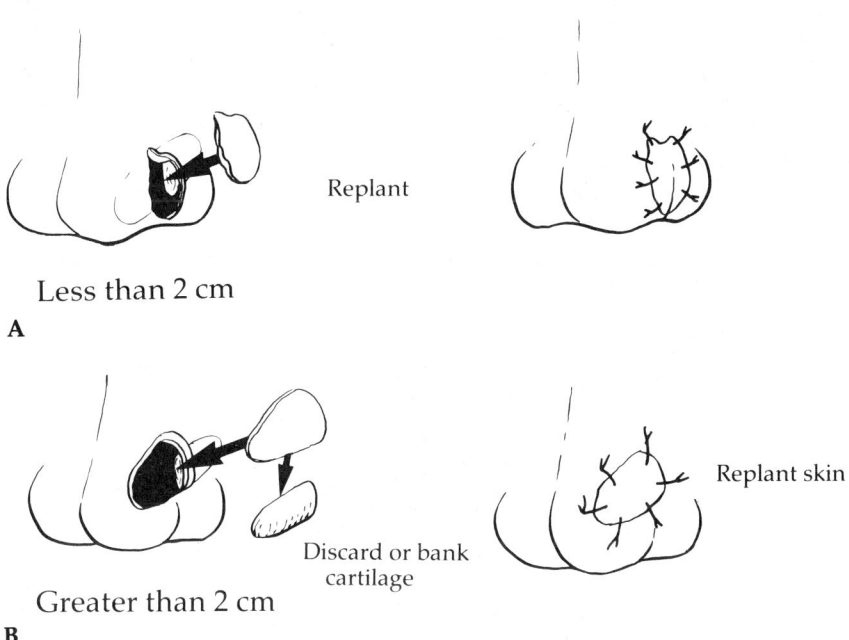

Figure 5-25. Small amputated segments of skin and cartilage of the dorsum or tip are replaced (A); larger segments are converted to a full-thickness graft (B).

 a. *Small defects* (less than 2 cm). The entire amputated skin and cartilage can be replaced as a free composite graft.
 b. *Larger defects* (greater than 2 cm). It is advisable to remove the cartilage from the underside of the amputated skin and bank it in the abdomen or another inconspicuous site. The skin can be replaced as a full-thickness graft.
3. Amputations of skin, cartilage, and lining. These are through-and-through amputations including skin, cartilage, and/or bone and underlying intranasal mucous membrane (Fig. 5-26).
 a. *Small defects* (less than 3 mm). Adapt the skin edges and close primarily. If contaminated or badly contused, the wound can be dressed and the defect closed secondarily after resolution of infection and demarcation of nonviable tissue. If the amputated tissue is tidy, it can be replanted as a composite graft.
 b. *Intermediate defects* (less than 2 cm). These can be replaced as a composite graft with a potential for survival of approximately 50 to 75 percent.
 c. *Large defects* (greater than 2–3 cm). Amputations of greater than 2 to 3 cm rarely survive when replanted as a composite graft. The alternatives are as follows:
  (1) Defects of 2 to 3 cm. Make the composite graft smaller (2 cm or less in diameter) by excision of tissue from the edges, and then replant.
  (2) Defects larger than 3 cm. If the defect is tidy and the part is only "slightly" more than 3 cm, replant the amputated nasal tip (even though survival is unlikely). For larger defects, consultation and referral for operating-room reconstruction should be obtained. The plastic surgeon may attempt to add additional blood supply

Figure 5-26. Amputation of skin, cartilage, and lining.
A. Small, through-and-through amputations of less than 3 to 4 mm are closed by direct approximation.
B. Composite replantation grafts are used for defects larger than 3 mm and smaller than 2 cm.
C. Larger defects may require a slight reduction of the replanted part.

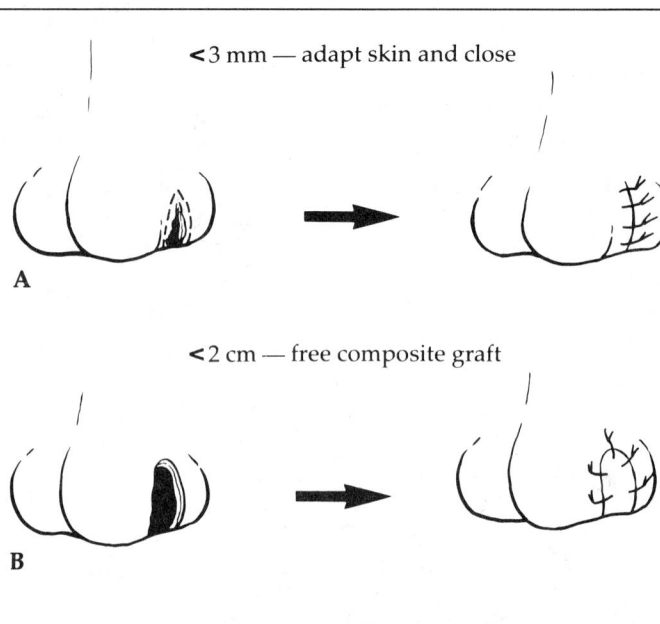

to the replanted nose. The mucous membrane (or vestibular skin) and cartilage are excised, creating a raw subdermal surface on the entire amputated part of the nose. A thin flap from the inner surface of the arm or cheek is elevated. The flap is then used for the inside lining of the nose. This pedicle flap provides blood supply to the entire inner surface of the amputated nose rather than just its margins.

AMPUTATIONS OF THE EAR
1. Amputations of skin only. These are rare injuries, and a simple full-thickness graft suffices.
2. Amputations of skin, cartilage, and posterior skin (Fig. 5-27). Most amputations involve both the anterior and posterior surface of the ear, including the interposed cartilage.
    a. *Small defects* (less than 3–4 mm) can be closed directly, producing a somewhat smaller ear. The closure is facilitated by excising small triangles in the antihelical fold, as illustrated in Fig. 5-27. If the triangles are not excised, the ear will severely "lop" or the wound edges will be subjected to excessive tension.
    b. *Intermediate defects* (5 mm–3 cm) can be treated by replacing the amputated ear as a free composite graft.
    c. *Large defects* (greater than 3 cm) usually do not survive replantation. Therefore, additional blood supply should be added to the am-

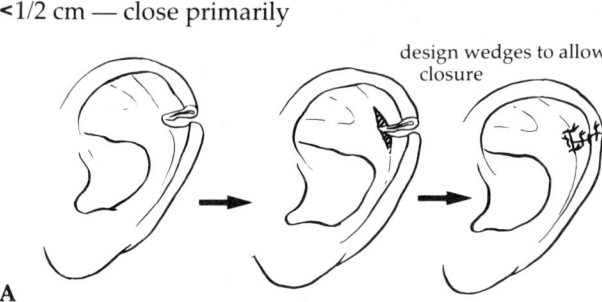
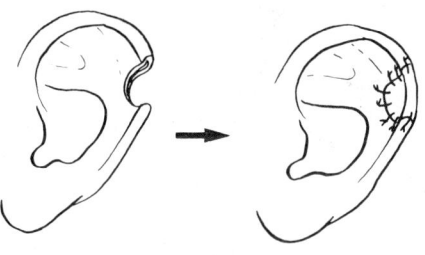

Figure 5-27. Amputation of ear skin, cartilage, and posterior skin.
A. Small amputations are repaired by direct closure, facilitated by excising wedges in the antihelical fold.
B. Medium-sized defects are repaired by replacing the amputated segment as a graft.

putated part by dermabrasion or flaps. If this is not possible, the ear cartilage should be salvaged and the wound closed to allow primary healing. These techniques should be performed in an operating room by a plastic surgeon.

(1) Figs. 5-28 and 5-29 illustrate two methods useful in adding blood supply to the posterior surface of the reattached segments. These techniques are best for amputations of one-half or more of the ear.

(2) Salvage and banking of ear cartilage (Fig. 5-4) is a method used for the severely injured ear or when the surgeon has not had experience with flaps and dermabrasion. The method was described earlier in this chapter. If replantation can be done within several days, the amputated ear can be refrigerated rather than banked in the abdomen.

LIP AMPUTATIONS

Lip amputations (Fig. 5-30) are commonly caused by animal or human bites and therefore are usually untidy and contaminated. Some debridement of wound edges is required. Antibiotics are usually indicated. Small- and medium-sized defects are closed either by direct advancement or with a composite replantation graft.

A lip with a large defect (3 cm to one-half of the lip or more) is difficult to reconstruct. Therefore, salvage of the lip tissue should be attempted, which is an operating-room procedure. If replantation fails, however, the lip can be reconstructed more effectively than the ear or nose.

There are two alternatives for replantation of large segments of an amputated lip:

1. Composite graft of a 2-cm portion of the lip, discarding the remainder
2. Microvascular anastomosis (labial artery)

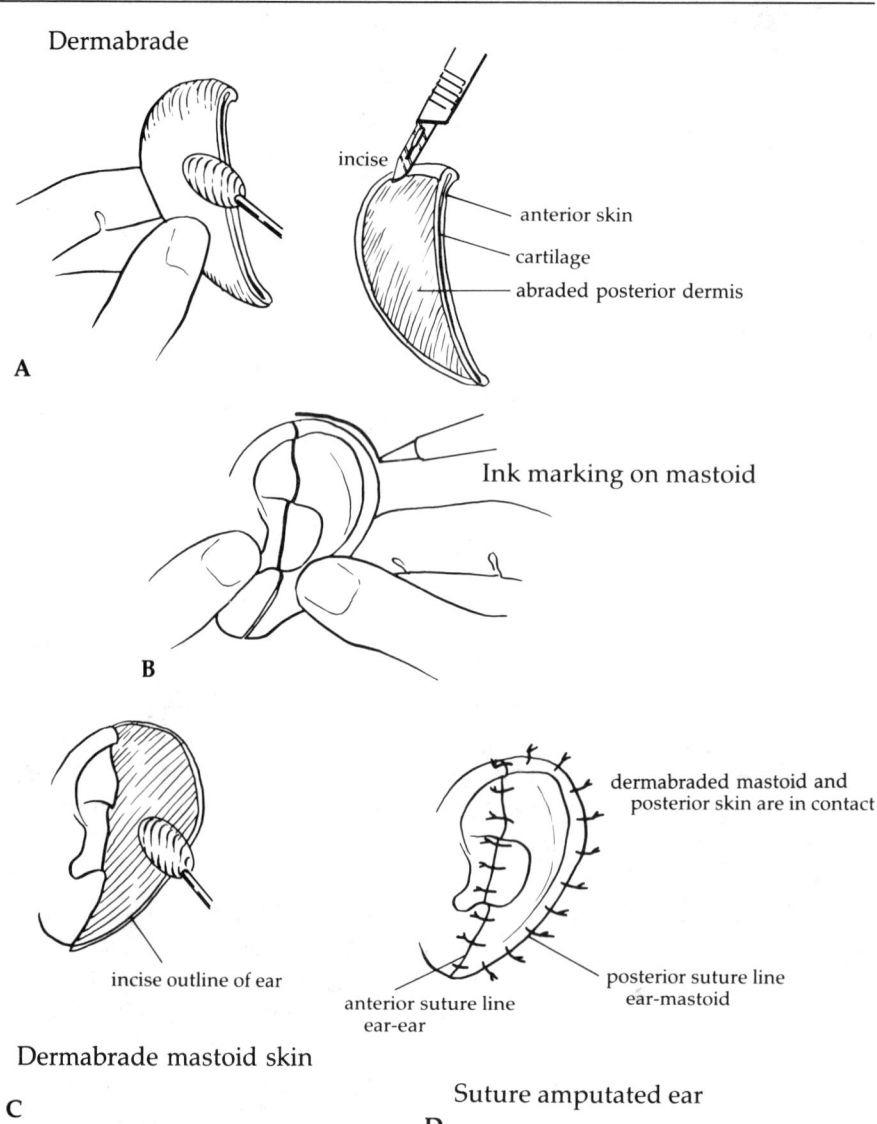

Figure 5-28. Dermabrasion.
A. Dermabrade the posterior surface of the ear epithelium, leaving the dermis exposed. Incise the junction of the dermabraded posterior skin and the intact anterior skin. Undermine the anterior skin slightly.
B. Position the ear in its normal anatomic site and press against the mastoid skin. Outline the ear with an ink marker, and incise this outline.
C. Dermabrade the area within the ear outline.
D. Suture the amputated ear along its posterior border to the mastoid skin with the dermabraded posterior aspect of the ear against the dermabraded mastoid skin. Carefully suture the ear as a three-layer closure to the ear stump. Apply a dressing as indicated in Fig. 8-16.

Of these alternatives, only composite replantation is commonly performed, although microvascular surgery offers the greatest potential for maintaining viability.

SCALP AND FOREHEAD AMPUTATIONS
1. *Small defects* (less than 2 to 3 cm) usually can be closed directly following undermining and advancement of these tissues.
2. *Intermediate defects* (3–4 cm) may require skin replacement. A thin split-thickness skin graft is preferred, because color match is not important and the thin split graft allows for wound contraction, thus reducing the size of the defect. A composite graft could be tried, but success is not likely.
3. *Large defects* (greater than 4 to 5 cm) cannot be closed and cannot be repaired with composite grafts. Therefore, the wound must be skin grafted or an attempt should be made at microvascular anastomosis. Total scalp avulsion from entanglement in machinery is a situation par-

AMPUTATIONS AND SKIN LOSS

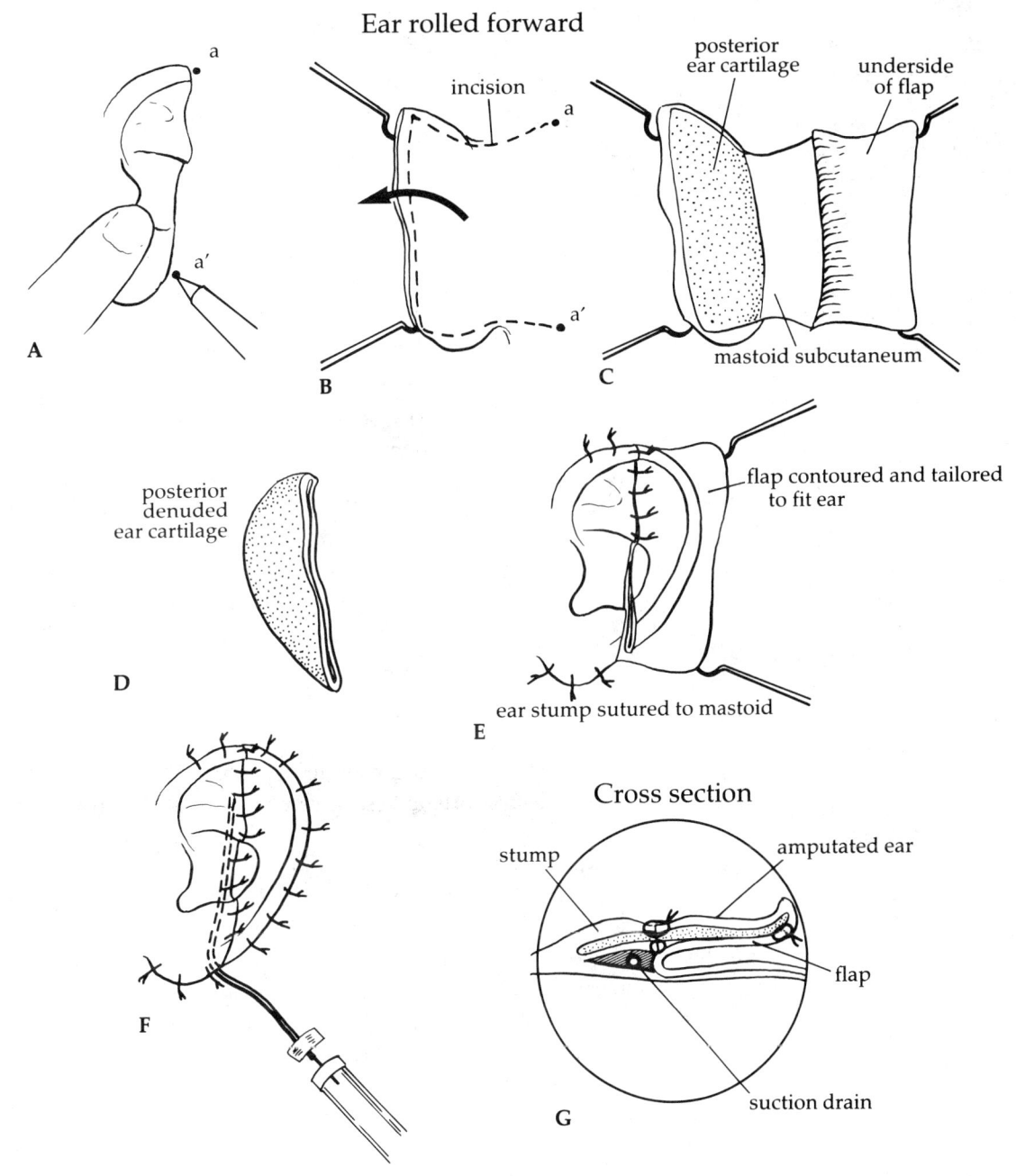

Figure 5-29. The skin flap method is useful when one-half of the ear or less has been amputated.
- A. Pin the ear against the mastoid skin, and mark the upper and lower margins (a and a').
- B. Roll the ear forward, and outline a skin flap. The base of the flap is between a and a'. The upper and lower borders extend from these points along the mastoid skin, onto the ear, and to the amputated stump.
- C. Elevate the flap.
- D. Denude the posterior aspect of the amputated ear of epithelium by surgical excision.
- E. Suture the ear stump to the mastoid skin at the superior and inferior borders. Also suture the stump and amputated part together.
- F. Carefully contour the flap onto the posterior side of the ear (denuded) and suture along the rim. Tailor the flap to fit the ear.
- G. Insert a small suction drain so that the flap will adhere to the replant. This is made from a #23 scalp vein set with additional holes cut in the tubing. Suction is achieved through a red-top vacuum tube for blood drawing.

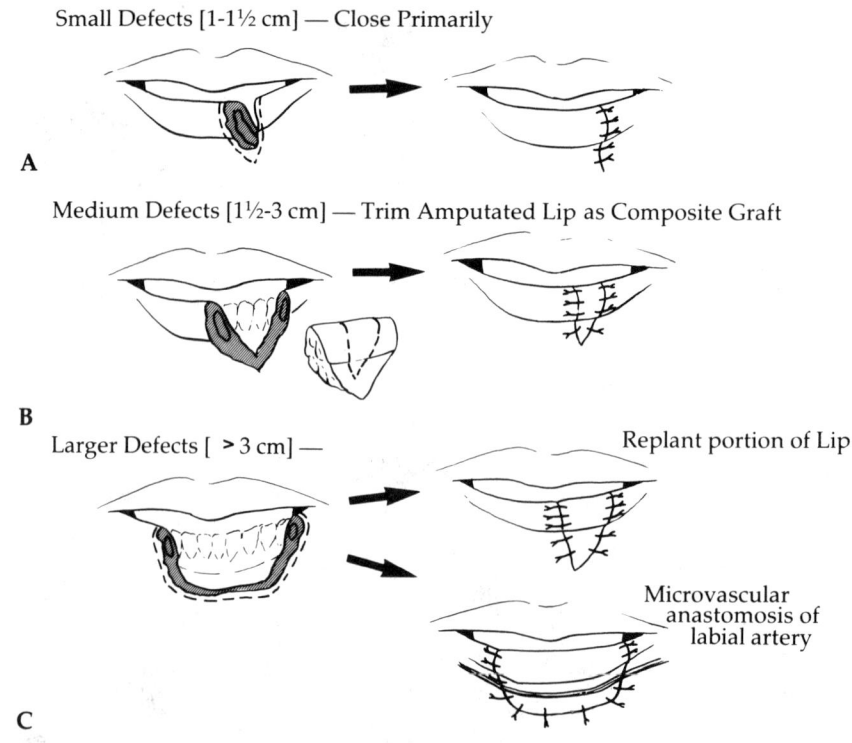

Figure 5-30. Lip amputations.
A. Small defects (1–1½ cm). One-fourth to one-fifth of the lip can be *primarily closed* by debridement of the skin edges and careful closure of the anatomic layers.
B. Medium-sized defects (1½–3 cm). One-fifth to one-third of the lip can be closed by either debridement of edges and replantation or direct closure. If the lip is too tight (2- -3-cm amputation), the amputated lip can be trimmed to 1 to 2 cm and replanted as a smaller composite graft.
C. Large defects (> 3 cm) can be treated by replantation of 2 cm of the lip or by microvascular anastomosis.

ticularly suited for microvascular repair. The superficial temporal and retroauricular and supraorbital vessels can be used for the anastomosis.

FACIAL SKIN AMPUTATIONS

The amputated skin of the part, if not severely traumatized, can be defatted and used for a full-thickness graft. Depressions related to defatting the healthy facial skin and replacing it as a full-thickness graft are of minimal importance and usually are self-correcting.

If the tissue is unhealthy or unavailable, defects should be covered with free skin graft. There is no advantage to using the severely damaged, amputated part as a composite graft.

EYELID AMPUTATIONS

The eyelid is a critical structure for protection of the globe and is extremely difficult to reconstruct adequately. Therefore, preservation of as much eyelid tissue as possible is paramount.

The anatomic relation of the lids to the levator muscle and nasolacrimal apparatus is discussed in Chapter 6, Penetrating Injuries and Deep Transections. These structures must also be considered when evaluating the eyelids. The importance of careful examination and ophthalmologic consultation for globe injuries must be given highest priority.

1. *Small defects* (less than 5 mm, or one-sixth of the lid) (Fig. 5-31). These defects can be debrided and the lid closed by direct approximation, as described in Chapter 4, Fig. 4-9. Careful attention must be taken to reattach the levator muscle of the upper lid.

AMPUTATIONS AND SKIN LOSS

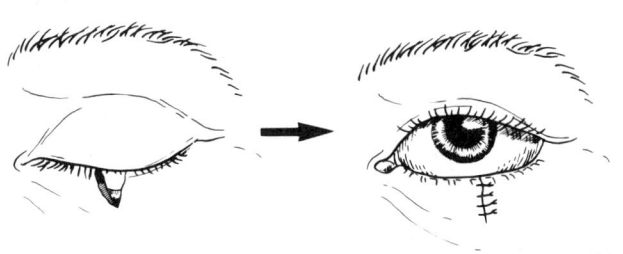

Small Defect [< 5mm] Adapt and Close

Figure 5-31. Eyelid defects of 5 mm or less can be debrided and closed by a layered technique, similar to that illustrated in Fig. 4-9.

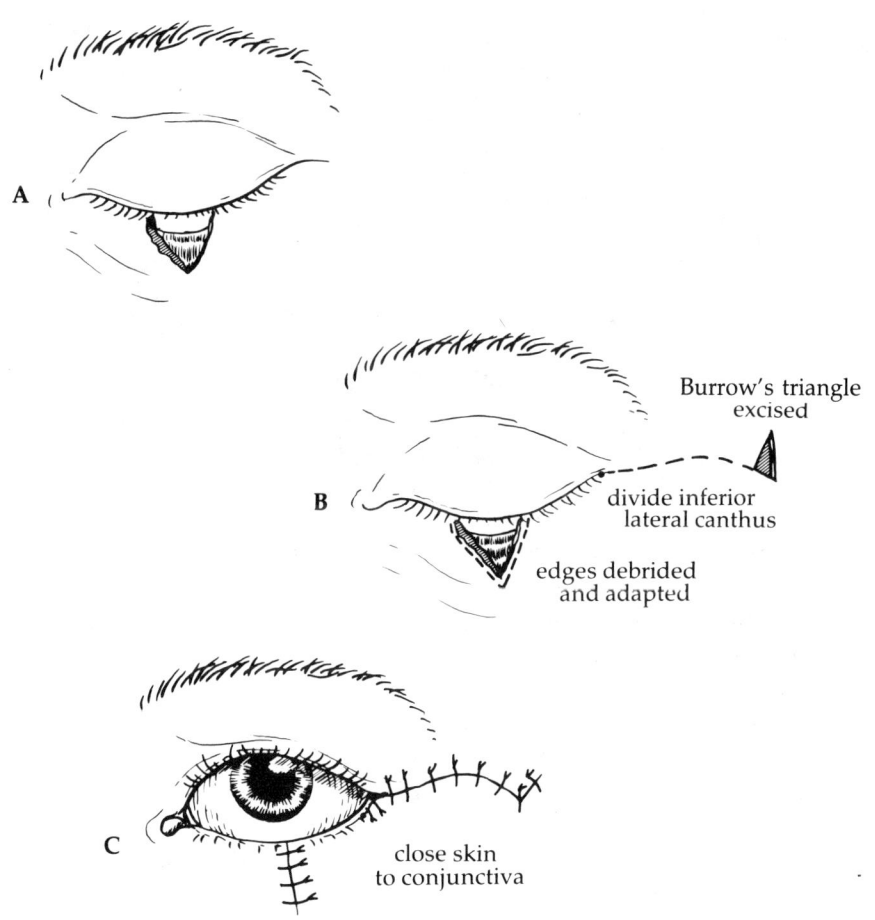

Figure 5-32.
A. Medium-sized eyelid defect (1½ cm or one-half of lid).
B. Debride the edges and make a skin incision in the lateral canthal wrinkle line. Separate the lateral canthus from the skin flap (but the canthus remains attached to the upper lid and bone), and remove a surrounding triangle to facilitate medial advancement.
C. Close the wound.

2. *Intermediate defects* (1½ cm, or one-third of the lid) (Fig. 5-32). Adapt edges, release lateral canthus from lateral orbital rim, and close (canthoplasty). These defects can be closed by direct approximation, but with considerable tension. The tension can be relieved and an adequate result achieved by sliding the lateral lid medially after releasing the lateral canthus. This technique should be done by an ophthalmologist or plastic surgeon.
3. *Large defects* (1½–2 cm or more, or one-half or more of the lid) (Fig. 5-33). The amputated segment is replaced as a composite graft; conversely, if

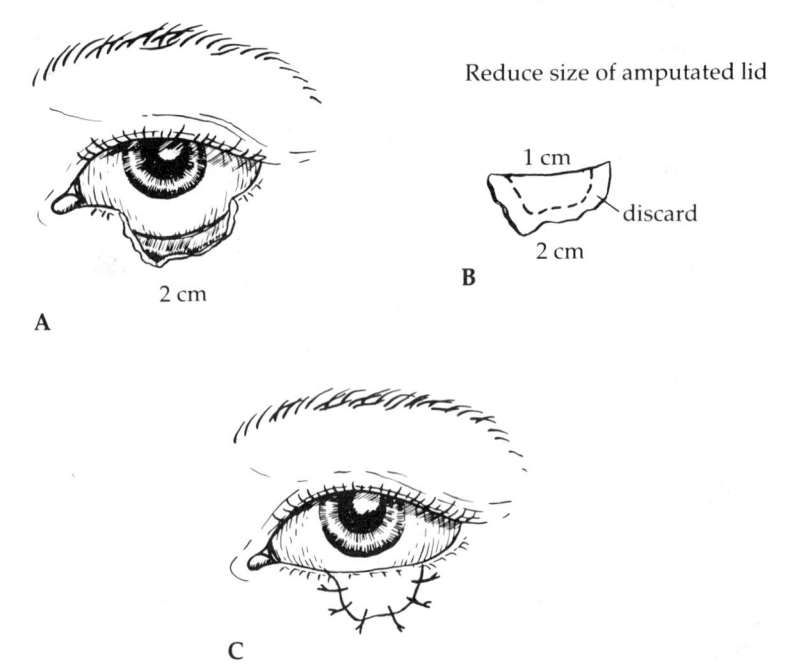

Figure 5-33. Large eyelid defect (A). An eyelid composite graft should be about 1 cm in length and height. If it is much larger it can be trimmed (B). The composite graft is sutured accurately to the defect with as few sutures as possible (C).

suitable vessels exist in the part, it may be replaced by microvascular techniques. These injuries require a secondary reconstruction.

An attempt at reattachment as a composite graft can be justified as long as the adjacent tissues are not injured or can be minimally debrided. An eyelid composite graft should be approximately 1 cm in width to survive. Therefore, if the amputated part is larger than 1 cm in width, it should be reduced in size. It is preferable to save some of the lid rather than replant the entire piece and have it fail to survive.

4. *Complete eyelid avulsion* (Fig. 5-34). Loss of the entire lower lid is a serious problem. Reconstruction is extremely difficult and ultimately less than ideal because of functional and cosmetic limitations of reconstruction.

The difficulty of reconstruction is related to replacing muscle, lid margin mucosa, and tarsal plate. The skin is removed, therefore, and the other tissue salvaged for replantation as a composite graft. Additional blood supply is added with a skin flap from the upper lid and/or cheek skin depending on the size of the defect.

If conjunctiva can be advanced by dissection of the fornix conjunctiva, the conjunctiva of the amputated part can also be removed. This is preferable whenever possible because new blood supply is brought in from both sides, and the composite is sandwiched. All eyelid procedures require postoperative immobilization, with a suture tarsorrhaphy and light eye-pad dressing.

Upper Limb Amputations

GENERAL PRINCIPLES

1. Skin distribution and anatomy. Because there is minimal surplus skin on the hand or digits, whether the result of injury or wound debride-

AMPUTATIONS AND SKIN LOSS

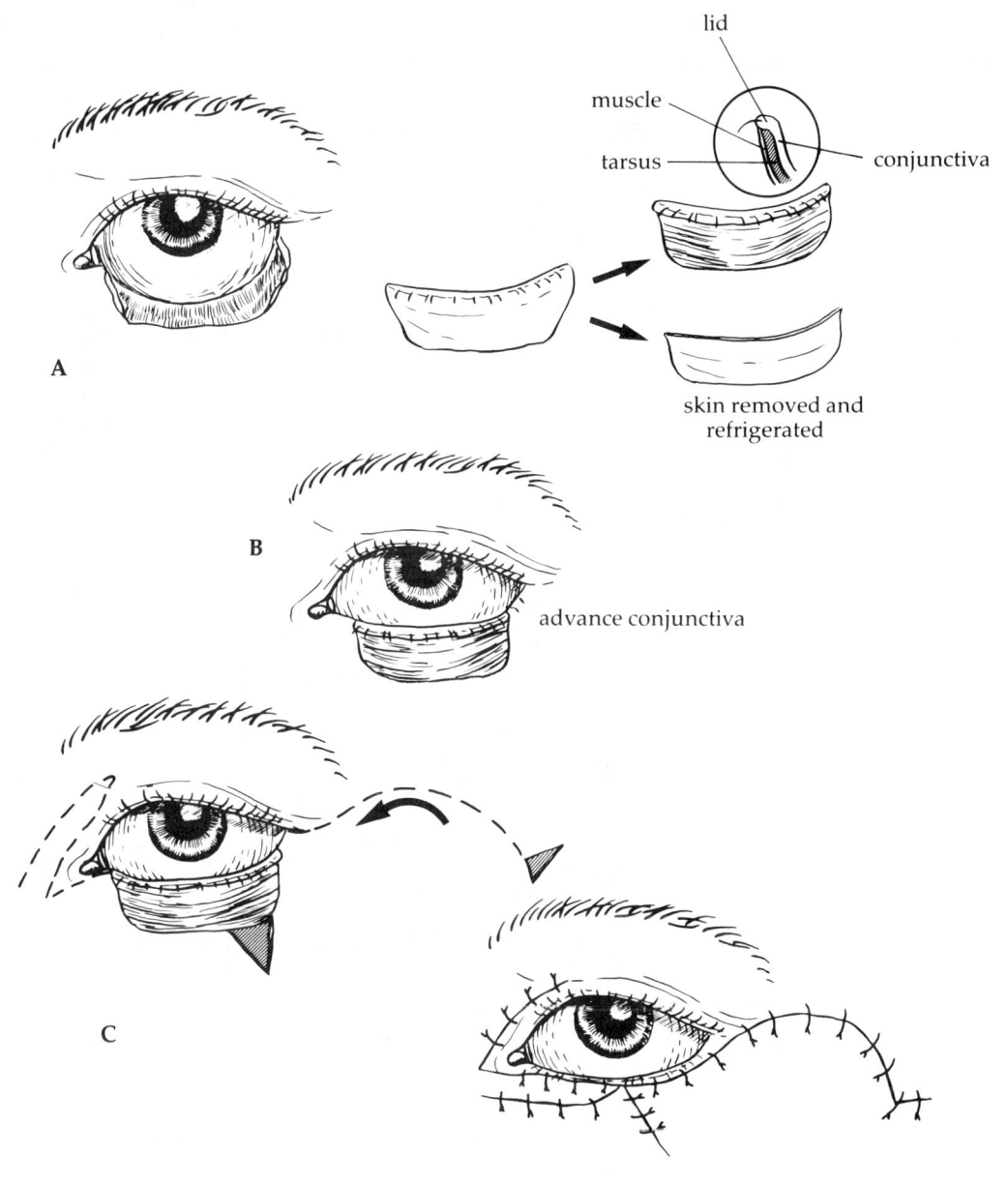

ment, the amputated skin must be replaced or reconstructed and must have sufficient sensibility and pliability for optimal function. A raw wound left to heal by secondary intent (contraction and epithelialization) produces a tight, tender scar with thin epithelium that is inadequate for good function. The small defects in the loose skin of the forearm tolerate some tension. The dorsal hand skin appears to tolerate a great deal of skin loss. However, with a closed fist it is apparent that there is little excess skin. The palm skin has strong attachments to underlying palmar fascia. This attachment prevents shifting of the skin. The fingertip has almost no reserve tissue. Skin loss here rarely can be managed by advancing the wound edges, unless underlying bone is shortened.

Figure 5-34. Complete eyelid avulsion.
A. Remove skin from the defect; save the skin in the refrigerator.
B. Debride the margins of the remaining segment and suture this into the defect. Conjunctiva can be advanced from the sulcus to overcome tissue shortage.
C. Transpose an eyelid flap and/or a cheek flap to add blood supply to the anterior surface. Small excisions of dog-ears facilitate flap movement.

2. Microvascular replantation. With the development of microsurgical skills and technology, digital and hand and arm vessels can be reanastomosed successfully. Replantation of totally or partially amputated parts, especially digits, requires special equipment and expertise that is usually found at medical centers. However, almost all amputation injuries are initially seen at local clinics, hospitals, or physicians' offices, where primary care begins. The primary management of such injuries frequently determines whether replantation can or should be attempted.

Guidelines can only influence, not dictate, management. The following guidelines have been established as indications and contraindications for consideration of replantation of amputated parts in the upper limb.
   a. Indications
      (1) Most amputations between the elbow and metacarpophalangeal joints
      (2) Amputated prime digits (e.g., the thumb)
      (3) Multiple digital amputations
      (4) Most amputations in a child's hand, including single digits
   b. Contraindications
      (1) Presence of serious medical problems
         (a) Cardiovascular disease
         (b) Active gastric ulcers
      (2) Local considerations
         (a) Severe crush or contamination of the amputated part
         (b) Warm ischemic time too prolonged (greater than 6 hours for digits)
         (c) Single digit amputations, especially those amputated proximal to the proximal interphalangeal joint

If any question exists as to whether a patient is a candidate for replantation, the final decision should be left to the microsurgical team. Contact should be made with and protocol obtained from a regional center. The management of amputated parts is discussed earlier in this chapter.

Proximal amputations at the metacarpal, wrist, or arm level are similarly managed. If hemorrhage is persistent in spite of adequate pressure dressing, a proximal tourniquet will control bleeding while major vessel ends are ligated as atraumatically and distally as possible. A pressure dressing and elevation usually control venous and small arteriole bleeding.

Partially amputated digits, hands, or other parts that have questionable viability also can be salvaged by microvascular anastomosis.

MANAGEMENT OF SPECIFIC SITES
1. Finger and fingertip amputations
   a. Partial amputation. When a sufficient pedicle remains attaching the partially amputated tip, accurate approximation of the wound edges may allow survival of the tip. Judgment is required to determine when a pedicle will not provide adequate vascularity—in those instances the partial amputation should be treated as a complete am-

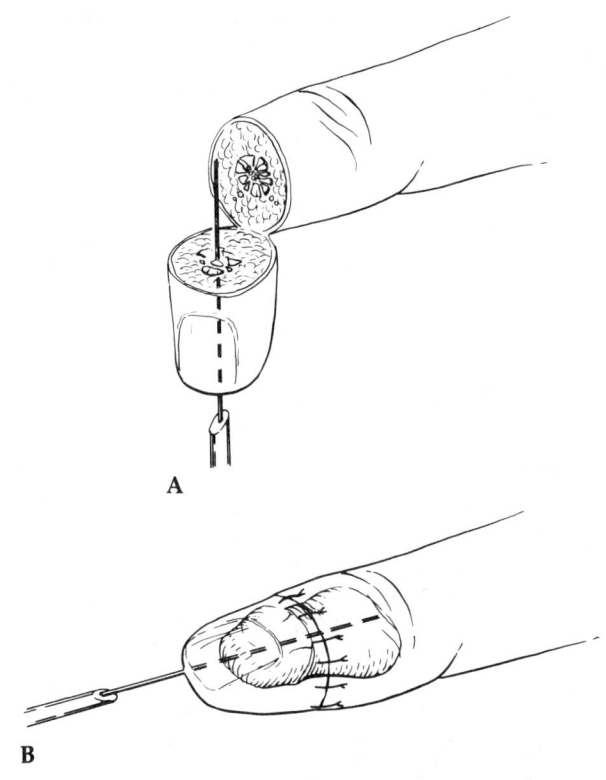

Figure 5-35. Bone stabilization is beneficial when there is loss of bone or when alignment cannot be achieved by skin sutures alone. This frequently occurs at the fingertip if the partial dorsal amputation is between the more proximal extensor and more distal flexor insertion.
A. First pass the wire or pin into the bone of the nearly amputated segment.
B. Following reduction of the fracture, advance the pin into the proximal segment.

putation. Unless it is absolutely certain that the pedicle is inadequate, however, it is best to be conservative and accurately approximate the wound edges. Microvascular anastomosis should be considered for partial proximal amputations of critical digits or the hand when the question of viability cannot be answered. If the amputation is beyond the insertion of the flexor or extensor tendon (base of the distal phalanx), there are no deforming forces on the amputated tip, and bone fixation is not usually necessary. Accurate soft tissue closure usually results in acceptable bony alignment. If the tip is displaced, a small Kirschner wire (0.035 in) or a fine needle (21 gauge) can be threaded across the bone fragments. This should be done percutaneously through the tip as atraumatically as possible (Fig. 5-35). Skin edges can then be approximated.

b. Composite replants
   (1) Free replanting. The urge simply to replace the completely amputated fingertip as a composite graft should be resisted in almost every instance. Success in an adult is very uncommon. If any crush component of the amputated part exists, the chance of survival plummets. Free replanting of the amputated part should be considered only in clean amputations in children. Complete survival when the part is not crushed is still unlikely, but it happens with sufficient frequency to warrant its attempt.
   (2) Method. The amputated part should be minimally debrided of any ragged pulp tissue, although ragged edges less seriously contused should not be debrided. Very accurate approximation

with as few sutures as possible, followed by absolute immobilization, may succeed. In a small child, a long arm cast is necessary.

(3) Postoperative management. The wound should not be disturbed for at least 7 to 10 days unless local or systemic signs or symptoms of infection occur. The longer one can temper the curiosity, the better. Gentle dressing removal usually reveals some blackening or darkening of the skin. Unless the part appears desiccated and shriveled or very purulent, it should not be disturbed. The epithelium and superficial dermis may slough while the deep dermis or epidermal elements survive to regenerate a new epithelial cover. In 2 weeks this degenerated layer should have separated. If the amputation is through the nail, the nail should be maintained to act as a splint. A suture through the two divided nail parts helps orient and stabilize the closure.

c. Closure of fingertip amputations. Fingertip injuries resulting in skin loss are the most common amputations anywhere on the body. These amputations are often caused by kitchen knives or power saws, or the fingertip is crushed in closing doors or windows. Such injuries may be divided into those causing full-thickness skin loss, those causing finger pulp loss, distal amputations with bone exposed, and complete finger amputations.

The surgical strategy for treatment of finger amputations depends on many factors. Moreover, there are several satisfactory alternatives for each type of injury. The therapy for digit amputations is determined primarily by anatomic factors, such as defect size, location, and contour; the ultimate decision, however, varies with patient age, work, general health, associated injuries, condition of the wound, and mechanism of injury.

The methods suggested below assume a clean tidy wound and no other complicating factors. If the wound is untidy and contaminated, the best treatment is to debride the unhealthy tissue and cover the open wound with a thin skin graft, or shorten a "noncritical" digit to a healthy level.

The treatment of digit amputations and tissue deficits is based on two functional concepts. (1) *All possible length must be saved for the pinch digits* (Fig. 5-36)—the thumb and index finger (or the most radial finger if the index is beyond salvage). Length can be sacrificed in nonpinch digits to achieve primary closure. (2) The "working surface" of the fingers must have adequate sensibility and durability. A tender or nonsensible fingertip is a hindrance rather than a help. Fingertip tissue deficits require different treatments to provide a good working surface, depending primarily on the site and amount of tissue loss. We have classified these injuries based on the type of injury: skin deficit only; skin and pulp deficit; skin, pulp, and bone deficit (of equal amounts); and skin and pulp deficit greater than bone deficit.

They also are divided according to the area of the deficit (Fig. 5-37): dorsal deficit, volar deficit, and transverse deficit.

Finally, the level of injury for each fingertip should be considered in the therapeutic decision.

AMPUTATIONS AND SKIN LOSS

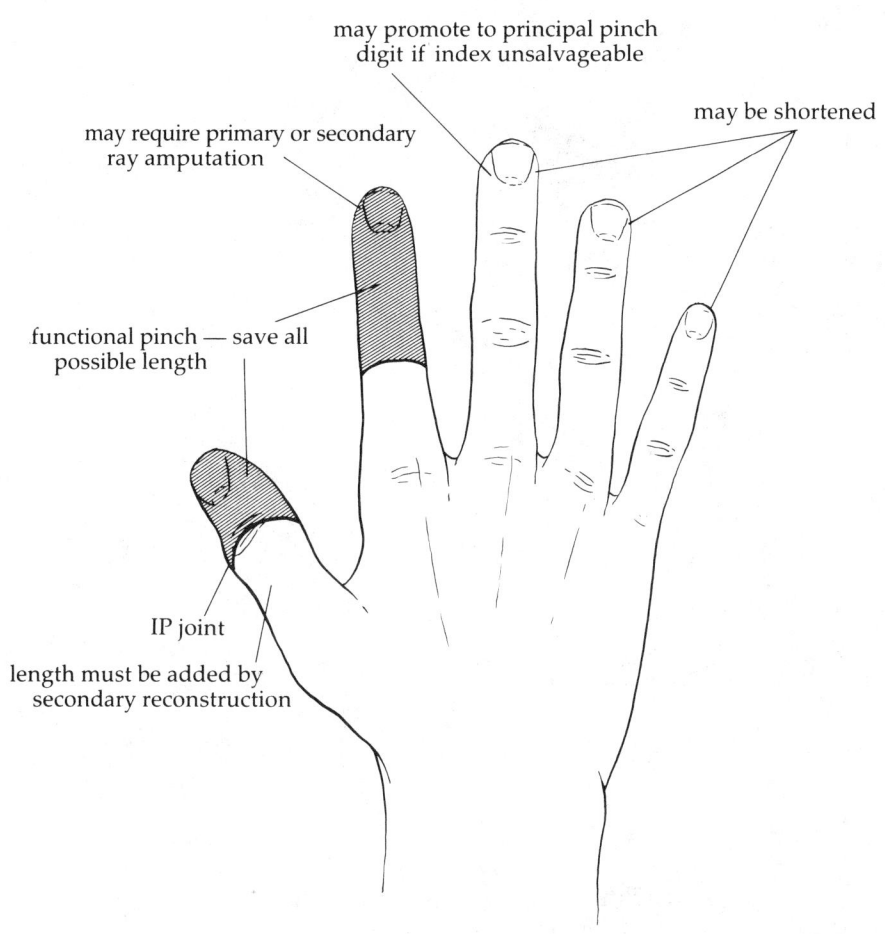

Figure 5-36. The level of amputation is a major determinant of therapy. The cross-hatched areas show the functional level that allows pinch function.

(1) Skin deficit only
  (a) Lateral or dorsal defect (use medium- or full-thickness graft). The medium-thickness graft gives adequate protection, yet does not distort the nail bed.
  (b) Volar defect. The volar pad is the functional area of the fingertip. Therefore, maximum protection and durability are required. A full-thickness graft should be used.
  (c) Transverse defect. The transverse defect removes the padding over the end of the phalanx. This can be a quite tender site if there is not adequate protection. A thin split graft allows wound contraction, pulling the padded volar skin over the tip, simplifying postoperative care, and reducing risk of infection. This contraction is effective only for defects less than 1 cm in diameter. The tip of the phalanx can be rongeured if slightly exposed.

  An exception to the above would be a child with a transverse tip injury of less than 5 mm. Taking a graft and maintaining immobilization and elevation may present difficult management problems.

  The wound will heal by reepithelialization and contrac-

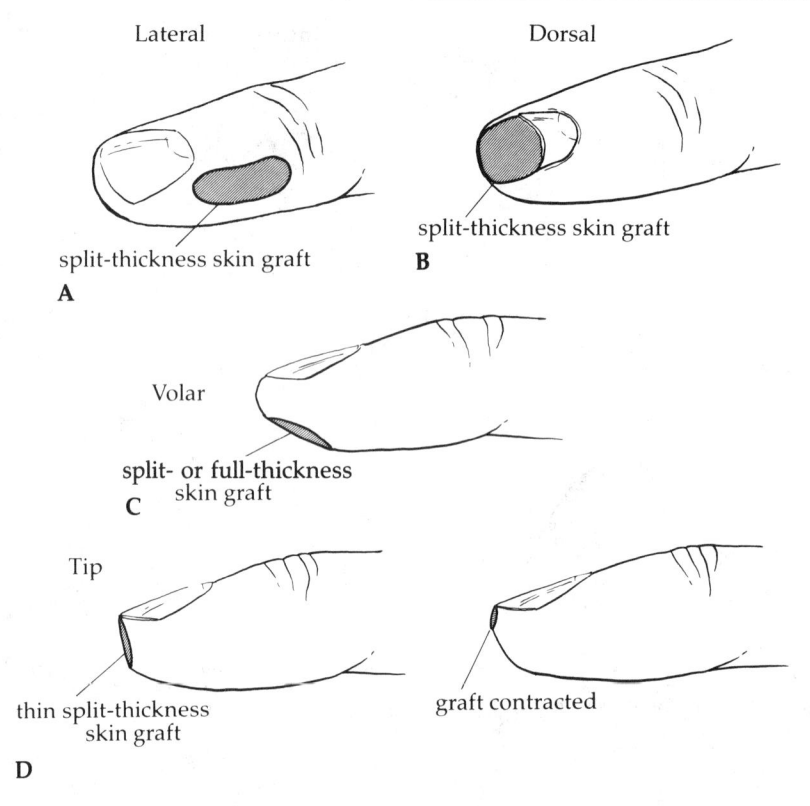

Figure 5-37. Fingertip grafts depend on an area of deficit. A and B. Medium split-thickness grafts are used for the dorsal and lateral areas. C. Full-thickness grafts are used for the volar areas, which require more padding, durability, and sensitivity. Full-thickness grafts should be reserved for ideal wounds, e.g., those with no crush or significant contamination. D. Thin split grafts can be used for small (< 1 sq cm) transverse defects. These will contract and pull the intact skin over the bone end.

tion, with essentially the same final appearance and functional result as if it were covered with a thin split-thickness skin graft. The difference is that with a graft, the hand must be elevated until revascularization occurs, generally 7 to 10 days. Social and economic considerations must be included in the decision-making process, as well as size and site of defect.

(2) Skin and pulp deficit. A more severe fingertip tissue injury occurs with loss of the important volar pulp. This pulp, composed of fibrous tissue and fat, acts as a pad to bolster the gripping surface of the skin, protecting the underlying bone and neurovascular architecture. Pulp loss exposes the terminal phalanx and may expose flexor tendon insertion. Skin grafting does not provide durable skin and frequently results in an unsightly, tender wound. Pulp loss must be replaced, particularly in critically functional areas for grasp and prehension, such as the thumb, index finger, and long finger pulps. Lateral oblique wounds may result in some pulp loss but may be managed with a full-thickness skin graft with good result.

Larger wounds, especially of the volar pulp, require local flaps or flaps from adjacent fingers. It should be stressed that unless bare bone or tendon bare of its paratenon makes up the base of the wound, a split-thickness skin graft can always be used to promote rapid healing. Referral to a specialist can then be done less urgently. A secondary flap reconstruction provides a good

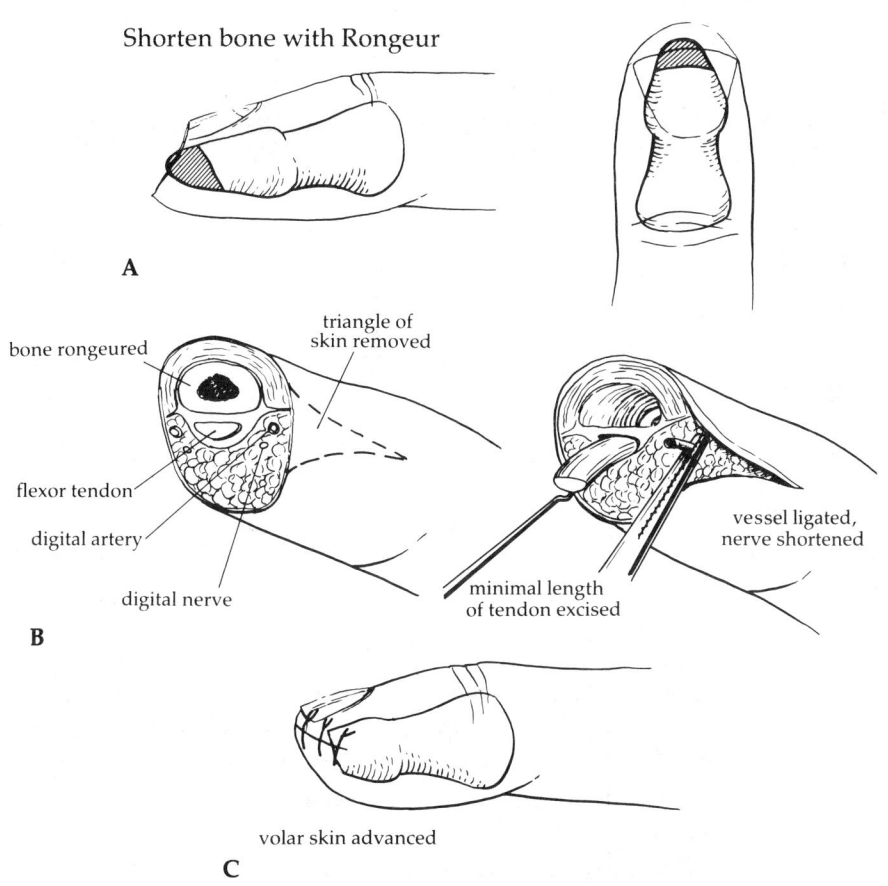

Figure 5-38. The "amputation closure" is the most commonly performed procedure of complete amputation at almost any level in the digit.
A. Rongeur the bone back a sufficient amount proximal to the soft tissue wound to permit relatively loose skin approximation.
B. Identify both neurovascular bundles; tie arteries with plain catgut or coagulate; and gently pull digital nerves distally and cut sharply, allowing the ends to retract well into uninjured soft tissues. The flexor and/or extensor tendon ends may need to be trimmed but should never be sutured to each other over the stump.
C. Trim sufficient pulp fat to allow skin closure.

result and can be performed safely if the wound has been healed by judicious application of thin split-thickness skin graft. When bone is exposed on the thumb or index finger, particularly if the wound is untidy or contaminated and debridement would shorten the bone, a thin split graft can be applied directly to the periosteum or to exposed medullary bone. The patient can then be referred for definitive flap reconstruction.

(a) Rongeur and close (Fig. 5-38). If the amount of exposed bone is minimal and most of the skin loss is on the dorsal surface, then shortening of bone and primary skin closure are indicated. This is particularly useful for the ring, middle, and little fingers. Even if the defect cannot be closed completely, it is helpful to cover the working surface of the digits with good padding placed over the bone. If the amount of exposed bone is so great that removal compromises pinch function, then flap soft tissue cover is eventually mandatory.

The bone is rongeured just inside the remaining pulp. Most of the bone is removed from the volar side to allow the volar skin to be rotated upward.

(b) Kutler flap (Fig. 5-39). The Kutler flap can be used in transverse tip avulsions with loss of pulp tissue when digital bony length must be preserved. This is often required on the thumb and index finger.

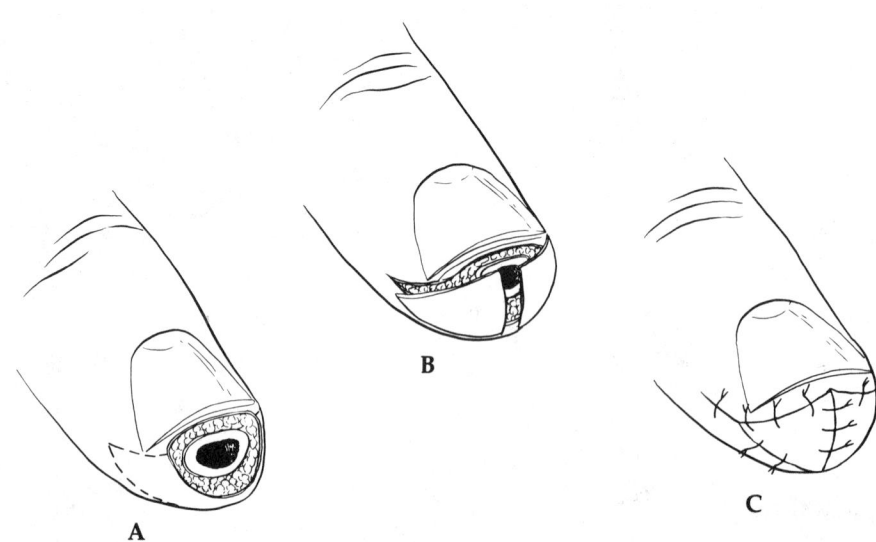

Figure 5-39. The lateral advancement flap, or Kutler flap.
A. Design triangular flaps such that the length is about twice that of the tip defect.
B. Elevate flaps on a wide subcutaneous pedicle containing the terminal branches of the digital neurovascular bundles.
C. Final position.

The basic design consists of two opposing lateral advancement flaps based on subcutaneous blood supply coming up through the pulp and deep attachments. The flaps are small and cover a defect no larger than 1 to 1.5 cm in diameter. The donor sites for the two lateral flaps can be closed in a V-Y advancement.

Because these flaps are usually closed under some tension, if the tip tissues have been crushed, such surgical manipulation frequently results in death of the various parts of the flap. Thus, the procedure is dangerous when a large crush element is present. The subcutaneous flap is richly vascular if designed and mobilized properly. Adequate mobilization is crucial for success. The septa attaching the flap to the periosteum of the volar aspects of the terminal phalanx are sharply divided. After the skin on the lateral sides is incised, a spreading motion is used to mobilize the flap without injuring the neurovascular connections. Approximately 5 mm of advancement per flap are possible.

The disadvantages of this method are the following:

(i) Subcutaneous pedicle flaps are technically demanding, and minimal error in design or technique causes flap necrosis.
(ii) There are scars at the tip of the finger that can become tender.

(c) Volar advancement. Two distinct designs are possible: a V-Y advancement on a subcutaneous pedicle and an island advancement (Fig. 5-40). The V-Y is more commonly used for small transverse defects (less than 10 mm) and, like the Kutler flaps, is based on a subcutaneous blood supply. This is an exacting procedure that must be designed and performed with precision. Inadequate mobility and slough of the flap can easily occur.

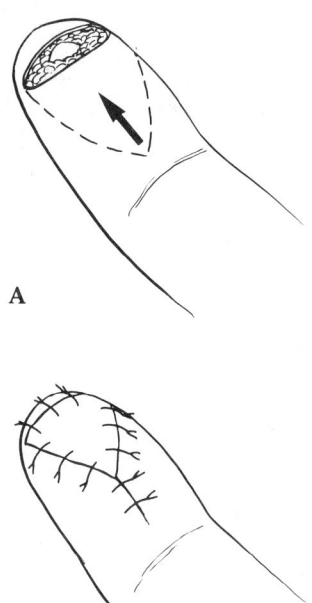

Figure 5-40. The volar island flap, which is technically similar to the lateral island, or Kutler flap, shown in Fig. 5-39.
A. A volar island is created by incising the skin and dividing all septae between pulp and bone.
B. The neurovascular bundles are "teased" and stretched so that the island can be advanced distally.

The arterial island bipedicle flap is used for larger defects of 1.0 to 1.5 cm.

The volar island arterial pedicle (Fig. 5-41) can be used for any finger. The method is based on advancing skin and subcutaneum of one or both neurovascular bundles. The maximum lengthening is about 1.5 cm. With this amount of advancement, the donor area at the base is covered with a full-thickness graft. If less than 5 mm of advancement is required, only distal interphalangeal finger flexion may be necessary for coverage of this defect.

(d) Cross-finger flap (Figs. 5-42 and 5-43). The dorsal skin and subcutaneous tissue is transferred on a pedicle from an adjacent donor finger. The donor and recipient fingers are immobilized for a minimum of 10 days, preferably 2 weeks, before division of the pedicle and inset of the flap are completed. The donor site is covered with a thick split-thickness skin graft or a full-thickness skin graft. The design of a cross-finger flap varies with the finger that is injured.

In general, cross-finger flaps are used for large volar defects of 1 to 2 cm on the thumb or index finger, but they can be used for any digit. Excellent padding and sensibility is achieved. This technique is particularly useful when the digital injury is so extensive that local advancement flaps cannot be safely used, when the defect is large, and when length and function of the digit must be preserved as much as possible.

Figure 5-41.
A. The volar arterial island is elevated as was described in Fig. 5-40. Careful dissection of the neurovascular pedicle is required.
B. By carefully stretching the neurovascular bundles, the arterial island can be advanced 1 to 1½ cm. This procedure is best performed in the operating room under tourniquet control.

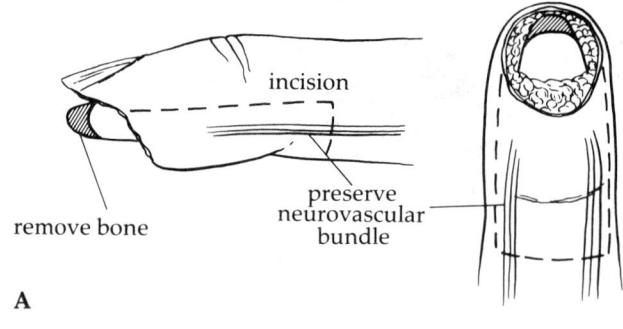

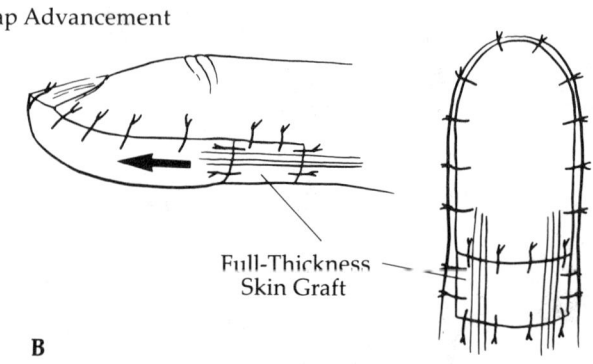

Figure 5-42. The cross-finger flap, which is useful for thumb defects of 1 cm or more.
A. Elevate volarly based rectangle of skin and subcutaneous tissue from the middle finger.
B. Suture this flap to the volar side defect. A few sutures approximates the dorsum of the thumb to the donor defect.

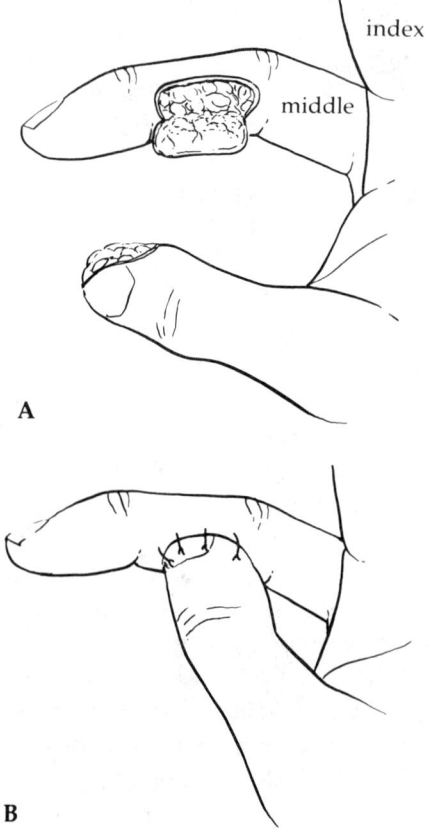

AMPUTATIONS AND SKIN LOSS

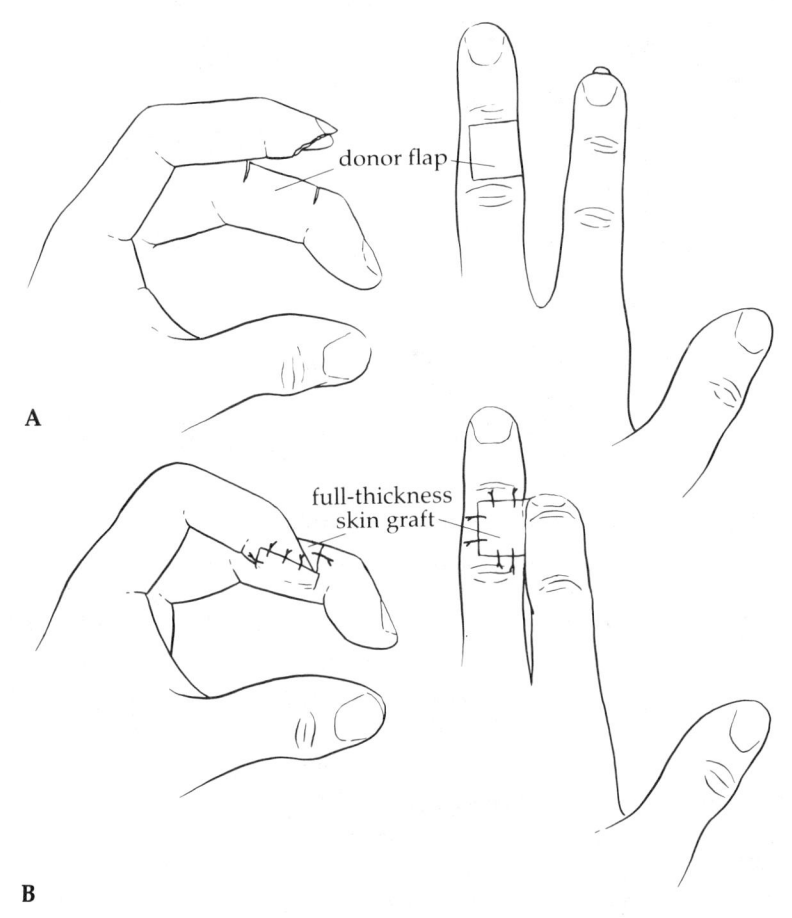

Figure 5-43. Cross-finger flap for an index finger defect, using dorsal skin.
A. Raise a laterally based flap. Adjust the positions of the donor and recipient digits so that excessive flexion at either proximal interphalangeal joint is avoided.
B. Cover the donor defect with a full-thickness skin graft. After division of the pedicle, it is frequently possible and advisable to allow the remaining wound to heal by secondary intention.

(e) Extensive bone exposure of thumb—tubed distant flap (Fig. 5-44)

  (i) Thumb. When there is a circumferential loss of soft tissue with a long segment of exposed bone (and tendon and nerve), a tubed distant flap is required for adequate soft tissue cover. This is only necessary for a thumb avulsion or to salvage the remaining digit from a 3-digit amputation. Later, an innervated flap will be needed to provide better sensibility. The island pedicle flap or radial nerve neurovascular island are common flaps used when tissue with better sensibility is required.

  These distant tube pedicle techniques should be performed by a plastic surgeon in the operating room. If a specialist is not available, a thin split skin graft as a temporary cover is indicated.

  (ii) Index finger. An index digit amputation proximal to the proximal interphalangeal joint leaves a stump too short to oppose effectively to the thumb pulp. Most people so injured automatically and very successfully transfer their pinch function from the index to the middle finger. The index stump frequently is a hindrance and often is treated by secondary ray amputation. The necessary

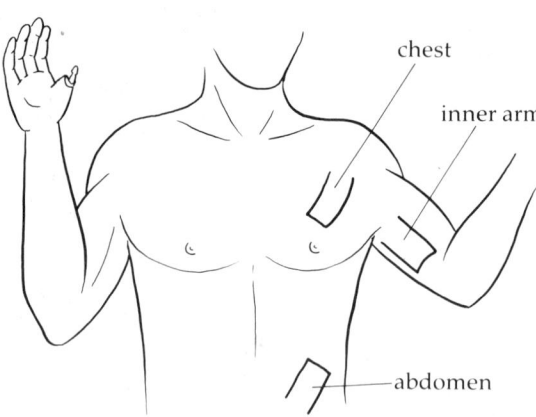

Figure 5-44. Donor sites for a tube pedicle flap.

length of the pinching finger or thumb remaining after amputation is of critical importance.

The middle finger must be treated like an index finger if the index finger is amputated proximally. When length is not a concern, the usual and best method of repair for a transverse amputation of the three ulnar digits is additional shortening of the bone to provide sufficient soft tissue to close the top without tension.

(iii) Ring avulsion injuries. Degloving injuries frequently result when a ring becomes hooked on a protruding object. The force usually is transmitted through the ring, circumferentially tearing the skin and stripping all the soft tissues distally. Tendons usually remain intact, but both neurovascular bundles and all dorsal veins are interrupted. Tendon sheaths and joint soft tissues are exposed. Occasionally, the distal phalanx becomes disarticulated at the distal interphalangeal joint, often with avulsion of a portion of the profundus tendon. These are serious injuries and usually require treatment by a specialist, usually with hospital admission.

Initial amputation at the metacarpophalangeal level may seem radical treatment for a digit exhibiting full motion. However, salvage of such a digit, especially if the injury is isolated, is usually very difficult. The functional result is usually poor. Salvage involves reanastomosis of the avulsed distal vessels (which has a very poor prognosis because of the damage over a great length of the vessels with avulsion injuries), a split-thickness skin graft of the remaining digital surfaces, or burial of the digit in abdominal or chest pedicle. The distally attached soft tissues cannot simply be replaced.

2. Hand amputations
   a. Skin defects (Fig. 5-45)
      (1) Dorsal skin. Loose dorsal skin is easily avulsed in accidents involving presses, chains, or belt drive. These are frequently associated with lacerations that are ragged and untidy.

AMPUTATIONS AND SKIN LOSS

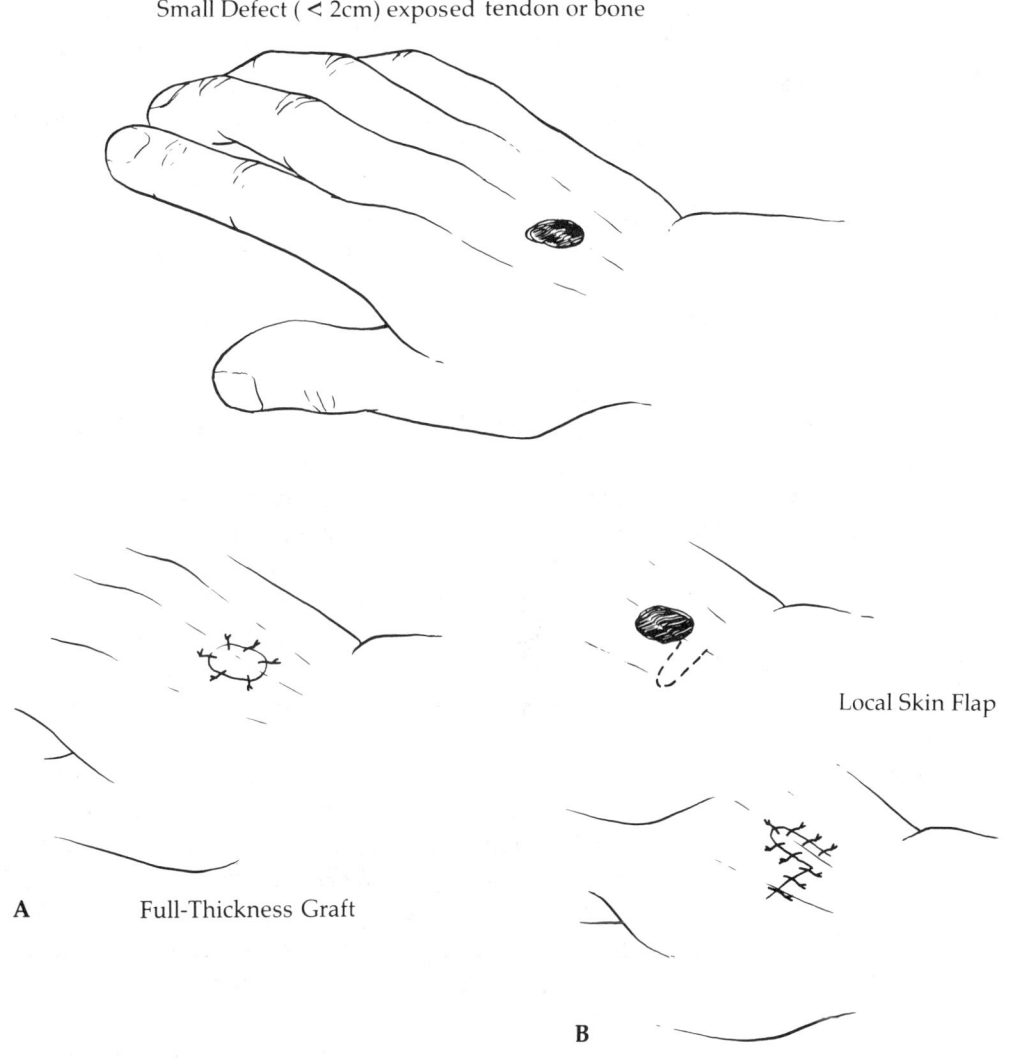

Figure 5-45. Small defects with exposed bone and tendon can be repaired with either full-thickness grafts, which can bridge small grafts (A), or local transposition flaps, which can be smaller than the defect and should be no more than 1 to 1½ cm wide (B).

The wound should be cleaned and debrided. Small defects of several millimeters in size can be sutured without tension. Larger skin defects should be grafted primarily, if possible, or in 2 to 3 days with an intermediate-thickness graft.

The type of graft used on a full-thickness wound of the hand is generally determined by the character of the graft, local wound conditions, and ultimate function of the area to be grafted. Medium-thick grafts should be placed on tidy wounds, and thin grafts should be placed on untidy contaminated wounds.

   (2) Palmar skin. Coverage of a larger palmar wound with a very thin split-thickness skin graft may allow prompt take of the graft but may not provide adequate functional skin cover. Here a very thick split- or full-thickness skin graft provides the best result.

 b. Exposed tendons or bone. *Small defects* (less than 2 cm) can be treated in two ways. A full-thickness skin graft accurately sutured to the edges of the defect may take well, eventually bridging this avascular bed. This is successful only if the greatest dimension of the graft is less than 2 cm, meaning no part of the graft is greater than 1 cm from any edge.

A local skin flap should be transposed over the bare tendon and the flap donor area covered with a skin graft.

Large defects (greater than 2 cm) should not be treated with local flaps because of paucity of tissue. A temporary split graft will protect the wound and may take, but it is likely that a later reconstruction with a distant flap will be required. This is particularly necessary if tendons are avulsed and tendon transfers or grafts are contemplated.

3. Forearm amputations
   a. Skin loss only
      (1) *Small defects* (1–2 cm) can be managed adequately by undermining at the level of the antebrachial (premuscular) fascia and a layered closure.
      (2) *Larger defects* (3 cm) (full-thickness losses) must be skin grafted, although occasionally well-placed, moderate-sized defects may be closed by various local flaps. The avulsed skin can be used as the graft if it is tidy and clean.

      If the base of the wound is on fascia, a medium-thickness split-thickness skin graft can be expected to take. Where subcutaneous fat forms the surface of the defect, a thinner graft may be needed.
   b. Skin and fat loss (with exposure of vital structures). Wound coverage is more important where structures vital for function are exposed (particularly, gliding structures such as tendons or joints) or where tissue is unlikely to support a skin graft (e.g., bone devoid of periosteum). Gliding mechanisms generally must be separated from overlying dermis by areolar or fatty tissue. Their definitive ideal management requires flap coverage. Such wounds should be temporarily covered with a split-thickness skin graft or a moist sterile dressing and the patient referred to a specialist for permanent flap coverage.
   c. Complete amputations. A complete amputation of a forearm should be considered for replantation. Even with severe crush or avulsion injury it may be possible to debride large segments and have a functional but short forearm. Consultation should be obtained.
4. Nail injuries. Fingertip injuries are among the most common hand injuries, and injuries to the nail structures frequently complicate such injuries, especially distal injuries or crush injuries. The important elements are the nail plate, underlying sterile matrix (nail bed), proximal germinal matrix, and underlying bony phalanx, which provides support for the nail. Severe loss of bony support and injury to the germinal matrix may well result in an altered nail. Reconstruction of the injured nail element must be considered in fingertip injuries. Nail injuries may be classified into avulsions, lacerations (including amputations through the nail), and crush injuries.
   a. Avulsions (Fig. 5-46)
      (1) Adults. The nail plate usually detaches itself from the germinal matrix in adults. If the nail plate is completely avulsed and either lost or destroyed, a nonadherent gauze dressing is placed over

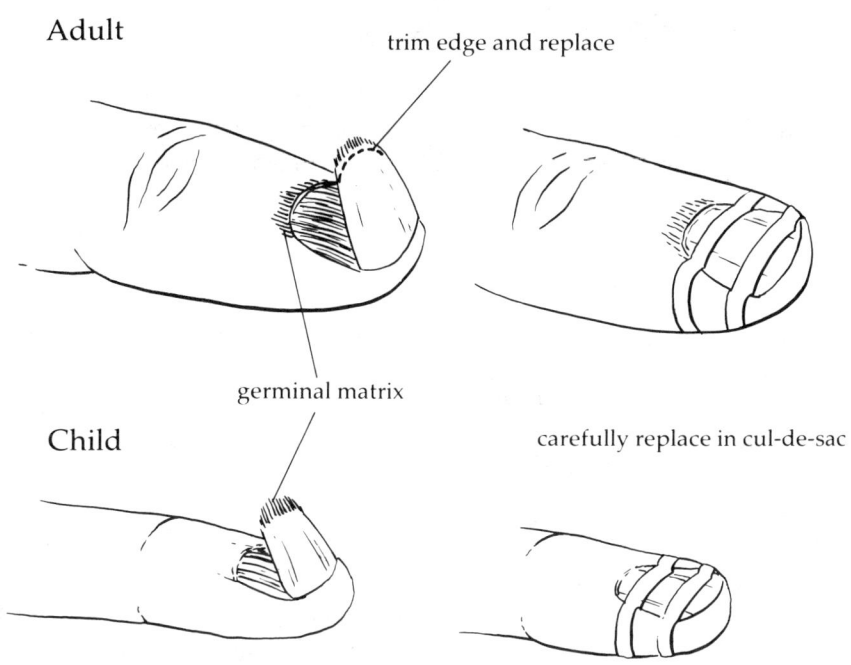

Figure 5-46. Nail avulsion. The detached nail should be repositioned and taped in place. The nail germinal matrix is more likely to be avulsed in a child.

the exposed sterile matrix and left in place for 7 to 10 days. A flexible piece of plastic or a properly shaped piece of suture pack, introduced into the cul-de-sac at the base of the nail, prevents adherence of dorsal and volar surfaces until the new nail begins to grow. The nail bed will have hardened sufficiently to be nontender. If the nail plate is attached distally or is available in complete avulsions, it may be replaced by trimming the edges and securing the nail plate with a small compressive dressing. The nail splints the distal tissues; it does not reattach to the nail bed. When a finger is caught in a door, a partial avulsion of the proximal edge of the nail from underneath the dorsal epithelial (epinychial) fold can occur. It is unnecessary to replace the nail border beneath the fold. The edge is trimmed and the nail plate splinted to the nail bed.

(2) Children. Management of the same injuries in a child may differ because a large portion of the germinal matrix may remain attached to the avulsed nail. Carefully replace the nail within the sulcus so that the germinal matrix may survive as a free graft. The same is true of all avulsions of the nail in children.

b. Lacerations (Fig. 5-46). Sharp blows may lacerate the nail plate as well as the bed. When the nail is completely avulsed, any laceration of the nail bed should be closed accurately with fine (6'0) plain catgut sutures. A nonadherent dressing is applied to provide optimum healing of the bed so that future nail growth may be as normal as possible. Allowing the wound to heal by secondary intent usually results in greater scarring of the bed and a poor nail contour. Avulsion of the nail bed should be treated like any full-thickness injury, by split-thickness skin grafting. If the nail remains attached on either side of the laceration, the sutures may be passed through the nail, the nail bed thus approximating these structures. The nail acts as a splint during healing.

    c. **Amputations.** If sufficient bony support remains (generally at least half the length of the nail), the fingernail may grow to be aesthetically and functionally worthwhile. If less than half of the bony support of the nail remains, the new nail will severely curve volarly during growth, be unsightly, and function poorly. The nail bed including the germinal matrix may require excision at a later time. Nail obliteration is a difficult procedure that should be performed as elective surgery. If any germinal matrix remains, it will generate a nail remnant or nail horn, which will snag on clothing and be unsightly. It must be remembered that the germinal matrix extends much more proximally than is usually realized, almost to the insertion of the extensor tendon on the distal phalanx.

5. **Postoperative care of finger amputation.** Two to three weeks are required before a skin graft or flap is stable enough for day-to-day wear and tear. It may be protected by a small finger guard of plastic or aluminum that allows the patient to work. However, prolonged use of a finger guard is to be condemned. The fingertip has to become accustomed to minor trauma or the initial sensitivity of injury persists unduly. The patient should be advised that there is an initial period of somewhat uncomfortable accommodation before the fingertip becomes nontender. The finger also suffers a more or less prolonged period of cold intolerance, and the patient should be so advised.

    Persistent tenderness may be secondary to a neuroma from the amputated digital nerve. This pain is described as an electric shock and usually can be localized by the patient to a small area in which a nodule representing the neuroma may be palpable. Persistent tenderness seems more frequently related to the scar of wound closure or to the site of split-thickness skin graft attachment to the well-innervated periosteum at the bone amputation site. This pain is not electric-like and is less well localized. Treatment differs according to the cause of tenderness. Painful neuromas should be identified and removed from contact surfaces by one of many procedures. The persistently tender stump, secondary to scar or graft adhesion to periosteum, is more difficult to treat. Usually it requires revision of the stump with better soft tissue closure by placement of a full-thickness skin graft and local or distant flap coverage.

6. PENETRATING INJURIES AND DEEP TRANSECTIONS

Penetrating injuries cause unique initial problems related to the diagnosis and treatment of disruption of nerves, ducts, vessels, and other structures. Moreover, the penetrating object presents secondary problems, e.g., the prevention and treatment of infection, and localization and removal of the object.

Penetrating injuries from objects such as glass, splinters, knives, and bullets can cause transection of nerves, tendons, blood vessels, or other anatomic structures within the soft tissues and of vital organs within the body cavities. A careful diagnostic examination based on a knowledge of the regional anatomy must be performed to identify injury to these deep structures. Transection of deep structures also can occur from lacerations or even severe crush injuries. The diagnosis and repair of these injuries is discussed here.

Infection is a frequent complication because of the combined effect of foreign bodies, contamination, and tissue devascularization. Animal bites present unique problems because of tissue loss, infection, and toxins. Penetrating injuries, often caused by criminal assault and vehicular, industrial, and home accidents, may have forensic and compensatory implications. Therefore, photographic or x-ray documentation, careful observation and recording of findings, and salvage of debrided tissue or extracted foreign bodies should be part of the management.

After emergency care is given and initial diagnostic evaluation is completed, the physician must decide which injuries require definitive care in the emergency department and which require consultation or operating-room surgery. This decision is based not only on the type of wound, but also on the experience of the surgeon, quality of facilities and instruments in the emergency department, and availability of a consulting specialist.

INITIAL MANAGEMENT

Bleeding

SUSPICION OF INJURY

Penetrating injuries can include vascular injury, with blood loss and shock. Penetrating injuries adjacent to major vessels should be explored in the operating room if the patient remains stable. However, the absence of pulsatile bleeding, shock, or expanding hematoma should not dissuade the emergency physician from suspecting vascular injury and requesting consultation and exploratory surgery. This is particularly true in anatomic sites in which large hematomas can go unnoticed for prolonged periods and terminate in sudden shock. The neck, mediastinum, groin, axilla, abdomen, and chest are common sites of hidden injury.

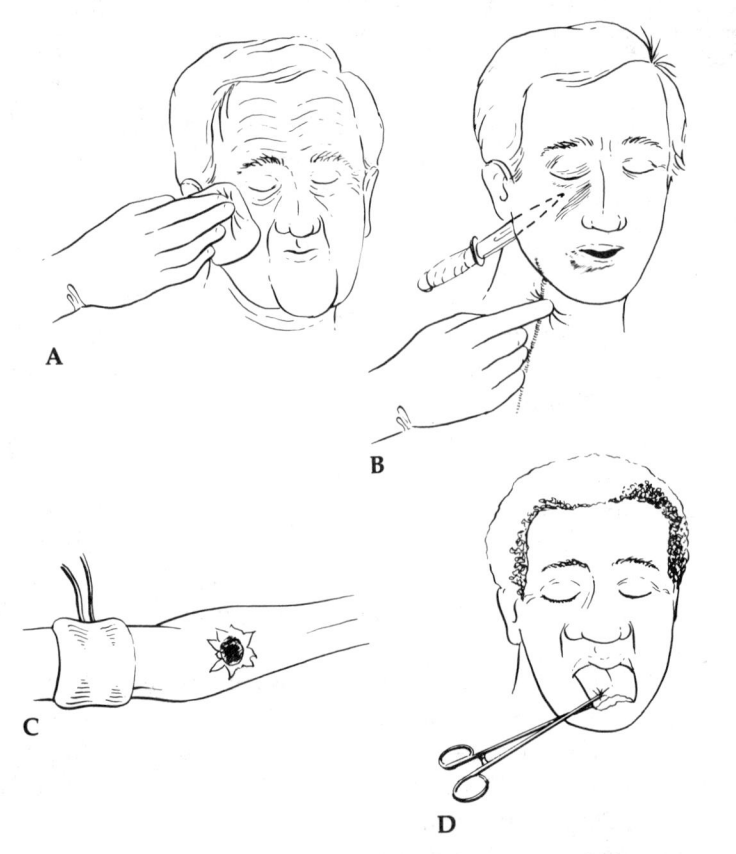

Figure 6-1. Alternative methods of achieving hemostasis of penetrating injuries.
A. Direct pressure is used for most wounds.
B. Pressure points are rarely used except for inaccessible deep penetration of the face (or body cavities).
C. Tourniquets can be used for extensive wounds of the extremity.
D. Clamping is occasionally used for accessible large vessels of the face that do not require microvascular repair.

INITIAL HEMOSTASIS

The usual therapeutic steps to stop hemorrhage by compression or tourniquet (Fig. 6-1) are of prime importance, as is replacement of blood volume with electrolyte solutions, colloids, and blood.

1. Compression of injury site. Massive bleeding from a wound over a great vessel of an extremity or the neck usually can be controlled by direct pressure over the site of injury; this is ineffective only when the vessel is deeply situated in a body cavity.
2. Proximal pressure points. Pressure over the proximal major vessel diminishes the flow of blood to the distal site of injury, allowing pressure at the wound to be more effective in controlling hemorrhage. Pressure points are useful primarily for on-site care when tourniquets are unavailable. Frequently useful sites include the carotid artery at the base of the neck or in the midneck, axillary artery in the axilla, brachial artery at the antecubital fossa, femoral artery in the groin, and popliteal artery in the popliteal fossa.
3. Tourniquet. If direct or proximal pressure is ineffective for extremity injuries, a tourniquet should be placed proximal to the site of hemorrhage. On-site temporary cloth or elastic tourniquets are quite effective but are less desirable because the narrowness and indeterminate pressure can cause direct compression damage to underlying structures. If the patient arrives with a belt, cloth, or rope tourniquet, this should be removed and either a commercial pneumatic tourniquet or a blood pres-

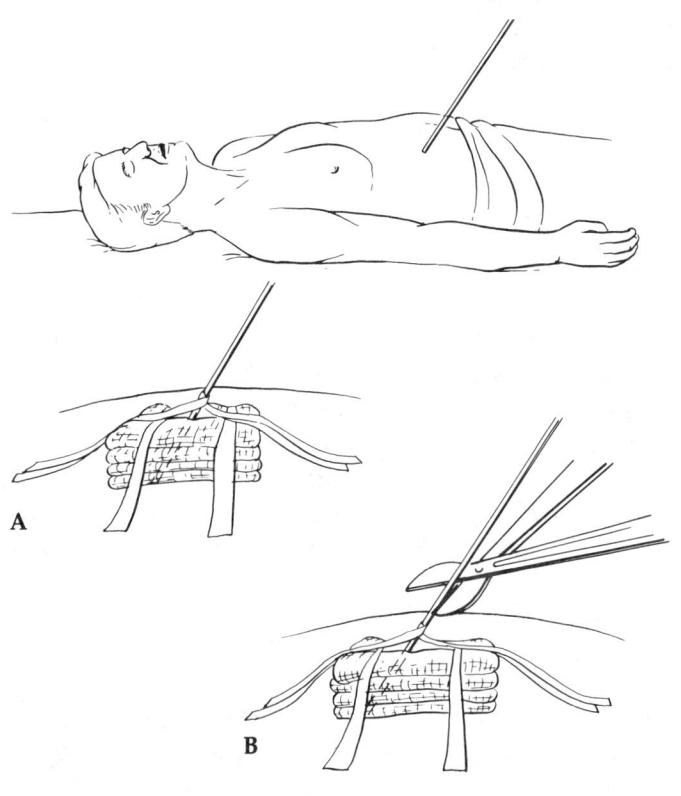

Figure 6-2. Prevention of additional damage from embedded objects.
A. Penetrating object is thoroughly immobilized with gauze and tape.
B. Excessive length of wood or thin metals can be cut off to simplify immobilization and ensure that the object is not moved through contact with a protruding end.

sure cuff applied. For the arm, approximately 200 to 300 mm Hg is sufficient to control bleeding distal to the tourniquet. For the leg, a pressure of 350 to 450 mm Hg is required.

The most frequent pitfall is too low or too high a pressure. Too low a pressure allows arterial inflow but venous blockage, which causes venous congestion and thrombosis. Too high a pressure damages underlying tissues, especially major peripheral nerves.

Any tourniquet should be removed totally or deflated for several minutes every half hour while pressure is exerted on the wound.

4. Clamping. Large vessels that are easily visible and accessible can be clamped to avoid life-threatening bleeding. This is particularly true for the head and neck (except the carotids). The major disadvantages of clamping are inadvertent *damage to adjacent nerves* and damage to vessels that should be repaired by microvascular surgery. Clamping can be used on unconscious patients with intraoral or facial wounds.

Prevention of Additional Damage

Penetrating metal fragments, arrows, and knives are often impaled in the tissue. *The deeply embedded object should not be removed!* Rather, it should be immobilized with gauze, tape, or wraps until it can be removed carefully and the wound explored in an operating room (Fig. 6-2).

The reasons for removal in the operating room include the following:

1. Movement of the object can cause injury to vessels, nerves, or other structures. Immobilization prevents additional damage.

2. The object may be tamponading a major bleeding site, and when it is removed, bleeding can be profuse.
3. The diagnostic assessment of the actual depth and tract of the wound can be more easily made in the operating room by the operating surgeon.

Antibiotics and Other Prophylaxis

Many penetrating injuries are contaminated and associated with ischemic tissue destruction, which predisposes to secondary infection; prophylactic antibiotics and tetanus toxoid are always required for animal bites and often for other wounds. Antibiotics should be started as soon as possible. Guidelines for choice of antibiotics are discussed in Chapter 1, Tables 1-2 and 1-3. Subsequent treatment requires removal of all foreign material, debridement, copious antiseptic irrigations, and the decision either to leave the wound open or to close it. Additional antisepsis or antitoxins may be required for animal bites. Tetanus and rabies prophylaxis are discussed in Chapter 2.

Diagnostic Radiology

Deeply penetrating injuries require surgical exploration by the consulting surgeon in the operating room. However, preliminary radiologic examination is usually helpful *if the patient is stable and x-rays are readily available.* This should be discussed and ordered by the emergency department physician after discussion with the operating surgeon.

HEAD AND NECK AND SOFT TISSUE FILMS

A standard soft tissue x-ray or CAT scan can identify the following:

1. Subcutaneous emphysema. This may be caused by penetration of a hollow organ (e.g., esophagus, trachea, or pharynx). At the entrance site of an isolated skin wound, a small amount of air can be seen. Air deep in the tissue or in fascial planes should raise suspicion of damage to either digestive or respiratory structures (or the rampant growth of anaerobic gas-forming organisms).
2. Abnormal soft tissue shadows. Hematoma can occur in the absence of severe external bleeding. A widened mediastinum or other soft tissue plane or shift of the trachea or esophagus may be caused by bleeding. Exploration in the operating room is usually indicated.
3. Foreign body. Look for the presence and location of foreign bodies.

CHEST AND ABDOMEN

The management of thoracic and abdominal injuries is not discussed in this book, although diagnostic evaluation should be performed by the emergency physician.

Careful evaluation is required for signs of hemothorax, pneumothorax, tension pneumothorax, and cardiac puncture. Appropriate consultation should be obtained.

Supine, upright, and cross-table lateral films of the abdomen can show air in the peritoneal cavity. Peritoneal lavage, "stabograms," and arteriograms are favored by some physicians. However, the use of these diagnostic techniques should be determined by the consulting surgeon.

CLASSIFICATION OF PENETRATING INJURIES

Penetrating injuries can be classified according to the mechanism (high or low energy) and anatomic depth of injury (superficial or deep). A special category is given to bites because of the unique problems of infection and toxins and to wounds with established infection.

High-energy Penetrating Injuries

High-energy injuries are likely to have additional damage at a distance from the entrance wound, whereas low-energy penetration results in damage adjacent to the tract only. High-energy sources are bullets, grenades, and exploded fragments. Tissue injury is often caused by propagation of a shock wave. Most wounds of this type require operating-room management.

Low-energy Penetrating Injuries

Except for stab wounds involving major vessels, low-energy injuries from objects such as splinters, hooks, and glass are usually minor. The primary objectives of treatment are removal of the foreign body to prevent infection and evaluation for compound injury to nerves, vessels, and other structures. Except for some stab wounds, treatment can nearly always be carried out in the emergency room.

Superficial Penetrating Injuries

Wounds of the skin only are usually associated with a low-energy penetrating source and have the same treatment implications (i.e., removal of foreign body and prevention of infection).

Deep (compound) Penetrating Injuries

These wounds must be examined carefully for damage to deep structures, and a decision must be made whether definitive care is to be carried out in the emergency room or operating room. Guidelines for this decision are discussed with each specific injury, although most deep compound injuries are better managed in the operating room.

HIGH-ENERGY INJURIES

Bullet Wounds

1. These injuries usually require hospitalization and surgical exploration in the operating room. Hemostasis and physiologic stabilization are the primary emergency department objectives.

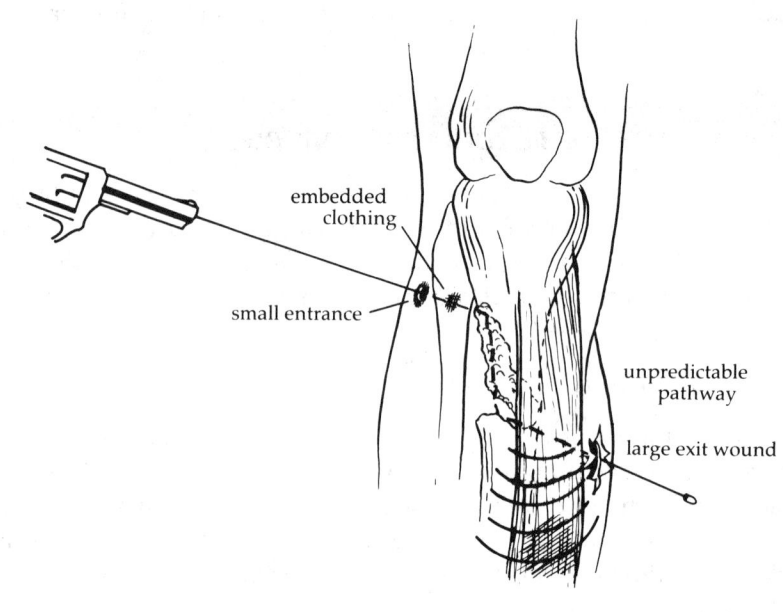

Figure 6-3. Bullet wound, characterized by small entrance site; larger, stellate exit site; and unpredictable intervening pathway. Muscles, nerves, and vessels can be injured from direct impact of the bullet, bone fragments, or shock waves.

2. X-rays and diagnostic assessment are carried out after the patient is stable.
3. Photographs and pathologic examination of debrided wounds are required for medicolegal purposes.
4. Antibiotics should be started.
5. The wound of entrance is usually regular and smaller than the wound of exit. The exit wound is usually irregular, stellate, and larger (Fig. 6-3).
6. Deposits of gunpowder and clothing must be removed. This can be initiated in the emergency department before operating-room exploration.
7. The pathway of the missile may not be a straight line between entrance and exit sites, and unexpected injuries can occur because of the irregular pathway.
8. Deeply embedded bullets are removed in the operating room. The severity of injury has a stronger relation to the velocity of the missile than to any other factor.
9. Shock waves from high velocity bullets can cause extensive tissue necrosis at a distance from the actual tract. Muscle necrosis and vascular thrombosis are particularly dangerous.

Shotgun Injuries

Although muzzle velocity and gauge are important, the critical factor for the most commonly used shot guns is the distance from gun to victim (Fig. 6-4). Severity of injury can be predicted by this distance:

Type 1 Range greater than 7 to 10 yards causes minimal penetration into subcutaneum.
Type 2 Range of 3 to 7 yards usually involves injury of deep structures.
Type 3 Close range—less than 3 yards—causes massive damage and results in death or tissue loss.

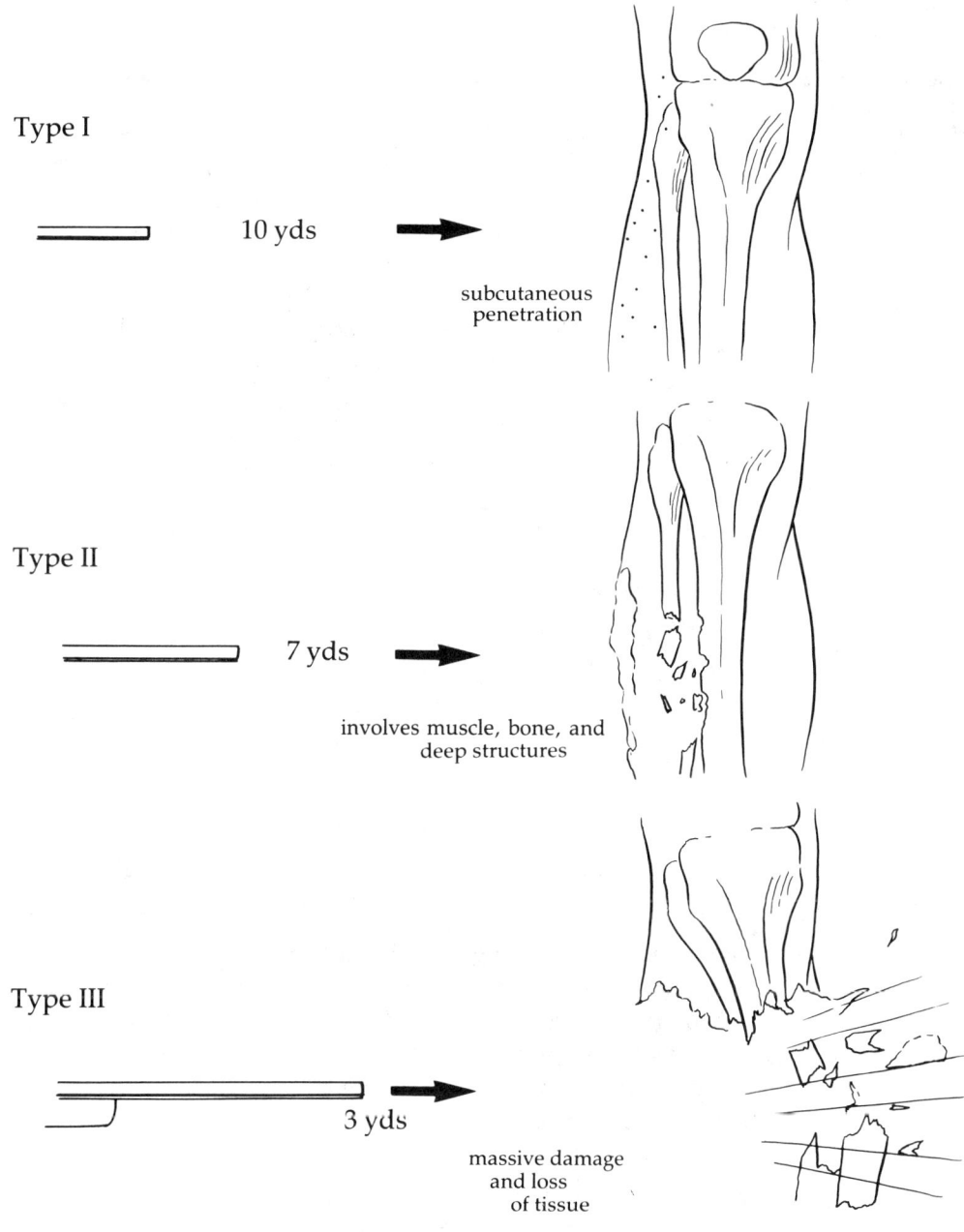

Figure 6-4. Types of shotgun wounds. The severity of shotgun injuries is most dependent on the distance from gun to tissue rather than shot size or type of gun.

Thorough operative exploration and debridement are critical to successful management. The emergency department and operating-room responsibilities are the same as for bullet wounds.

Pressure Injections from Paint Guns

PATHOPHYSIOLOGY

These injuries are the result of inflammatory reaction and secondary infection from the paint or grease in the tissue and, to a lesser extent, are the direct result of the energy of injection.

Paint can be injected at a pressure of up to 3000 lbs per square inch, most

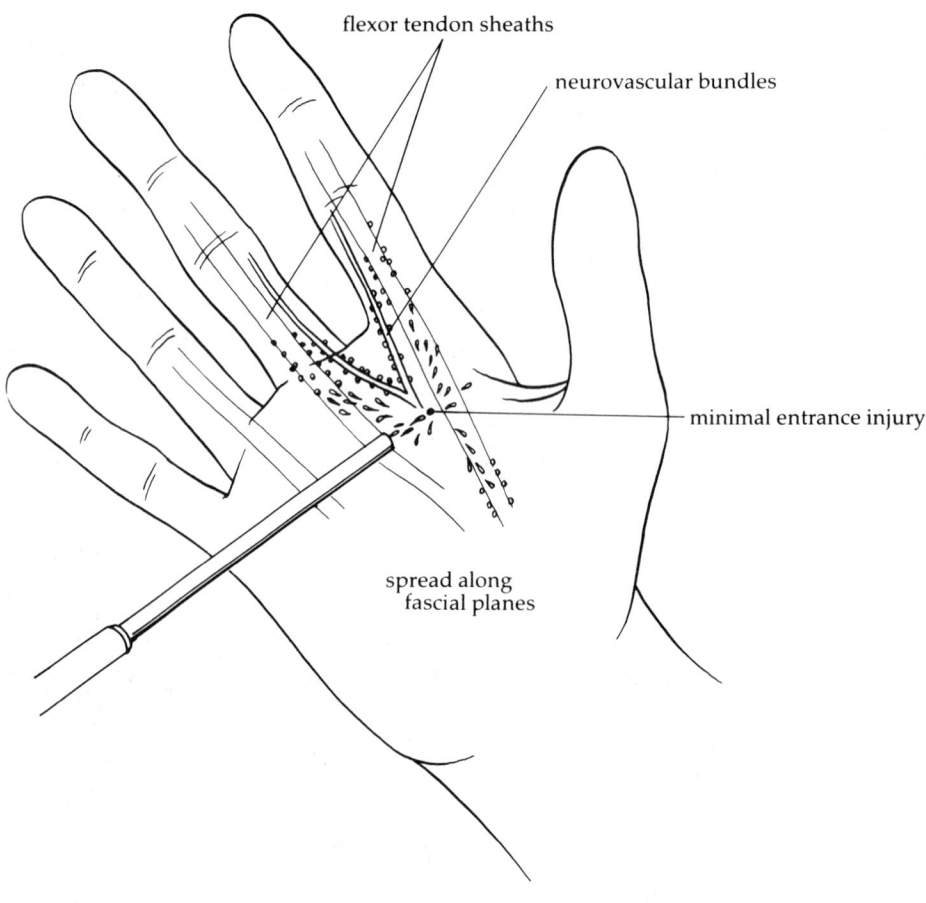

Figure 6-5. Paint and grease gun injuries have a tiny, often inconspicuous, entrance site, but extensive chemical infiltration occurs subcutaneously and along fascial planes and tendon sheaths, causing severe inflammation.

commonly, into the fingers or hand (Fig. 6-5). At this pressure, the paint *spreads along the fascial plane.* The injury may seem trivial initially, but severe inflammatory reaction to the paint and secondary bacterial infection usually lead to necrotizing effects and mandatory amputation, or at best, a severely fibrotic, poorly functioning extremity. Paints have varying intensity of inflammatory reactions:

Most severe reaction—Soya Alkyd and mineral spirit bases
Moderate reaction—turpentine base
Least reaction—xylol, acrylic, and titanium oxide based paints

TREATMENT
This is an operating-room problem. Although the best treatment has not been clearly delineated, we recommend:

1. Surgical consultation for emergency incision and debridement
2. Dexamethasone, 40 mg IM, followed by 10 mg qd for 3 to 5 days
3. Prophylactic (broad-spectrum) antibiotics

Do not attempt closed wound irrigation; it may spread the paint and bacteria and does not seem to have any benefit in diluting or washing out the paint.

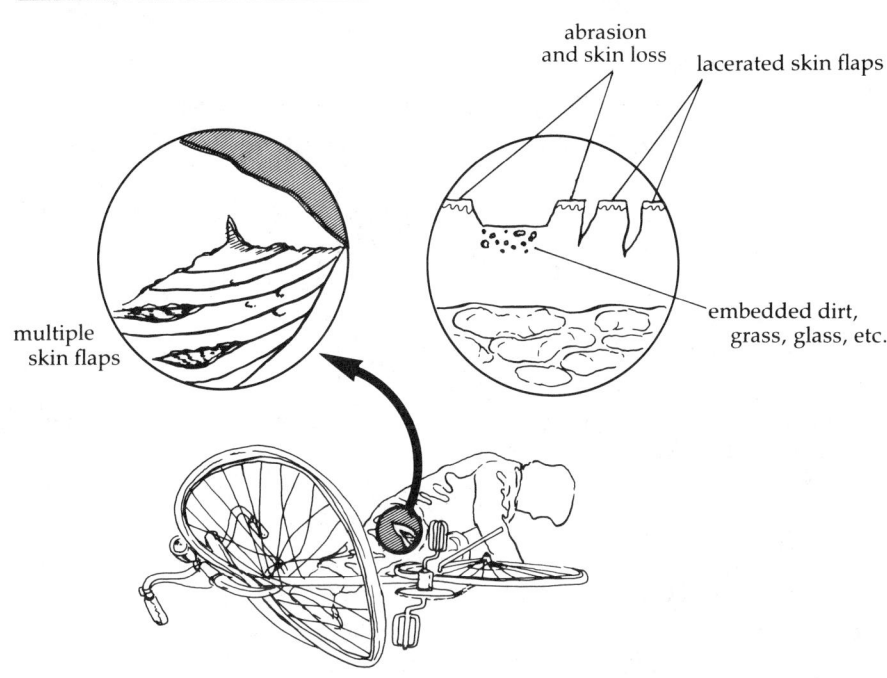

Figure 6-6. Road dirt abrasions, which frequently result from falls onto knee or elbow. The injury includes skin loss, lacerations, and penetration of debris to various depths. Deeply embedded debris, if not removed, results in "unsightly tattoos."

LOW-ENERGY INJURIES

Stab Wounds

Stab wounds are caused by long thin objects such as knives and fragments of wood, metal, or glass. The nature and severity of the injury depends primarily on the site and depth of the wound. As mentioned above, occasionally the patient arrives in the emergency department with the knife, arrow, or other impaled object still in place. The initial management of such a patient involves controlling hemorrhage, fluid resuscitation, stabilization of the patient's general condition, and preparation for definitive management in the operating room.

Penetrating wounds to the chest and abdomen caused by such objects are not discussed here. The management of such wounds to the extremities are discussed later in this chapter in terms of the evaluation and treatment of injuries to deep structures.

Foreign Bodies

Most low-energy penetrating injuries are from fragments of wood (splinters), glass, or objects such as hooks. There is rarely a problem of unsuspected deep damage. Removal of the foreign material, debridement, and other antiseptic measures are important.

ROAD DIRT ABRASIONS

The "road dirt abrasion" is from the scraping of skin on the ground, causing dirt, splinters, asphalt, rocks, glass, and other objects to penetrate (Fig. 6-6). Lacerations and skin loss may occur in addition to penetration. All penetrating foreign material must be removed before closure of lacerations and coverage of skin loss.

1. Pathophysiology. The problems associated with road dirt embedded in the skin are:
   a. Wound infection
   b. Wound tattooing—Foreign material is phagocytized by local macrophages and remains at the injury site causing skin discoloration (tattoo).
   c. Contour irregularity—Fragments of glass or metal can alter the surface contour.
   d. Skin loss—Epithelial abrasive loss can occur, or large full-thickness skin fragments can be avulsed.
   e. Foreign body reaction—An inflammatory response to foreign material can lead to fibrosis and pain.
2. Treatment. This can be carried out in the emergency department if there is adequate anesthesia and equipment.
   a. *Assess and palpate wound.* The patient may have localized tenderness at the site of foreign bodies in the skin. Therefore, identify foreign bodies by palpation before administration of anesthesia. This is particularly effective with glass or splinter injuries. The following maneuvers require topical or injection anesthesia.
   b. *Visualize and remove large particles.* An indirect, oblique light may be helpful in making shadows and irregular surfaces more obvious than they are under direct, flat light.
   c. *Feel the smaller particles* beneath the surface and remove them carefully with a forceps.
   d. *Scrape* the surface with the back of a forceps blade or knife handle. Metal or glass may produce a clicking sound, or you may feel the instrument catch on the foreign body.
   e. *Scrub* the surface with a bristle brush (surgical scrub brush or toothbrush). This is very effective for multiple small particles of dirt or asphalt. The brushing should be done firmly, much the same as you would scrub for surgery. Intermittently irrigate the surface to remove blood and particulate matter.
   f. *Emulsify* the wound if it is greasy. Use iodinated soap (e.g., Betadine) followed by a vaseline-based ointment (e.g., Neosporin), and repeat with soap. This helps remove water-insoluble dirt and grease.
   g. *Sand.* Very small foreign particles embedded in the dermis may require dermabrasion with medium-grade silicon carbide (Carborundum) paper. However, standard sandpaper of comparable grades is acceptable. Dermabrasion also smooths out tiny flaps and fragments of skin. The depth of abrasion can be judged by the size of and distance between punctate dermal bleeding sites. As you proceed deeper, the bleeding is from larger vessels that are more widely separated. Care must be taken not to remove excessive epithelium or dermis and produce a full-thickness skin loss.
   h. *Irrigate with a water spray.* The Water Pik wound lavage system produces a pulsatile high-pressure spray that can dislodge small particles and irrigate out surface bacteria. Low-pressure drip systems from IV bottles are not as effective.
   i. *Debride.* Nonviable or severely contused or heavily contaminated tissue should be excised.

j. *Suture.* Lacerations and flaps of skin should be treated as indicated by the nature, depth, and location of the laceration (see Chap. 4).
k. *Dress.* Because these abrasions are usually contaminated, a dressing with topical antibiotic ointment and gauze should be used. Frequent changes and reevaluation are usually indicated.
l. *Antibiotic prophylaxis.* Systemic antibiotics (penicillin or cephalosporins) and tetanus prophylaxis are often required for extensive injuries.

SINGLE, SUPERFICIAL SPLINTERS

The majority of punctures are caused by nails, broken needles, thorns, glass, or wood splinters that enter the hands or feet. Because of the unique fascial-aponeurotic anatomy of the palms and soles, surgical exploration, even in the operating room, can be frustrating to the physician and damaging to the patient. Therefore, *the presence and position of the foreign body must be determined before considering wound exploration.*

1. Determining the presence of a retained foreign body
    a. Visual inspection. The foreign body sometimes can be seen because of its color under the skin or blood in the tract. The thread from a sewing needle may be visible.
    b. Palpation. Tenderness along the tract can be elicited by palpation with a small blunt-tipped object (forceps or probe). Counterpressure over one end of a foreign body may allow palpation.
    c. X-ray. An x-ray localizes radiopaque foreign material or the lucency from air along the wound tract. Identify the puncture by taping on paper clips or other markers that relate the foreign body position with the skin surface.
    d. Xeroradiography. Although not readily available, this technique can identify radiolucent objects (wood, glass) not detectable on routine x-ray. A drawback to the use of xerograms is their much greater x-ray dosage.
    e. Metal detectors. Although a detector can help locate deeply embedded objects, these are not usually available, and a careful clinical examination and radiologic study provide more exact information.
2. Treatment
    a. Direct extraction (Fig. 6-7). After localization, the foreign body or splinter should be removed by the simplest method (i.e., direct extraction with forceps, without surgical incision). Only if this fails should an open method of surgical exploration be used. This is particularly true of splinters on the tactile area of the fingers or weight-bearing areas of the sole of the foot. Surgical scars at these sites can be functionally debilitating from pain.

    Thorns, cactus, and palm spines may penetrate, break off, and lodge in a joint space. This results in a surprisingly virulent synovitis with pain and great swelling, although the inflammation is usually sterile and responds only to removal of the foreign body. The patient presenting with a history and physical signs suggestive of this condition should be referred to a specialist for consideration of exploring the joint.

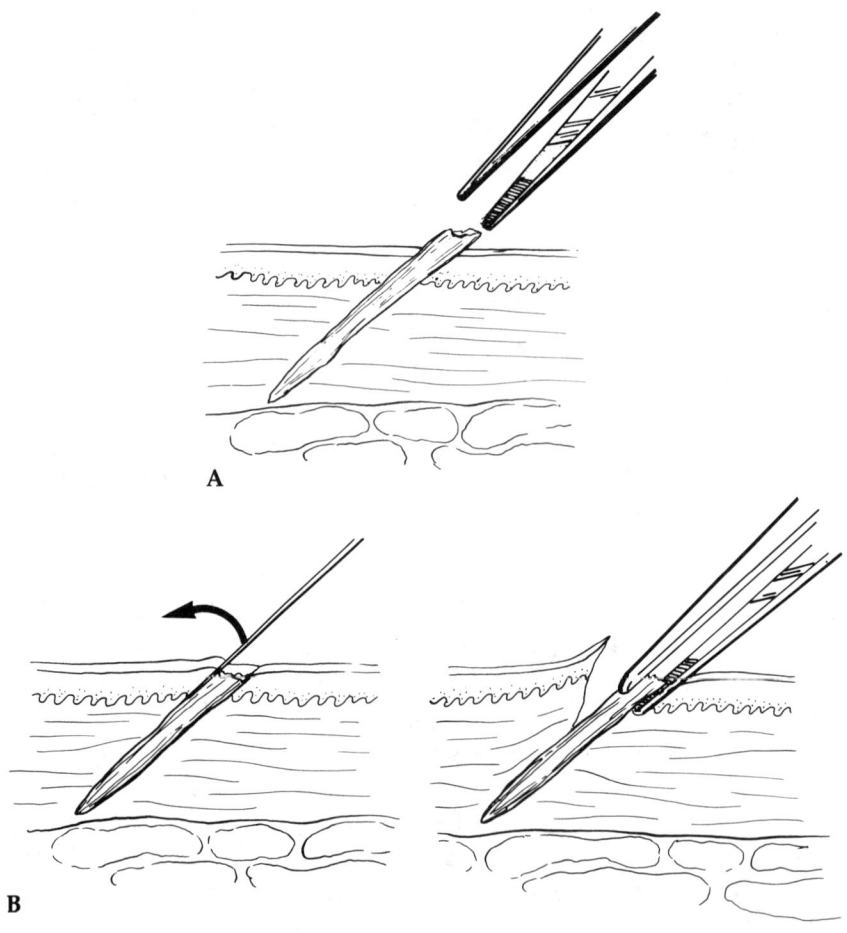

Figure 6-7. Extraction of superficial foreign body.
A. Identify the pathway by visual inspection and palpation. Tenderness can be elicited with pressure along the foreign body. Grasp and remove the object, pulling parallel to the long axis of the object.
B. If the foreign body is buried, unroof the overlying skin by elevating it with a needle to allow access to the end.

    b. Watchful waiting. If the splinter cannot be identified (particularly if not documented by x-ray), it is reasonable to consider watchful waiting rather than surgical exploration. Often the foreign body enters the skin and is extruded spontaneously. Watchful waiting is indicated if adequate, frequent reexamination is possible and if surgical exploration is likely to cause unwarranted scars or tissue damage.
    c. Surgical exploration. Exploration for seemingly easily accessible foreign bodies can be extremely difficult, and more tissue injury can occur from the exploration than from the foreign body retention. A tourniquet and good anesthesia are essential to the success of exploration in the extremity. If any difficulty is encountered, it may be best to defer the procedure until the operating room is available.
       (1) The skin overlying the foreign body should be surgically incised with the *minimum exposure required to identify and extract the foreign body.*
       (2) If the foreign body is contaminated or a secondary infection has developed, the wound should not be sutured but allowed to heal by delayed closure if contaminated or by secondary intention if infected.

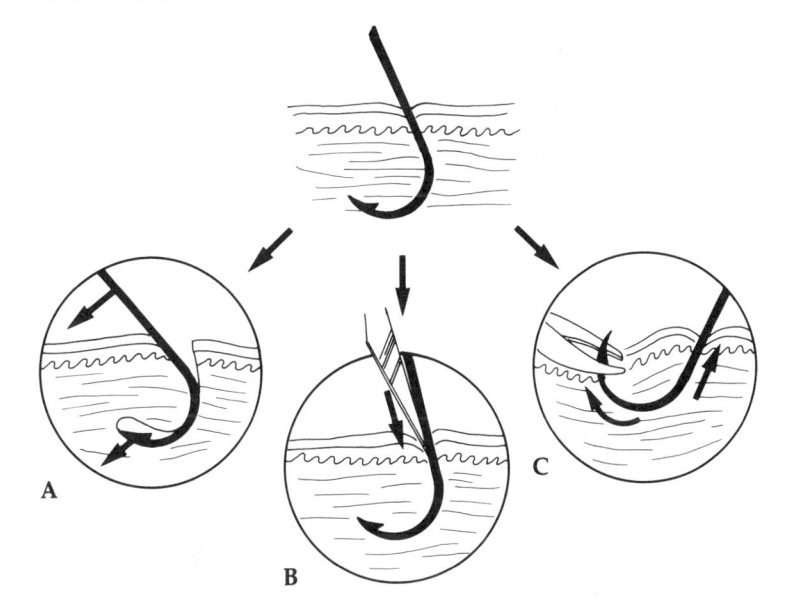

Figure 6-8. Fishing hook removal.
A. Retrograde extraction is used only when the barb is embedded very superficially and danger to local tissue is minimal. Even if the hook is extracted, there can be unnecessary damage by the barb. Pressing the non-barbed external curve against the tissue can minimize the effect of the barb.
B. Incision of overlying skin also can be used for a superficially embedded hook; it is primarily an adjunct to retrograde extraction but requires local anesthesia. Insert a #11 scalpel blade along the tract of the hook, and incise the overlying tissue adequately to allow hook retraction.
C. Advancement and cutting off the barb is the preferred method because of minimal tissue damage. Usually this method leaves no surgical scar. Advance the hook until the barb is fully exposed above the skin surface. Then remove the barb with a wire cutter; the hook can be removed in retrograde direction.

MULTIPLE GLASS FRAGMENTS

All windshields and some household glass in present-day use are made of laminated "safety glass," which tends to cause multiple punctate lacerations and skin flaps associated with embedded fragments of glass. Treatment is similar to that described for a single foreign body. Because visual inspection is not as helpful, palpation to induce tenderness and scraping with a metal forceps blade to hear the sound of metal-to-glass contact are required. Skin flaps and lacerations are treated in the appropriate manner, as described in Figs. 3-36, 4-5, and 4-6.

FISHING HOOKS

Because of the barbed end of fishing hooks, special methods are required for removal. This can be done by retrograde extraction, by skin incision (unroofing), or by advancement and cutting off the barb (Fig. 6-8).

SUBUNGUAL SPLINTERS

Wood splinters or metal shavings frequently penetrate under the fingernails. Surprisingly, the splinter can be driven well proximal to the nail tip and its end broken off. Therefore, it cannot be grasped easily even though it is visible through the nail. Direct extraction is used for protruding splinters and nail splitting for buried splinters (Fig. 6-9).

LARGE, DEEPLY IMPALED OBJECTS (KNIVES, ARROWS, POLES)

Rarely should these injuries have definitive treatment in the emergency department, but emergency effort should be made to stabilize the patient to prevent additional damage. Carefully assess for penetration into body cavities or other vital soft tissue structures.

The exception to this rule is the stab wound of the chest in which direct cardiac penetration has occurred and rapidly progressive pericardial tam-

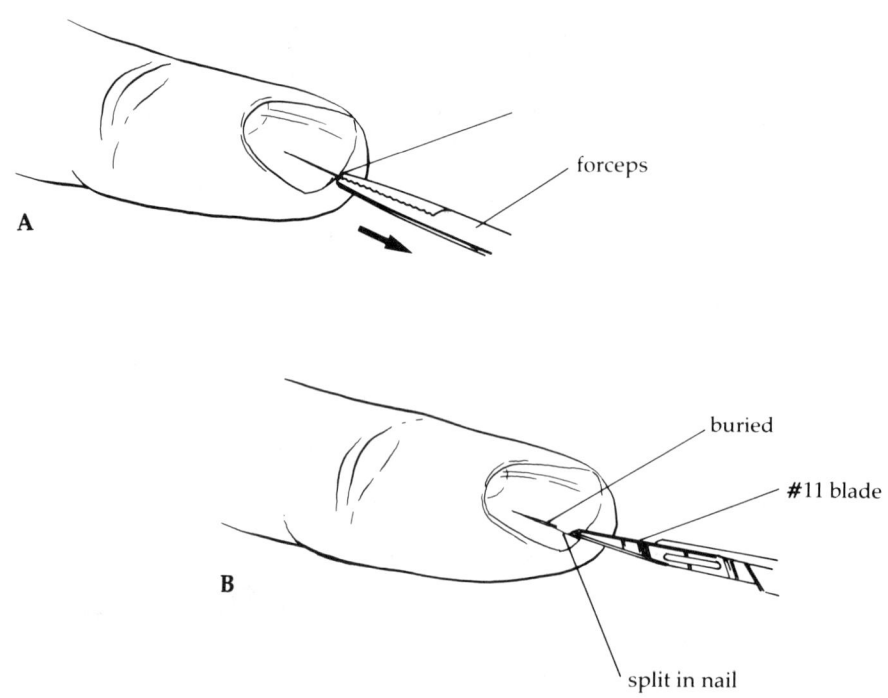

Figure 6-9. Extraction of sub ungual splinters.
A. Direct (retrograde) extraction. Occasionally the end of the foreign body tip is located close to the tip of the nail. By teasing the skin matrix away from the nail plate, a fine pair of splinter forceps can be inserted and the object grasped and withdrawn. Digital anesthesia may be necessary.
B. Nail splitting. If the object is deeply embedded, the nail can be split longitudinally to the level of the foreign body. Following removal, the nail can be splinted or even "spot-welded" with cyanoacrylate adhesive (Krazy Glue). When considerable contamination exists, prophylactic antibiotics should be considered.

ponade is highly suspected. Removal of the impaled object or pericardiocentesis may be necessary to relieve the tamponade.

DEEP INJURIES

The exposed areas of the body, such as the head and upper limbs, suffer a disproportionately high number of injuries. Because injuries to these parts occur so frequently, their diagnosis and management are discussed in detail in the following sections. Because deep injuries to the chest and abdomen are usually not treated in the emergency department, they are not discussed.

Any penetrating object can damage underlying tendons, nerves, ducts, vessels, or other structures. Although these compound injuries are most likely to occur from high-energy sources, even a small, seemingly superficial penetration or laceration can cause underlying injury. Therefore, a thorough evaluation must be part of management.

The diagnosis and treatment of deep injuries may be either independent or simultaneous processes. For example, a facial fracture can be diagnosed radiologically, with treatment taking place independently in the operating room. More commonly, clinical examination raises the suspicion of a deep injury that can be confirmed only by surgical exploration and intraoperative diagnostic techniques. For example, parotid duct transection can be diagnosed by duct cannulation, but this is also part of the therapy. Thus, diagnosis and treatment frequently are parts of the same process. Nerve and vascular injuries usually require surgical exploration for diagnosis and treatment.

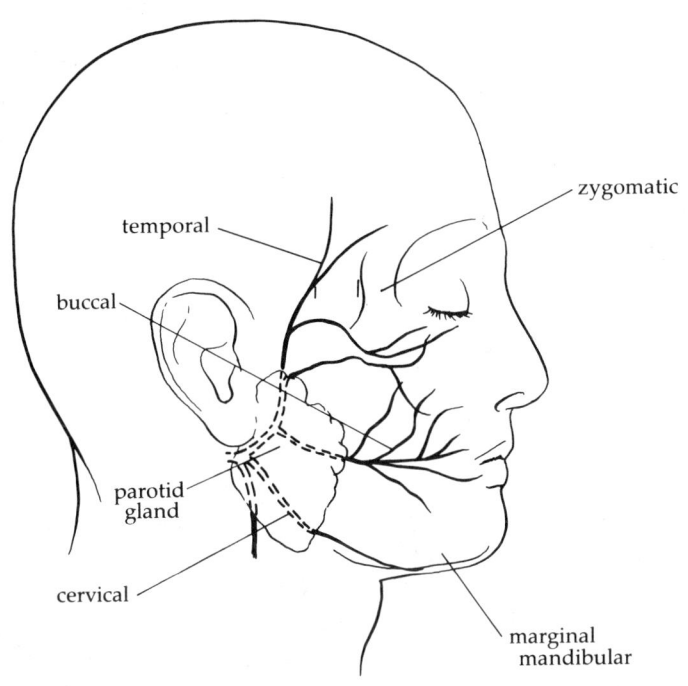

Figure 6-10. Anatomy of the facial nerve. The facial nerve exits from the stylomastoid foramen and immediately divides into a superior and inferior trunk. It then enters the substance of the parotid gland to ramify into five primary branches: temporal, zygomatic, buccal, mandibular, and cervical.

Deep Injuries of the Head and Neck

FACIAL NERVE

1. Diagnosis. The facial nerve (7th cranial nerve) innervates the muscles of facial expression and the sphincteric muscles around the eye and mouth. Any laceration or puncture wound of the face could injure a portion of the nerve. Thus, testing for nerve injury should be routine.
   a. Anatomy (Fig. 6-10). The facial nerve exits from the stylomastoid foramen in the sulcus between the mastoid process and the vertical ramus of the mandible as a single nerve trunk. The nerve bifurcates into two divisions, superior and inferior, and enters the substance of the parotid gland. In the proximal gland there are three main branches: the superior division gives rise to the zygomatic-temporal and buccal branches, and the inferior division continues as the mandibular-cervical branch. These three branches course through the parotid gland.

   There are many variations to this most common pattern. The portion of the gland superficial (closest to the skin) to the nerve is called the superficial portion of the parotid gland, and that part of the gland that is deep (closest to the oral cavity) is called the deep lobe of the parotid gland. Although these are not true anatomic lobes, the term is useful for descriptive purposes in parotid gland surgery. The major branches of the nerve exit from the parotid gland to the specific facial muscles. The region in which nerves exit the parotid can be identified by a line extending from the lateral canthus of the eye straight downward parallel with the anterior margins of the masseter muscle. As they leave the parotid, these branches are just below (deep to) the plane of the facial muscles.

The temporal branch from the parotid gland is at the level of the zygomatic arch, approximately 1 cm lateral to the orbital rim. The branches to the frontalis muscles, corrugators, and orbicularis muscles of the upper lid and some of the lower lid are from the temporal branch.

The zygomatic branch extends to the lower eyelid orbicularis muscle and to the muscles of the cheek and upper lip, including the buccinator, risorius, and caninus. The buccal branch can come from the upper trunk, lower trunk, or both.

The mandibular branch exits from the parotid gland at about the level of the angle of the mandible and 1 cm behind the mandibular rim. The marginal mandibular branch follows a course parallel with the mandibular rim to the region of the external facial artery and vein and then forms a 45° angle toward the oral commissure. The primary branch is to the depressor anguli oris and mentalis muscles. Additional branches to the platysma come from the main cervical trunk.

b. Tests of facial nerve injury

   (1) Frontal branch (Fig. 6-11). With the patient's head stabilized in a forward-looking position, the patient follows the examiner's finger. Move the finger in the superior direction. Observe for brow elevation and forehead wrinkling.

   Ask the patient to shut his or her eyelids tightly. The examiner attempts to elevate the upper eyelid against the resistance of the patient. This tests the orbicularis oculi muscle. A slight weakness of the affected side will be noted. Less wrinkling (crow's-feet) is noted.

   Ectropion of the lower eyelid may be noted, and the upper eyelid may not close completely. However, it is unusual to see ectropion in the emergency department, and this should alert the physician to the possibility of a previous nerve injury.

   (2) Buccal branch (Fig. 6-12A&B)

   (a) Ask the patient to smile or show the upper teeth and gums. Absence of a nasolabial crease or an asymmetric smile with shift of the mouth to the normal side are signs of injury.

   (b) Ask the patient to pucker the lips or to blow out an imaginary candle. This tests the orbicularis oris muscle. The patient may not be able to pucker the mouth and the teeth may be visible on the affected side. In addition, perioral wrinkles may not be formed.

   (3) Marginal mandibular branch (Fig. 6-12C). Ask the patient to show the lower teeth and gums. This tests the marginal mandibular branch to the depressor of the lower lip. The lip on the injured side will remain elevated relative to the downward movement of the contralateral side. The lower teeth may not be visible on the affected side.

   (4) Other tests. When there is a combined soft tissue injury with facial fracture or intracranial injury, a distinction must be made between a central nerve palsy (supranuclear) and a distal peripheral nerve palsy (infranuclear). The supranuclear palsy does not involve the temporal nerve branches to the frontalis and orbicularis oculi muscles because of intracranial crossovers.

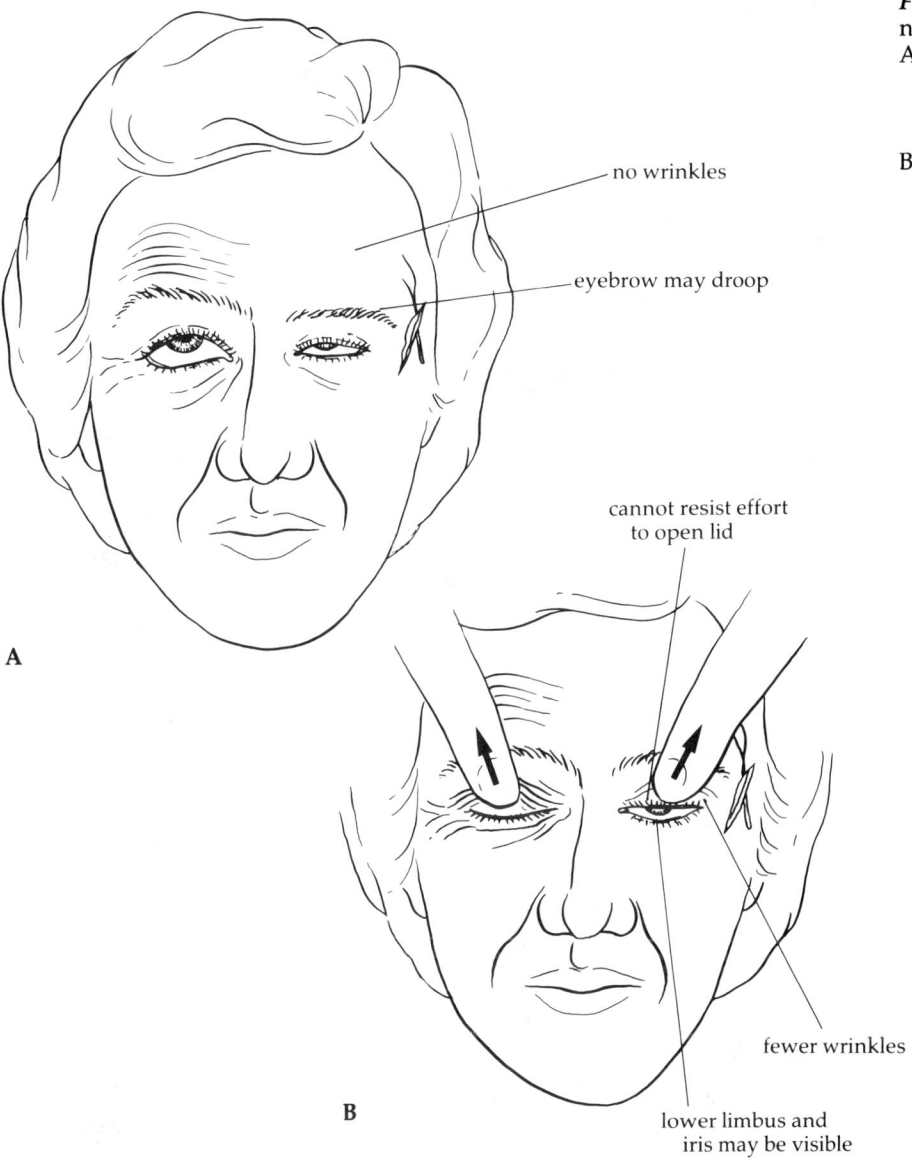

Figure 6-11. Testing frontal nerve paresis.
A. Ask the patient to look upward. Note absence of forehead wrinkles and ptosis of brow.
B. Pull upward on upper lids. Note absence of resistance to upward force on upper lid, fewer lateral (crow's-foot) wrinkles, and possibly, ptotic lower lid.

Central nerve palsies may show evidence of spontaneous involuntary movements, but there may not be voluntary muscle coordination.

Peripheral injuries involving the portion of the facial nerve within the temporal bone may show loss of chorda tympani function—lack of taste in the lateral portion of the anterior two-thirds of the tongue or dysfunction of the stapedius muscle with dysfunction of the tympanic membrane.

2. Treatment of facial nerve injuries (Fig. 6-13). Transection of a major branch to the facial nerve should be repaired with microsurgical techniques in the operating room. Identification of the transected branches may be easier if the wound is explored immediately rather than secondarily. In general, the major isolated trunks lateral to the line approximated by the lateral canthus and anterior margin of the masseter should

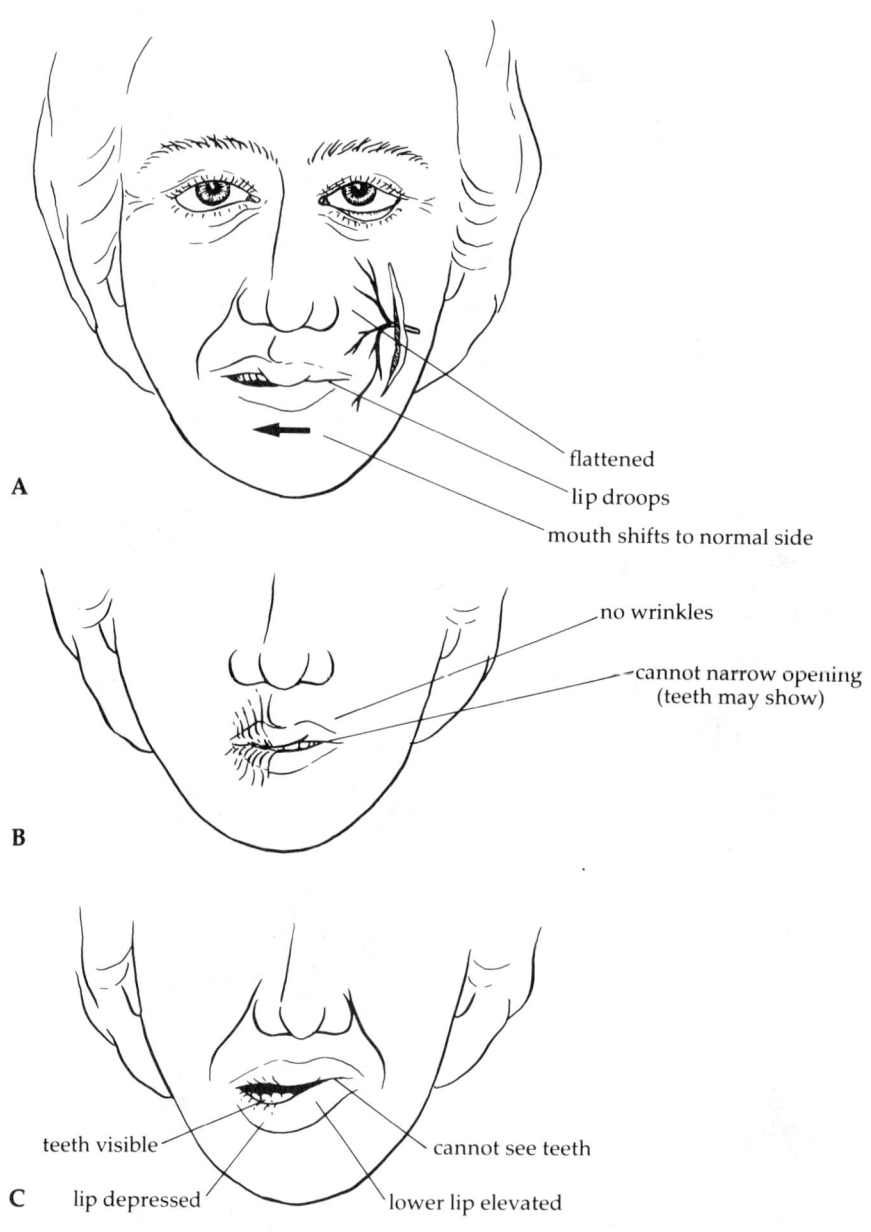

Figure 6-12. Testing buccal branch paresis.
A. Ask the patient to smile (or show teeth). Note flattened nasolabial crease and droop of upper lip.
B. Ask the patient to pucker lips. Note lack of wrinkles and lack of lip contact (teeth show).
C. The marginal mandibular branch is tested by asking the patient to show lower teeth. Note that lower teeth cannot be seen, and lower lip is elevated.

be repaired. Most of these are in the confines of the parotid. Centrally, the branches are small and have multiple crossovers that protect function. Moreover, the branches to the important eyelid and cheek muscles have received their innervation. These smaller peripheral branches should be repaired if identified, but good function may occur without repair because of crossover.

PAROTID DUCT

1. Diagnosis. A high degree of suspicion based on the anatomic location of the wound and confirmed by subsequent intraoperative wound exploration and duct probing leads to diagnosis.

   Injuries to the major salivary glands of the face (parotid and submaxillary) require surgical attention to prevent fistula formation or the ac-

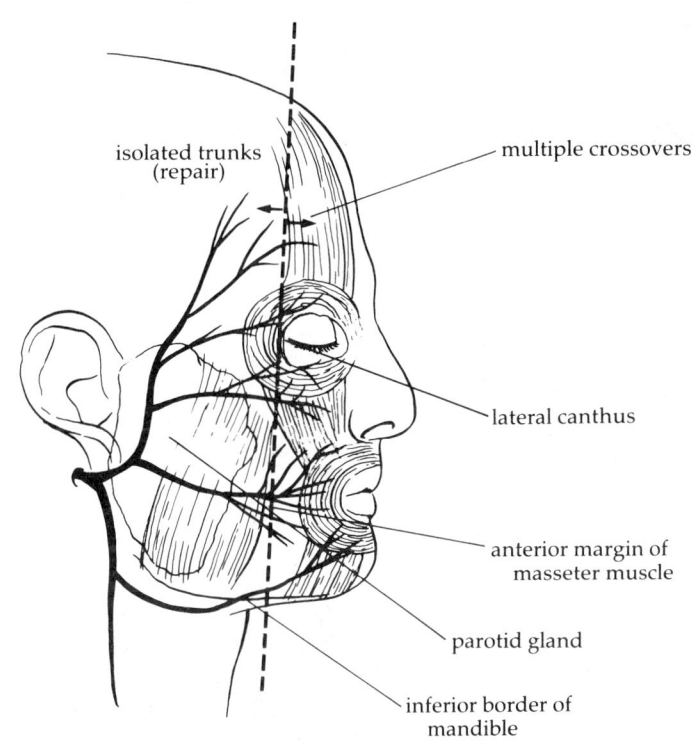

Figure 6-13. The facial nerve branches lateral to the line drawn from the canthus to the anterior masseter margin usually are major trunks that should be repaired. The buccal branches to the zygomaticus n., and risorious muscles usually are within the parotid gland.

cumulation of salivary secretion, which may act as a nidus for infection or retard healing.

a. Anatomy of the parotid duct (Fig. 6-14). The parotid gland is situated in the preauricular subcutaneous tissue. The boundaries are the vertical ramus of the mandible posteriorly; the anterior border of the masseter muscle anteriorly; the zygomatic arch superiorly; and the horizontal ramus of the mandible inferiorly.

The major parotid duct (Stensen's duct) courses anteriorly in a horizontal plane extending through the base of the nasal ala and the ear lobule.

The orifice is in the buccal wall just opposite the upper second molar tooth. The site can be identified by external landmarks. It lies at the intersection of the horizontal plane of the duct and a vertical line dropped from the lateral canthus.

After the orifice is identified, it should be probed with small lacrimal dilators. Care must be taken to allow the probe to slide through the duct and not create a false passage. The probe can then be seen in the facial laceration at the site of the distal end of the duct.

b. Tests of salivary duct transection

(1) Visual inspection. Occasionally it is possible to identify a transected parotid duct by visual inspection. A steady flow of salivary secretions may be visible in the wound. In many circumstances, however, there are extensive bleeding and ragged tissue ends that preclude adequate visualization. If duct transection is identified, the surgical repair should be performed in an operating room.

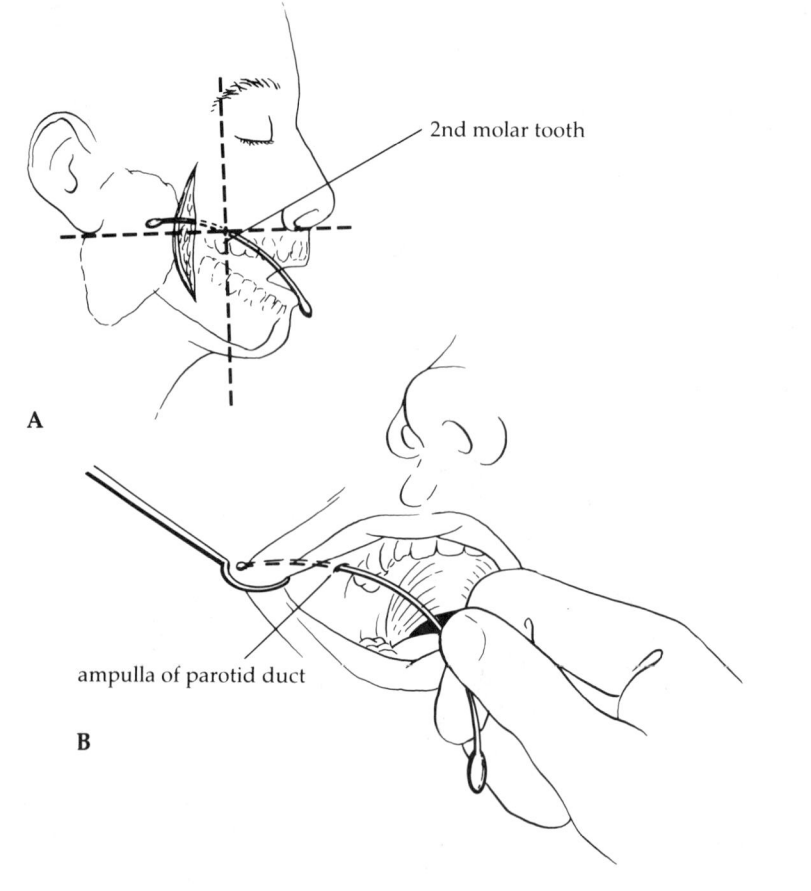

Figure 6-14. Parotid duct.
A. Several landmarks are useful for determining the location of the parotid duct. The duct generally runs along a line drawn from the ear lobule to the inferior alar border.
B. The orifice in the mouth is located opposite the second molar tooth. Externally, this can be located by intersecting the first line with a line perpendicular to the canthus.

  (2) Probing salivary ducts (Fig. 6-14B). Before closing a suspicious cheek laceration or penetrating wound in the region of the duct, a careful probing should be performed.
  Identify the intraoral papilla of the salivary gland orifice. The parotid duct is located adjacent to the maxillary second molar tooth. A slightly erythematous papular elevation may be identifiable. If it cannot be seen, the mucosa should be wiped dry, with careful observation for a small droplet of salivary secretion.
c. Treatment. A parotid duct transection can be treated in three ways: cannulation repair, internal drainage, or ligation. The choice of method is determined by the local anatomic conditions, other injuries, and availability of equipment and trained surgeons. Single, clean lacerations can be repaired (Fig. 6-15). The cannula should remain in place for at least 2 to 3 weeks. To lessen stenosis of the duct at the site of transection, the cannula should remain in place for up to 6 weeks.
  Multiple contaminated transections may need only internal drainage (Fig. 6-16). Lacerations involving the gland but not the duct require intraoral drainage only. Regardless of the method used, however, the injury must be recognized and treated to avoid cutaneous salivary fistula, wound dehiscence, and wound infection.

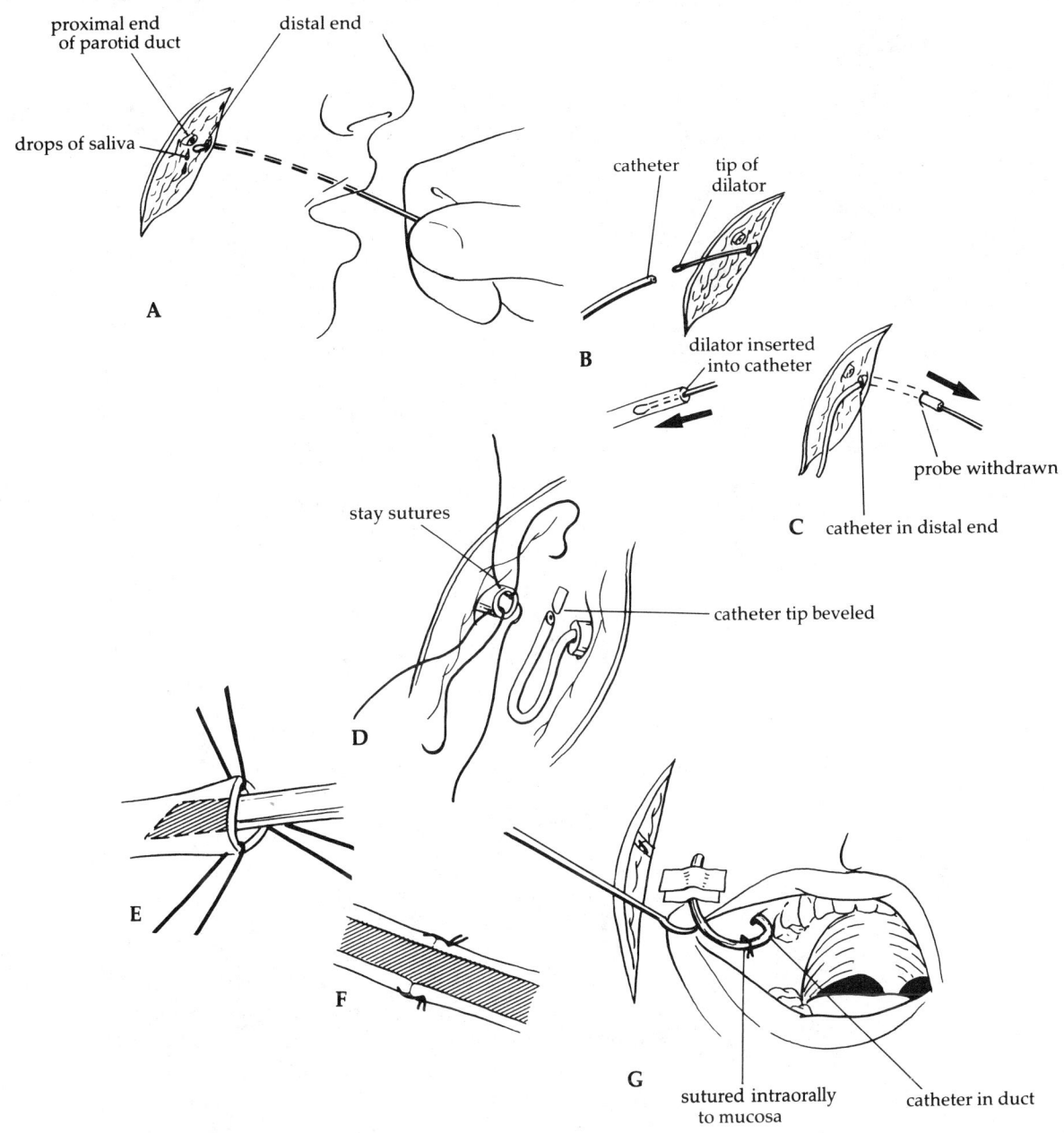

Figure 6-15. Repair of lacerated parotid duct.

A. Identify the proximal duct. (Its location is shown in Fig. 6-14.) Gradually enlarge the orifice so that the probe can be introduced. The lacrimal probe protruding through the distal portion of the transected duct is a helpful guide to identifying the approximate position of the proximal end. Visual inspection for saliva is required to identify the end precisely.

B. Place catheter over the probe.

C. Withdraw the probe. Thus, the catheter is carried with the probe through the distal end of the duct into the oral cavity.

D. A 7–0 or 8–0 chromic suture can be passed from the external surface of the proximal duct to the lumen in three separate points to triangulate the duct. The sutures can be used for stabilizing and spreading of the duct, which allows introduction of a catheter. The sutures are also used to anastomose the ends. The tip of the catheter should be cut to produce a beveled edge, allowing for more accurate placement of the tube.

E. Carefully introduce the beveled end of the catheter into the proximal duct. The duct can be dilated by careful probing with lacrimal dilators.

F. Pass the sutures previously used for traction through the distal duct from inside to outside and tie.

G. After the duct is repaired, suture the intraoral extension of the tube to the buccal mucosa so that it cannot slip out. Also, tape the end to the skin.

Figure 6-16. Drainage of parotid duct.
A. Place a small Penrose drain or catheter from the base of the glandular or ductile transection through the laceration into the mouth. If the laceration does not extend intraorally, communication should be established and the drain inserted in a similar manner.
B. Close the superficial portion of the gland and overlying skin and subcutaneous tissues.

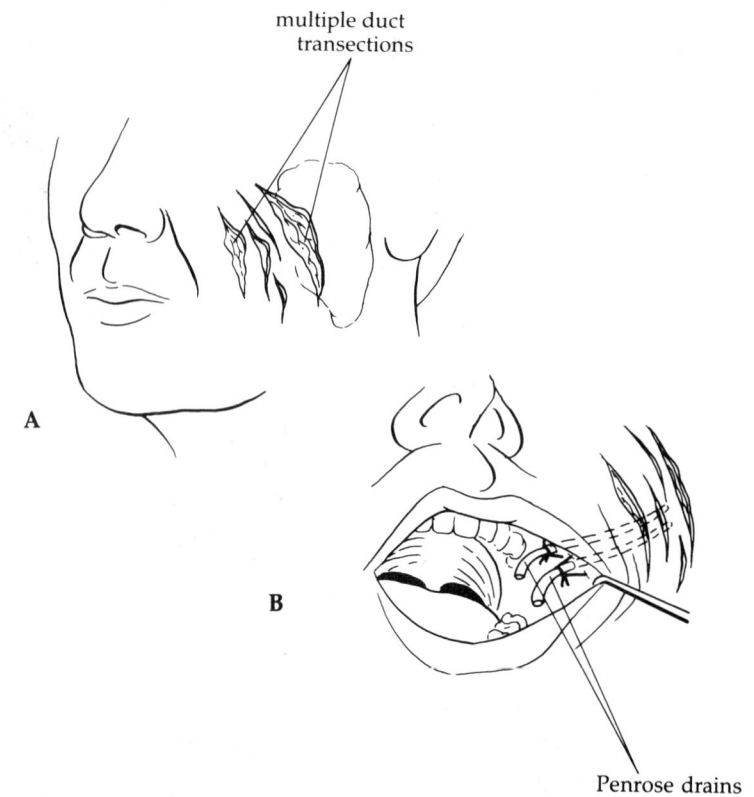

If there is an intraoral extension of the laceration, it should not be totally closed. Secretions from the transected gland can drain intraorally rather than externally through the cutaneous laceration. If the laceration is only cutaneous and not into the oral cavity, a drainage tract should be made. The drain should not be placed adjacent to the anastomosis.

NASOLACRIMAL DUCT
1. Diagnosis. An injury in the region of the medial orbit can transect the lacrimal apparatus. The initial diagnostic assessment should include visual inspection of anatomy and fluorescein tests, but definitive diagnosis may require lacrimal probing in the operating room.
   a. Anatomy (Fig 6-17)
      (1) The superior and inferior canaliculi pass behind the orbicularis muscle to enter the ampulla.
      (2) The ampulla is in the nasal bone behind the medial canthal tendon.
      (3) The nasolacrimal duct descends intranasally along the lateral nasal wall to exit below the inferior turbinate.
   b. Tests (Fig. 6-18)
      (1) Fluorescein, methylene blue, or other stains placed in the conjunctival sulcus can be identified in the transection site or intranasally with cotton gauze. Absence of fluorescein on the intranasal pledget suggests discontinuity because of complete transection or obstruction from clot, edema, or fractures.

PENETRATING INJURIES AND DEEP TRANSECTIONS

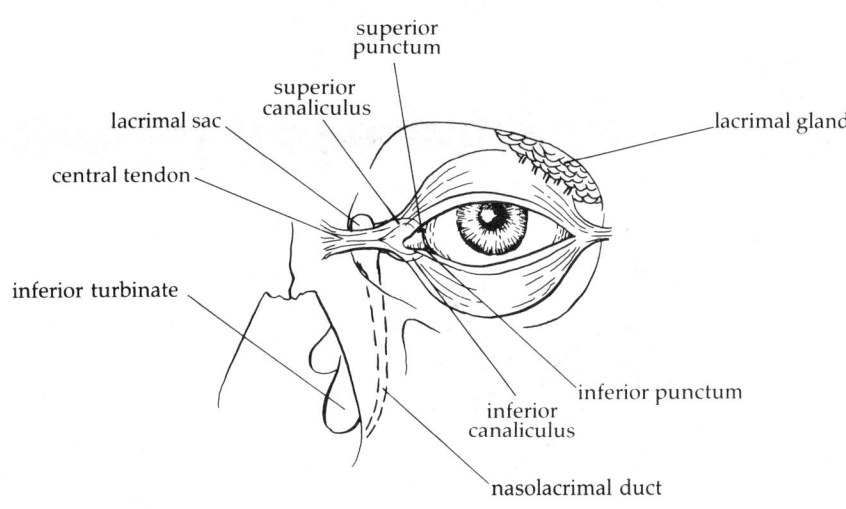

Figure 6-17. Anatomy of the nasolacrimal duct. The nasolacrimal apparatus is formed by the superior and inferior canalicular systems, which open onto their respective eyelids at the superior and inferior punctum. These canaliculi drain into the lacrimal sac located between the superficial and deep portions of the medial canthal tendon. The sac is drained by the intraosseous nasolacrimal duct, which opens under the inferior turbinate.

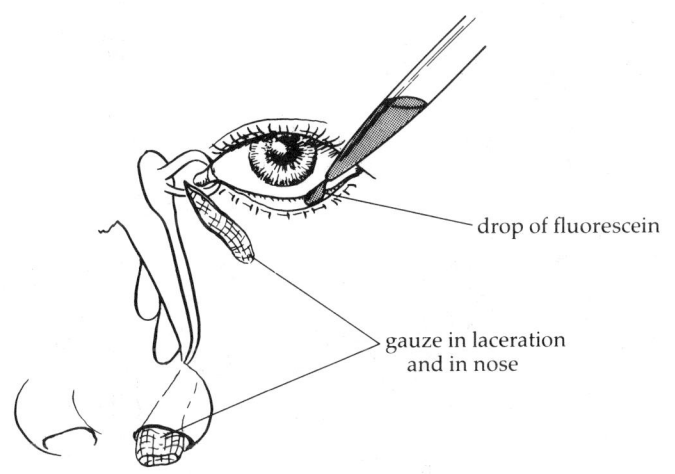

Figure 6-18. Testing for continuity of the nasolacrimal system. Place a dye that is compatible with the eye and conjunctiva, such as aqueous ophthalmologic fluorescein, over the inferior punctum. Place a gauze pledget in the laceration and also in the nose under the inferior turbinate. After several minutes, examine these pledgets under a Wood's lamp for fluorescence.

    (2) Dacryocystograms are not used for acute injuries.
    (3) Probing of the ducts is often required to confirm the diagnosis and treat the injury (Fig. 6-19). This should be done by the surgeon in the operating room. The methods of probing are discussed in the next section, along with treatment.

2. **Treatment.** The transection should be repaired at the time of injury. This can be achieved by either a straight tube stent across the anastomosis and into the ampulla or a stent loop through both canaliculi. Although either method can be used, the loop method is somewhat more difficult and requires a special instrument (pigtail probe), whereas the straight method is technically easier, although the stent is less easily immobilized and is therefore prone to be accidentally dislodged.

    It is estimated that 80 percent of tear drainage is through the inferior punctum. Thus, *it may not be necessary to repair superior canaliculus injuries.* Moreover, if the superior canaliculus is repaired, the straight stent method should be used to avoid inadvertent injury by the pigtail probe of the important inferior drainage system.

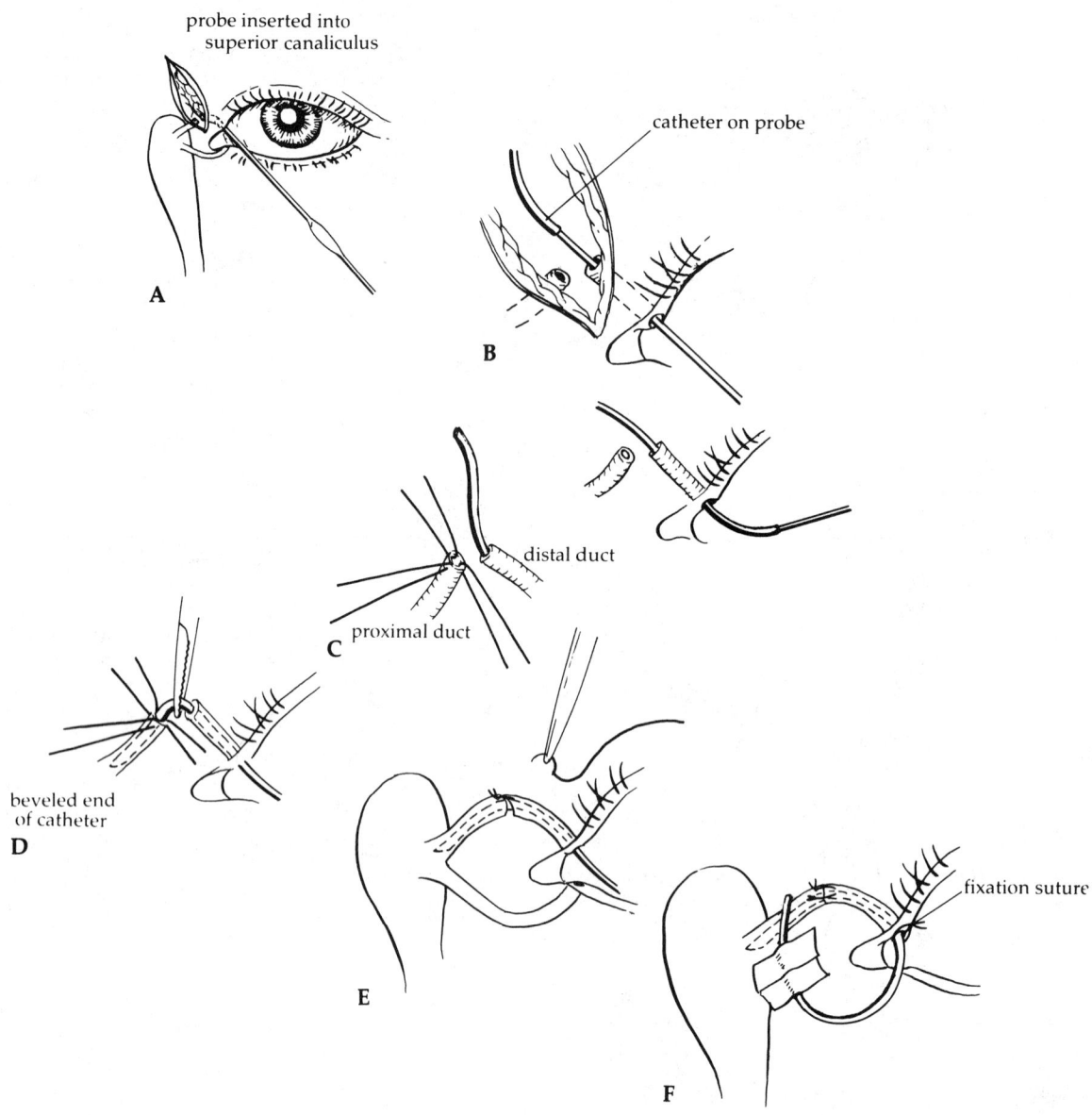

Figure 6-19. Probing the nasolacrimal duct.
A. Introduce the lacrimal probe via the punctum into the canaliculus. If there is a transected canaliculus, the probe will enter the open wound.
B. Place a catheter over the probe tip and pull back through the canaliculus.
C. Identify the distal canaliculus by careful examination. If it cannot be visualized, place a catheter in the inferior canaliculus and inject dye (methylene blue) into the ductal system until a droplet can be seen exiting from the transected distal end. Place traction sutures to triangulate the cut distal end of the canaliculus. Dilate the distal end with lacrimal probes.
D. Place the beveled end of the tube into the distal canaliculus. This is the most difficult and important maneuver.
E. Suture the canaliculus.
F. Fix the external tube with a silk suture and tape the end to the side of the nose.

The catheter stent should be left for 4 to 6 weeks to reduce the possibility of stenosis.

   a. Straight tube stent (Fig. 6-20). This method stents the injured canaliculus only and thus protects the uninjured canaliculus. The catheter tip is passed into the lacrimal sac and the end is sutured to the skin adjacent to the punctum. This method is used for superior canaliculus transections.

   A straight lacrimal dilator (beginning with the smallest size) is carefully placed through the punctum of the injured canaliculus. Progressively larger sizes are introduced until the duct is dilated sufficiently to allow passage of a catheter that is 1 or 2 mm in diameter. The larger probe is then advanced through the punctum at about 60° to 90° away from the lid margin and into the canaliculus. The probe is turned 90° and directed medially until it can be seen or felt in the laceration.

   b. Pigtail probe, or loop (Fig. 6-20). This method places a tube through both the superior and inferior canaliculi. It is commonly used for injuries to the inferior canaliculus. The main advantage of the pigtail probe is in identifying the distal cut end of the duct.

LEVATOR AND FACIAL MUSCLES

Lacerations of facial muscles should be repaired because muscle retraction causes sunken scars, aberrant scar movements, and decreased function (Fig. 6-21). More important, the levator and orbicularis muscles are essential for normal eyelid movements.

Diagnosis is made by careful observation before administration of local anesthesia so that movement of muscle ends can be seen and confirmed by intraoperative identification and repair. The repair is done with horizontal mattress sutures placed through the fascia.

VASCULAR INJURIES

The circulation to the head and neck is extensive, with multiple collateral vessels. Thus, vascular repair is not indicated except for injuries to the great vessels in the neck.

ORBIT AND GLOBE INJURIES

These injuries should be treated by the ophthalmologist. The responsibility of the emergency physician is to prevent additional injury by *immobilizing protruding foreign bodies and avoiding extrusion of globe vitreous or aqueous fluids*. Antibiotics and pain medications can be given after discussion with the ophthalmologist.

LARYNGOTRACHEAL AND PHARYNGOESOPHAGEAL INJURIES

These injuries are of major concern because of the *potential for spread of infection* from the intestinal tract or airway to the soft tissues and the mediastinum.

Voice changes suggesting laryngotracheal damage require evaluation by an otolaryngologist. These patients should be referred for consultation; only antibiotics or pain medication may be required.

Any stab wound of the neck is presumed to have injured the carotid artery and should be surgically explored in the operating room.

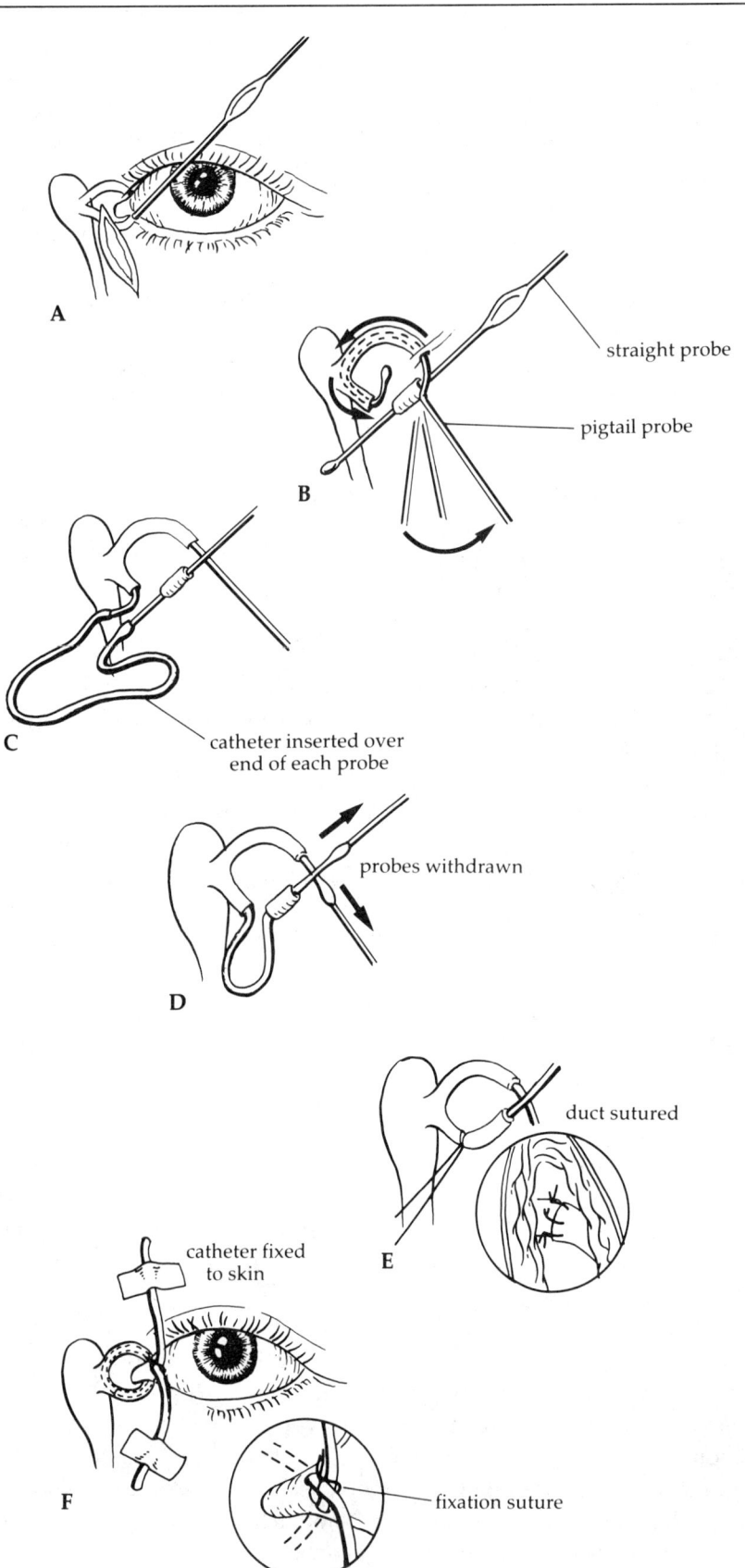

Figure 6-20. Cannulation of the lacrimal duct with a pigtail probe.
A. Place a straight lacrimal probe through the inferior punctum as described for the straight probe method.
B. Insert the pigtail probe through the superior punctum and carefully rotate the probe until it exits through the cut inferior canaliculus. (This is a technically difficult maneuver. The probe cannot be forced but should drop and slide by its own weight with minimal pressure.)
C. Place the ends of a catheter over the two probes.
D. Withdraw the probes, pulling the catheter through the puncta.
E. Suture the cut ends of the canaliculus, using a 6–0 or 7–0 nylon or absorbable suture (chromic, Dexon, or Vicryl).
F. Tie the catheter ends together and tape to adjacent skin.

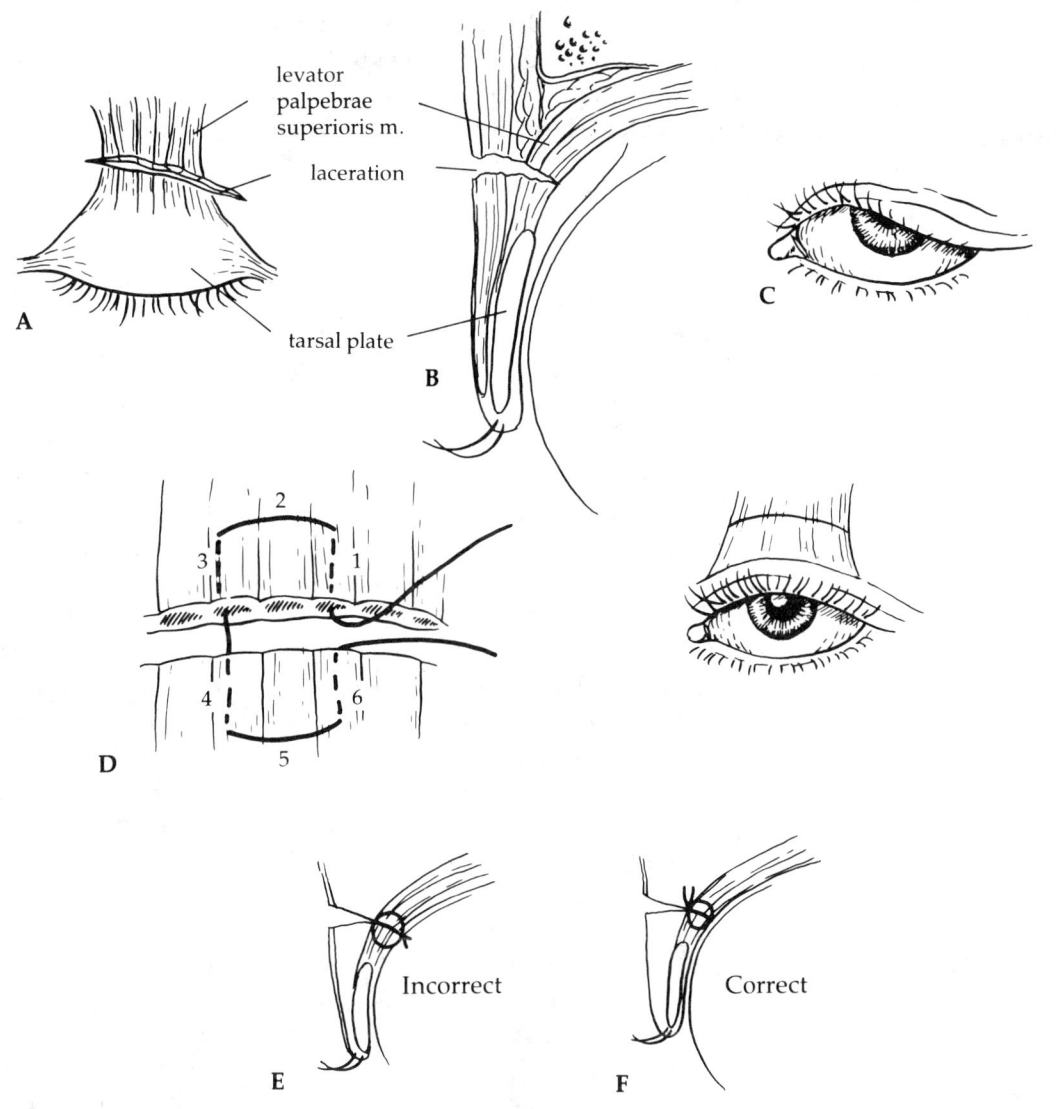

Figure 6-21.
A, B, and C. Transected facial muscles lead to sunken scars, dimpling of skin during muscle activity, and decreased movement and ptosis of distal attachment sites.
D and E. Facial muscles are repaired with a horizontal mattress suture. Care must be taken to avoid allowing suture ends to extrude into conjunctiva against globe.
F. Correct method of repair.

Deep Injuries of the Upper Limb

Injuries to structures in the distal arm and hand account for approximately one-third of all open injuries presenting to the emergency departments of metropolitan hospitals.

The priorities for care of compound injuries have been mentioned. This system of priorities also directs the sequence of the examination, with circulation evaluated initially, followed by skin cover, skeletal stability, and nerve and tendon function. The assessments for adequate skin cover and skeletal stability are discussed in Chapters 5 and 7. The emergency management of hemorrhage has already been discussed. What follows is a tissue-oriented approach to deep and compound wounds of the upper limb, presented in the order of preestablished priorities of care.

VASCULAR INJURIES
1. Diagnosis
    a. Anatomy
        (1) Arterial supply (Fig. 6-22). The hand gets its major blood supply from the radial and ulnar vessels and usually survives even if both vessels are transected at the wrist. Circulation reaches the hand through collateral vessels about the wrist. Although the hand survives, it is easily subject to poor healing and cold intolerance. If both vessels are transected, at least one should be anastomosed.
            A dual blood supply also exists in each digit. The same clinical circumstances of cold intolerance and poor healing are apparent for injuries to digital arteries.
        (2) Venous-lymphatic drainage. Venous and lymphatic drainage is primarily through subcutaneous vessels located in the *dorsum of the hand*. A constricting bandage or splinting in hyperextension at the wrist can easily inhibit venous and lymphatic draining from the hand. The vascular anatomy and the laxity of dorsal skin accounts for the ready swelling or edema in the dorsum of the hand. Injury or infection anywhere in the hand may manifest itself as dorsal swelling.
    b. Assessment of injury
        (1) Inspection
            (a) Bleeding. Injury to important vessels may be manifested by brisk arterial bleeding from the site of injury. Hemostats must not be blindly placed into the wound. These may damage adjacent uninjured tissues or additionally traumatize vessels that may later need to be anastomosed. Instead, direct pressure over the site of bleeding or an upper arm tourniquet inflated above arterial pressure may be lifesaving and avoids these potential problems.
            (b) Color. The other sequela of arterial injury may be a cool, pale, lifeless hand or digit. A bluish-red hand or digit with superficial venous engorgement indicates outflow obstruction.
        (2) Tests. Although final assessment must await intraoperative observation of the injured vessel, the following tests are helpful.
            (a) Pulse. The arterial system can be evaluated by such simple measures as palpating for radial, ulnar, or digital pulses.
            (b) Allen's test (Fig. 6-23) may localize the site of injury if this is not clear from observing the location of the wounds.
            (c) The Doppler test can both locate vessels and quantitate the flow.
            (d) Plethysmography also is useful in estimating flow.

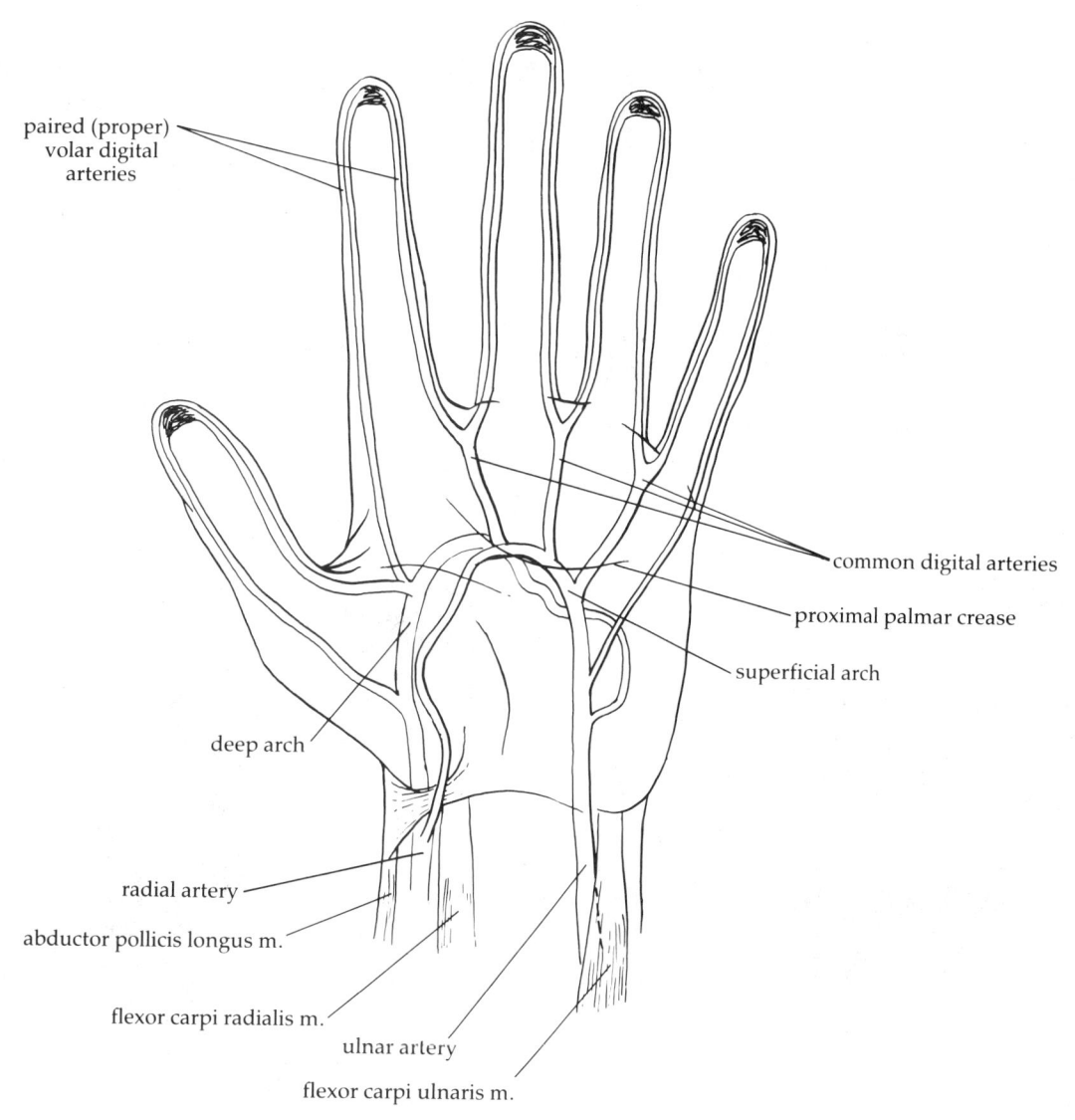

Figure 6-22. The vascular supply of the hand enters through the radial and ulnar arteries which interconnect via vascular arcades in the palm; the superficial arch gives off a common digital artery that provides the blood supply to the side of adjacent fingers. The relation of the wrist vessels to the wrist flexors is shown. The arcades are at the level of the distal palmar crease. The digital artery is 1 mm below the middigital axis.

(e) Vital dyes such as fluorescein act by staining tissues that are being perfused. Avascular tissue is not stained.

(f) Intracompartmental pressure. Circulation within some fascial compartments may be estimated by measuring the intracompartmental pressure, either directly, by placing a needle into the compartment (e.g., the interosseous muscle compartment), or indirectly, by radioactive scans.

2. Treatment of vascular injuries in the upper limb. We emphasize again that the emergency management of most injuries to major vessels consists of control of hemorrhage in the emergency room by direct pressure or tourniquet, followed by operative intervention. Occasionally, some definitive treatment of vascular injuries must be carried out in the emergency department. However, if a vascular injury is encountered, a therapeutic decision must be made whether the vessel should be ligated, repaired in the emergency department, or repaired in the operating

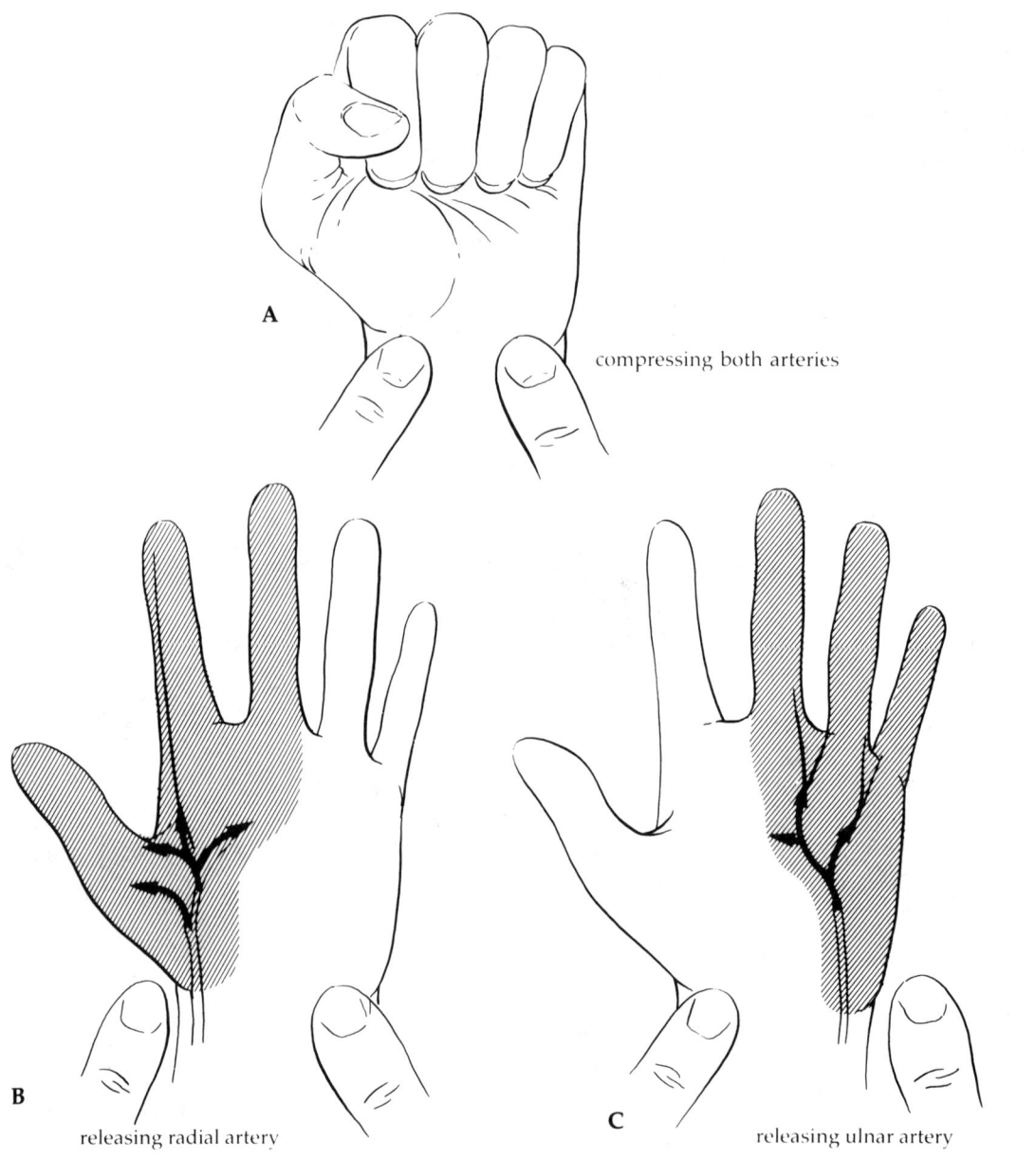

Figure 6-23. Allen's test. A. Both radial and ulnar arteries are simultaneously occluded at the wrist. What blood remains in the hand is milked out. B and C. Individually releasing either vessel and observing the hand for refill localizes a lesion to one or both vessels. If refill occurs through the radial artery, the hand must be reelevated and reoccluded before testing the ulnar artery (and vice versa).

room. The following guidelines are based on the assumption that the physician has sufficient experience and equipment.
  a. Emergency department ligation
    (1) Any veins except the femoral or brachoaxillary
    (2) Single, distal, small arteries (distal to wrist) of the extremity, if distal circulation is normal, there are *no other vascular injuries,* and *there is no physician available who can do microvascular surgery*
  b. Emergency department repair. Partial transections ("nicks") of large vessels may be repaired in the emergency department. The wound should be tidy and uncontaminated and have healthy distal tissues.
     Even these simple repairs require special instruments and should be done in the operating room whenever possible.
  c. Operating-room repair. The following injuries should be repaired in the operating room after control of bleeding by tourniquet, temporary ligature, or tamponade.
    (1) Complete or near-complete transections of major vessels (brachial, axillary, carotid, popliteal, femoral, iliac)
    (2) Complete or near-complete transections of medium or small arteries when there is distal ischemia

INJURIES TO THE MUSCLE AND FASCIA
1. The problems. Penetrating wounds or deep lacerations can transect major muscles and muscle fascia. Caution must be observed in repairing these injuries because of three major risks:
  a. Severe *necrotizing anaerobic infection* caused by gas-forming organisms (*Clostridium*) or mixed synergistic gangrene (*Staphylococcus, Streptococcus,* or *Pseudomonas*)
  b. *Pressure increase within an unyielding fascial compartment,* causing nerve and muscle ischemia and necrosis, or vascular compression with distal ischemia (Volkmann's contracture)
  c. *Muscle hernias,* causing discomfort and dysfunction
2. Diagnosis. Diagnostic examination is performed in the emergency department without anesthesia to determine function of major muscle groups in the region of the injury. Observe for:
  a. Oozing or hematoma. Muscle transection is associated with more bleeding than a comparable injury to fat or dermis. Moreover, the bleeding tends to recur with movement of that muscle group.
  b. Pain and tenderness. Muscle injuries are likely to be more tender than skin injuries because of hematoma in a closed compartment causing *nerve compression,* or because of *muscle spasm.*
  c. Limitation of muscle function. Muscle function may be decreased because of actual transection of the muscle or because of voluntary splinting or involuntary spasm.
  d. Deformity. A transected muscle may have an unusual bulge proximal and/or distal with a central depression at the injury site.
  e. Distal nerve or vascular dysfunction. Vessels or nerves within or adjacent to the muscle may be injured, the injury manifested by distal paresis, anesthesia, or ischemia.
3. Treatment. If only a fascial-muscle injury is noted, without nerve or vascular injury, the repair can be done in the emergency department.
  a. Fascial injuries (Fig. 6-24)

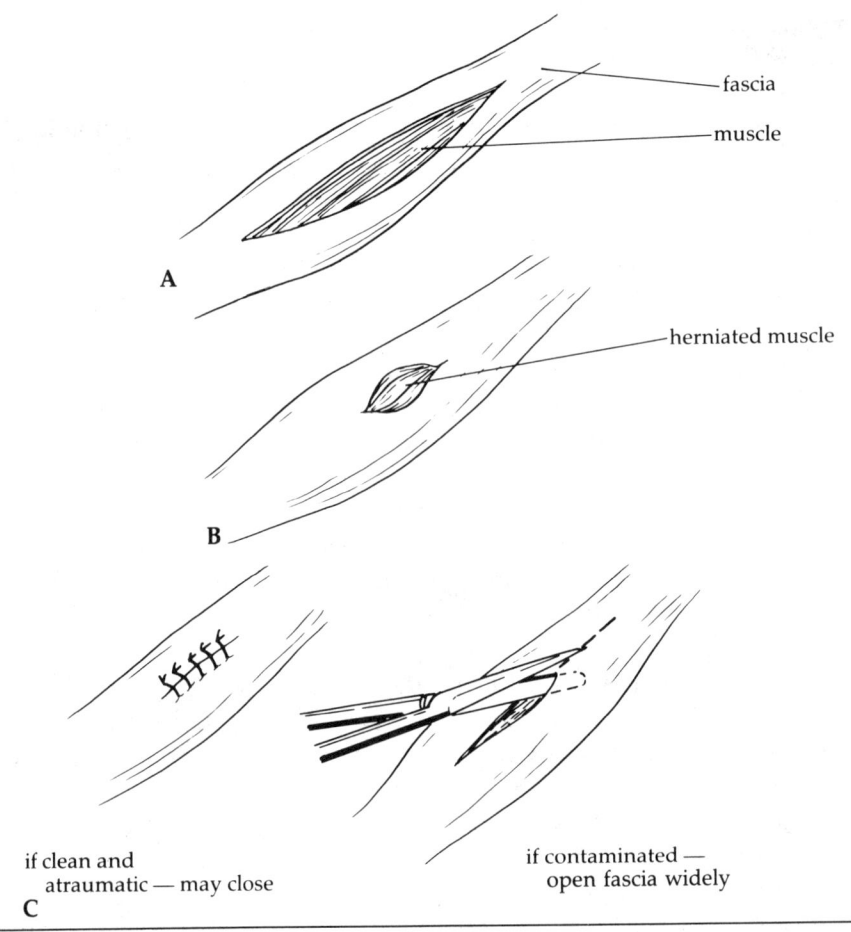

Figure 6-24. Fascial injuries.
A. Large fascial rents generally should not be repaired. The danger of repairing the rent is that undue muscle compression may occur.
B. Small rents may lead to symptomatic muscle herniations.
C. If it is a clean, atraumatic injury, it should be repaired with an absorbable suture such as 3–0 or 4–0 chromic catgut; if it is a contaminated traumatic injury, it should be broadened considerably by incising the fascia bluntly with the barely opened scissor tip.

(1) Large, atraumatic wounds. If only the muscle fascia is lacerated, without severe trauma to muscle and without herniation, the fascia need not be sutured because it will spontaneously reform.

(2) Small, traumatic fascial wounds. The fascia should not be repaired if there is major trauma or bleeding of muscle to avoid causing compartment compression. The fascial opening should be enlarged by pushing the slightly open blunt scissor tip down the fascia, which separates with ease.

(3) Small, atraumatic fascial wounds. A small fascial break can be repaired if adjacent tissue is healthy. A small fascial rent or unrepaired laceration may allow a muscle herniation.

b. Muscle injuries (Fig. 6-25). The objective is to debride devitalized tissue adequately and close healthy fascia but not to place sutures directly into muscle fibers. Incomplete laceration of muscle and fascia requires splinting for only 1 or 2 weeks before beginning gentle graded exercises. Complete lacerations require 2 or 3 weeks of immobility. The position of the arm and hand should relax the lacerated muscle group. It is unnecessary to splint uninvolved joints.

INJURIES TO TENDONS IN THE UPPER LIMB

Inherent to limb function is the independent gliding of tendons. In the profundus tendon, the excursion at the wrist is up to 7 cm from full wrist

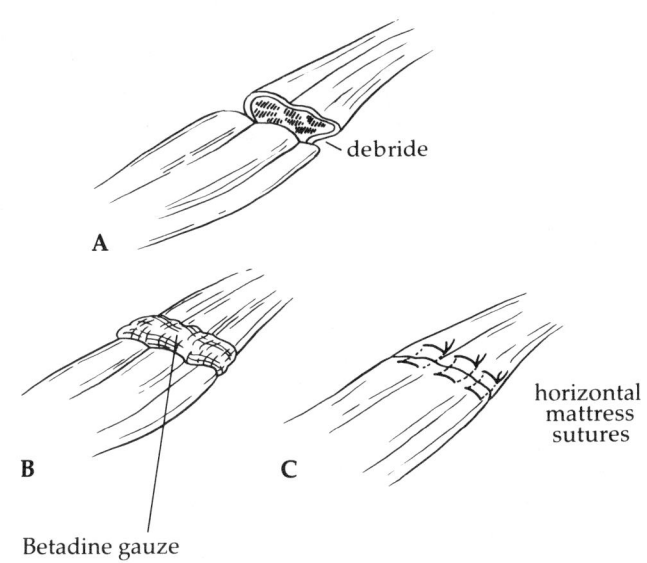

Figure 6-25. Muscle injuries.
A. Any contused or devitalized muscle must be debrided. If the muscle contracts as it is cut, it is likely to be healthy and unlikely to constitute a possible source of infection.
B. If doubt exists regarding muscle viability or there is severe contamination, pack the wound open with an iodophor (Betadine) gauze and perform a delayed closure or skin graft 3 to 5 days after the injury. Antibiotic prophylaxis should be used.
C. Because the structural integrity of muscle is very low, sutures placed in line with its fibers pull through with minimal tension. Close muscle lacerations by approximating the investing fascia with absorbable horizontal mattress sutures. Do not place sutures in muscle. They usually pull loose or increase the chance of infection.

flexion to full wrist extension. Trauma to a tendon or its sheath results in scar adhesions that resist motion. Therefore, a prime objective of a tendon repair is to avoid scar about tendons. Gentle technique, minimal dissection, and thorough cleansing and debridement (when necessary) are essential.

Although most tendons should be repaired by specialists in the operating room, there are circumstances in which specialists are not available or the injuries are not recognized until after emergency treatment has been instituted. Criteria for tendon repair in the emergency department include the following:

1. The physician has had previous experience with surgical method.
2. All surgical equipment is available.
3. The deep structure (e.g., nerve, tendon) is visible or easily accessible without need for extension of incisions, flaps, or undermining.
4. There is a clean, tidy wound.
5. The operating physician has no other emergency-department responsibilities that might require attention.
6. Delayed repair could jeopardize viability or function.
7. Delayed repair may result in foreshortening of the muscle belly, thus making direct approximation impossible or requiring extensive mobilization.
8. Repair is relatively simple and there is no advantage to using the operating room.

Not all these criteria need be satisfied, but in the physician's judgment there should be the potential for an outcome equivalent to what would be expected in the operating room.

For this reason, a brief review of tendon healing and the functional anatomy of this area follows.

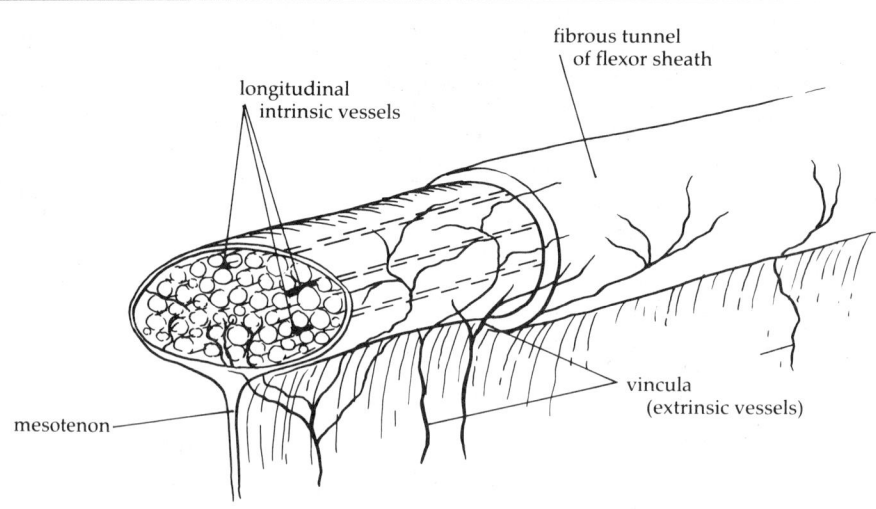

Figure 6-26. Vascular anatomy of tendons. In most areas a mesentery exists through which vessels pass to and from the tendon. In some areas, when the tendon passes through tight compartments such as the fibrous flexor sheath, the mesentery becomes more specialized, condensing into well-defined structures termed *vincula*.

1. Tendon healing
   a. Vascular anatomy of the tendon (Fig. 6-26)
      (1) The vascular supply of the tendon is through a unique mesotenon because of the tendon's specialized architecture and function.
      (2) For most of its length the tendon blood supply is derived from its mesotenon, which is a mesentery-like structure.
      (3) The mesotenon coalesces into filamentous strands (vincula) in the fibro-osseous sheaths of the digits and the carpal tunnels.
      (4) Most vessels from mesotenon and vincula surround the tendon surface. There are very few internal vessels.
      (5) Nutrition for the tendon is also derived from the synovial fluid.
   b. Mechanism of healing (Fig. 6-27). Tendon heals by the same sequence of hemorrhage, coagulation, inflammation, and scar formation as does skin. Because of the unique vascular anatomy, however, two patterns can occur, depending on the specific site and degree of immobilization.
      (1) Extrinsic pattern—"one wound, one scar." An immobilized tendon in continuity with the skin and other adjacent injured structures heals with scar adhesions. Capillary and fibroblast invasion comes from all surrounding tissues. Thus, scar incorporates all tissues as one wound.
      (2) Intrinsic pattern. Tendon can heal from fibroplasia within the tendon itself rather than from surrounding tissues. An injured tendon that has moved to an uninjured site or a repaired tendon not immobilized heals primarily from intrinsic sources. Peritendinous adhesions are lessened. For example, a flexor tendon transected with the finger in complete flexion, then repaired with the fingers in extension, results in tendon healing at a distance from the other injured tissues.
   c. Restoration of function. A balance must exist between tendon healing and gliding. Immobilization enhances healing and reduces the risk of early disruption by allowing initial ingrowth of scar, but it creates dense short scar adhesions that limit tendon sliding. Early

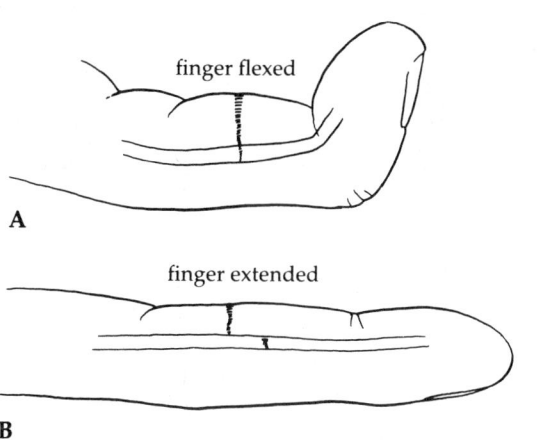

Figure 6-27. Healing of tendons.
A. A repaired tendon is allowed to heal in continuity with the cutaneous wound; healing is associated with fibrous adhesion among all parts of the wound.
B. A repaired tendon residing at some distance from the cutaneous wound, especially if the repair site lies within an undamaged flexor sheath, may heal with fewer scar adhesions.

mobilization allows for elongation of these fibrous adhesions and greater tendon sliding. However, mobilization performed too early or too forcefully may result in tendon disruption. The period of immobilization depends greatly on the location of injury and thus is discussed within the context of specific sites.

2. Diagnosis
   a. Flexor tendons
      (1) Anatomy (Figs. 6-28, 6-29, and 6-30). The flexor tendons cross the wrist joint volar to its axis. Usually 12 tendons function to flex the wrist and digits. Three tendons—the flexor carpi radialis, flexor carpi ulnaris, and palmaris longus (occasionally not present)—primarily flex the wrist and deviate the wrist either radially or ulnarly. The remainder pass into the digits through a tunnel—the carpal tunnel—formed by a dense ligamentous roof, and the bony sides and floor of the fixed transverse arch formed by the distal row of carpal bones. A single tendon, the flexor pollicis longus, inserts on the distal phalanx of the thumb, but two flexor tendons go to each remaining finger.

      The flexor digitorum superficialis tendon (Fig. 6-31A) inserts at the midportion of the middle phalanx and flexes the proximal interphalangeal joint. The profundus tendon lies deep to the superficialis tendon over most of their course from the forearm. At the level of the metacarpophalangeal joint, it perforates the superficialis tendon to become superficial to it over most of the proximal and middle phalanges. It inserts at the base of the distal phalanx and acts primarily to flex the distal interphalangeal joint.

      The intrinsic muscles of the thumb—the abductor pollicis brevis, flexor pollicis brevis, opponens pollicis, and adductor pollicis—act in concert with the long flexors and extensors to carry the thumb through its intricate range of motion. Hypothenar muscles act similarly at the ulnar border of the hand.

      On the flexor side, the median nerve supplies all flexors except the flexor carpi ulnaris and the two ulnar flexor digitorum pro-

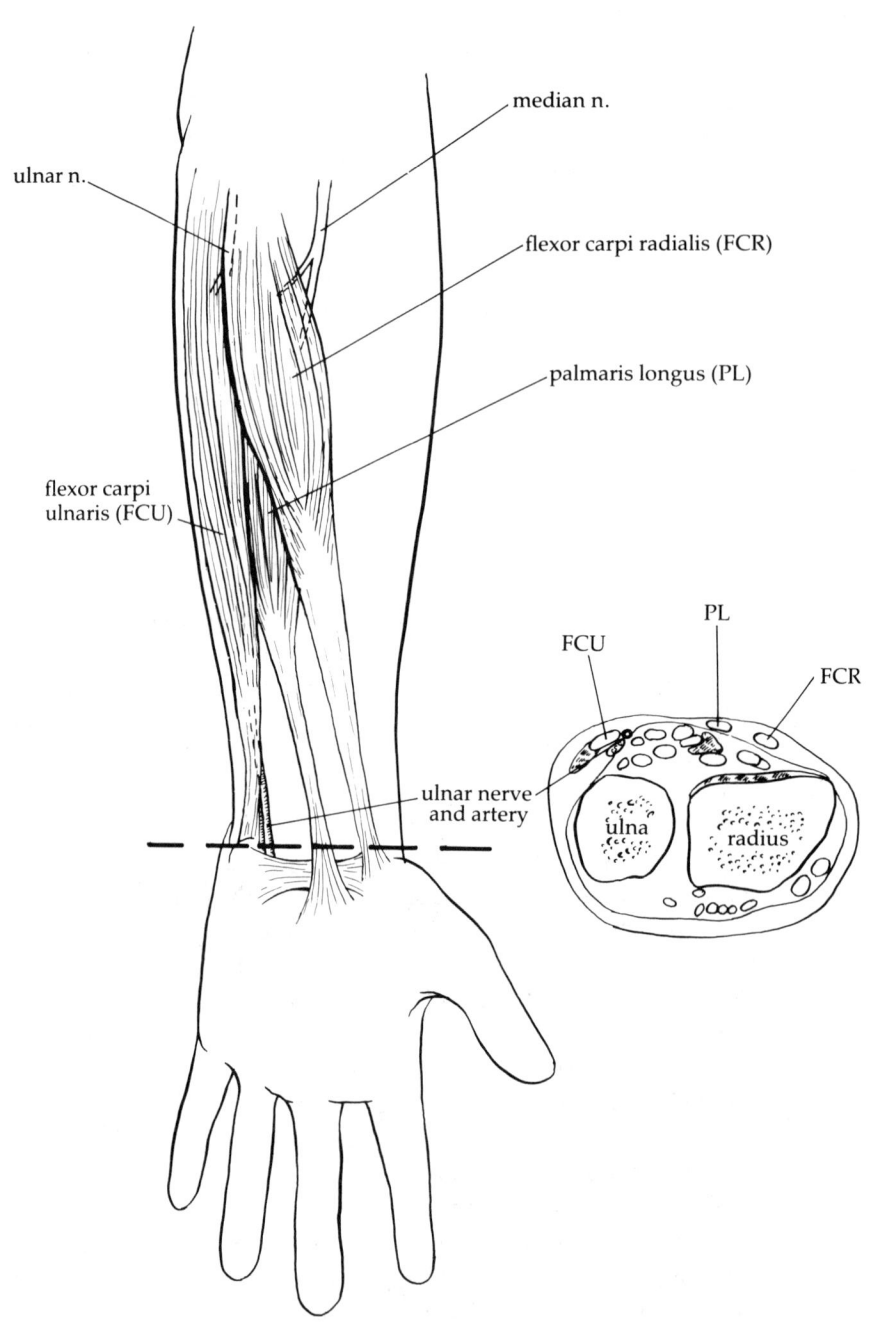

Figure 6-28. Anatomy of the superficial volar forearm muscles. The flexor carpi ulnaris (FCU) inserts onto the pisiform. It acts to flex and deviate the wrist ulnarly and is innervated by the ulnar nerve. The palmaris longus (PL) becomes continuous with the palmar fascia. It is absent in 20 to 40 percent of people, either unilaterally or bilaterally. The flexor carpi radialis (FCR) inserts on the volar base of the second metacarpal. It acts to flex and radially deviate the wrist. Both the PL and the FCR are innervated by the median nerve.

fundus muscles. These are innervated by the ulnar nerve. In the hand, the median nerve supplies all the thenar intrinsic muscles on the radial side of the flexor pollicis longus and the two radially located lumbrical muscles to the index and middle finger. All other intrinsic muscles are supplied by the ulnar nerve. These anatomic relations are discussed in detail in the following sections of this chapter.

Flexor tendon sheaths (Fig. 6-31B) begin at the level of the metacarpal head in the palm. The two flexor tendons become surrounded by fibrous tunnels, the flexor tendon sheath. This

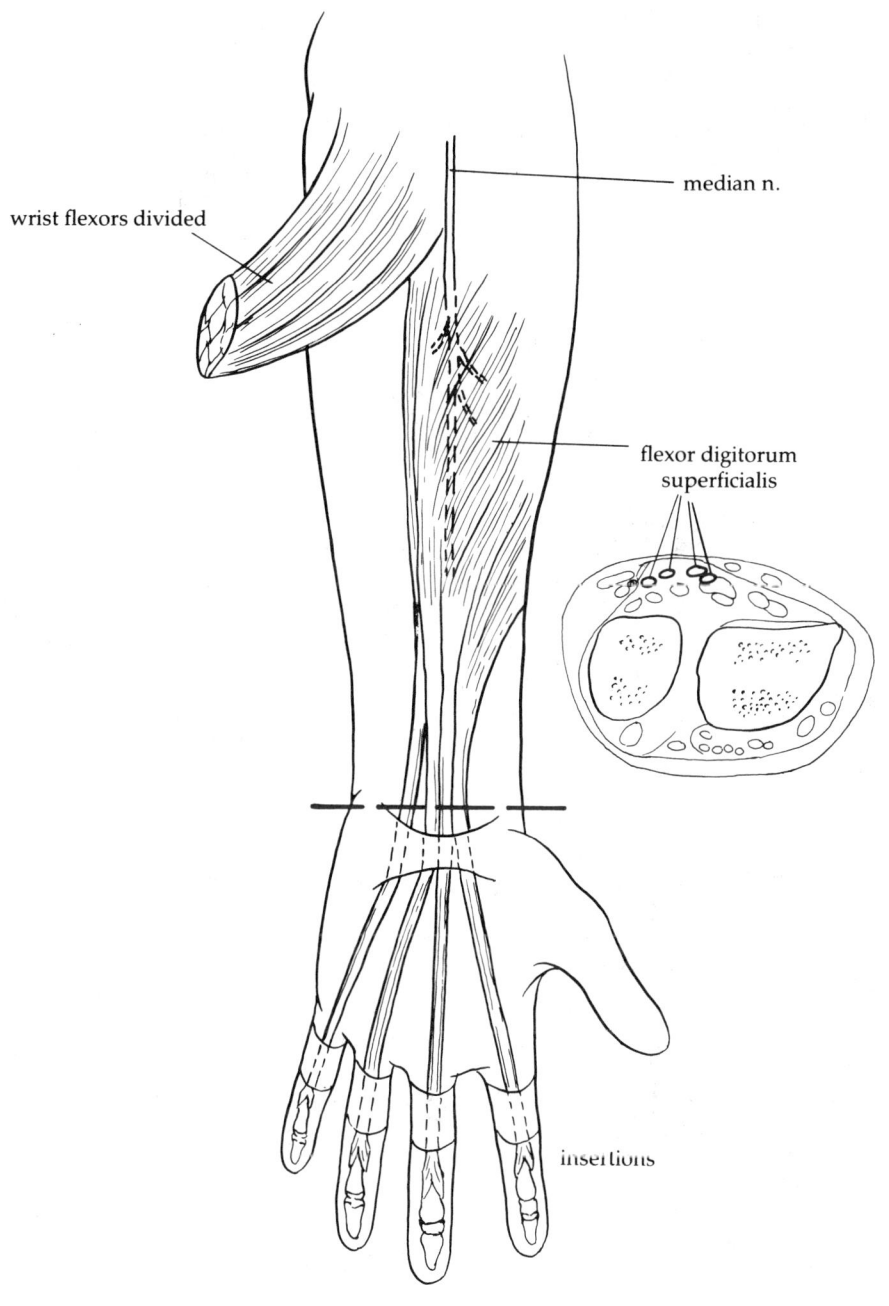

Figure 6-29. The middle group of flexor muscles is innervated by the median nerve—the tendons pass under carpal and flexor tunnels to insert on the middle phalanx.

sheath prevents bowstringing of the flexor tendons. The dense areas act as pulleys to increase the efficiency of movement.

(2) Testing of flexor tendons. All muscle groups in the area of injury should be tested. Loss of movement may indicate injury to the motor nerves supplying specific muscle groups or discontinuity anywhere between muscle origin and tendon insertion. It is useful to demonstrate with your own hand the exact motion you wish the patient to perform. This is particularly important when examining a child.

The wrist flexors are easily palpated as the patient forcefully

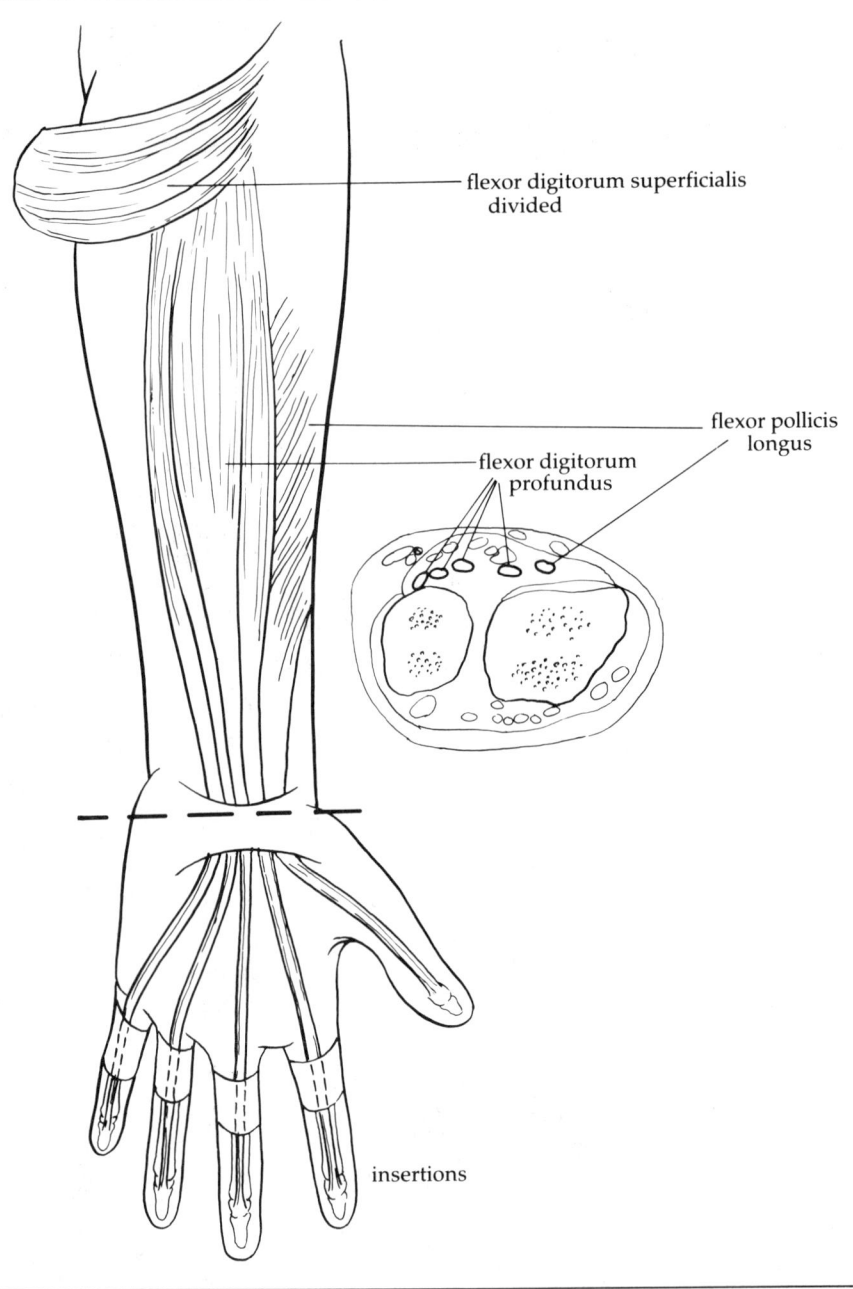

Figure 6-30. The deep group of flexors is innervated by both the median nerve, II and III, and the ulnar nerve, IV and V, and passes under the carpal and flexor tunnels. The median innervated flexor pollicis longus is included in the deep group.

flexes the wrist against resistance. The opposite uninjured limb is used for comparison.

Testing for independent function of flexor tendons is illustrated in Fig. 6-32. Several specific tests are helpful, particularly for evaluating tendon injury. A partial tendon laceration is suspected when pain is produced by resisting the normal extension of the tendon. If resistance produces minimal pain, a minimal laceration is present, whereas severe pain may indicate a nearly complete laceration. It is important to splint the wound while testing to eliminate wound pain.

The flexor superficialis and profundus tendons are tested for each finger in sequence as shown in Fig. 6-32. This requires

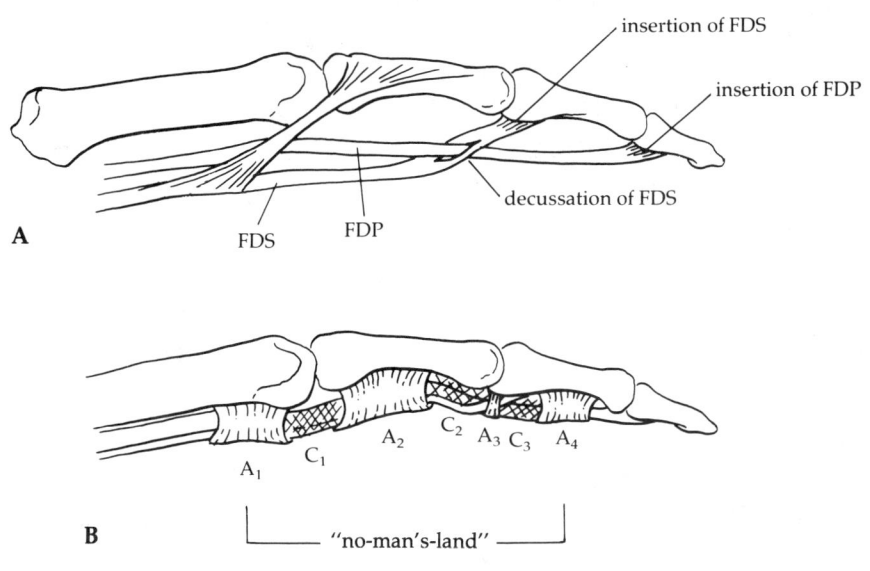

Figure 6-31. Anatomy of the flexor tendons in the digits.
A. The decussation of the flexor digitorum superficialis (FDS) at the level of the proximal phalanx allows the flexor digitorum profundus (FDP) to assume a more superficial position on its way to insert at the base of the distal phalanx.
B. The arrangement and location of the annular, or pulley, portions of the fibro-osseous flexor sheath. This area, A1–A4, is termed *no-man's-land* because of the poor results of primary tendon repair within this sheath.

immobilization of the other parts of the flexor system by the examiner.
b. Extensor tendons
   (1) Anatomy (Fig. 6-33). The extensor tendons cross the wrist joint dorsal to its axis of rotation and are separated on the dorsum by six compartments. The fibrous roof of these compartments prevents the tendons from bowstringing when the wrist extends.
   On the dorsum of the fingers (Fig. 6-34), the extrinsic digital extensors are assisted in extending the interphalangeal joints by tendinous contributions from several of the intrinsic hand muscles, primarily the interosseous and lumbrical muscles. Here the extensor tendon becomes a broad fibrous sheet or aponeurosis. Because of the various attachments and interrelations, the prime extensor function of the intrinsic muscles is at the interphalangeal (IP) joints, whereas the principal function of the extrinsic extensor tendons is to extend the metacarpophalangeal (MP) joints.
   (2) Testing of extensor tendons (Figs. 6-34 and 6-35). Extensor tendons are tested by evaluating the excursion of the joints about which the tendons display their prime function.
      (a) The primary function of the extrinsic extensor is to extend the MP joints.
      (b) The intrinsic extensors extend the IP joints.
      (c) Injury to isolated portions of the extensor mechanism presents characteristic clinical findings. The prime action of the extrinsic extensor is MP extension. Division of this tendon proximal to the MP joint results in inability to extend the MP joint *fully*. Laceration of the central slip results in inability to extend the proximal interphalangeal (PIP) joint fully, and laceration of the extensor mechanism beyond the PIP joint may result in a dropped tip (mallet finger or baseball finger).

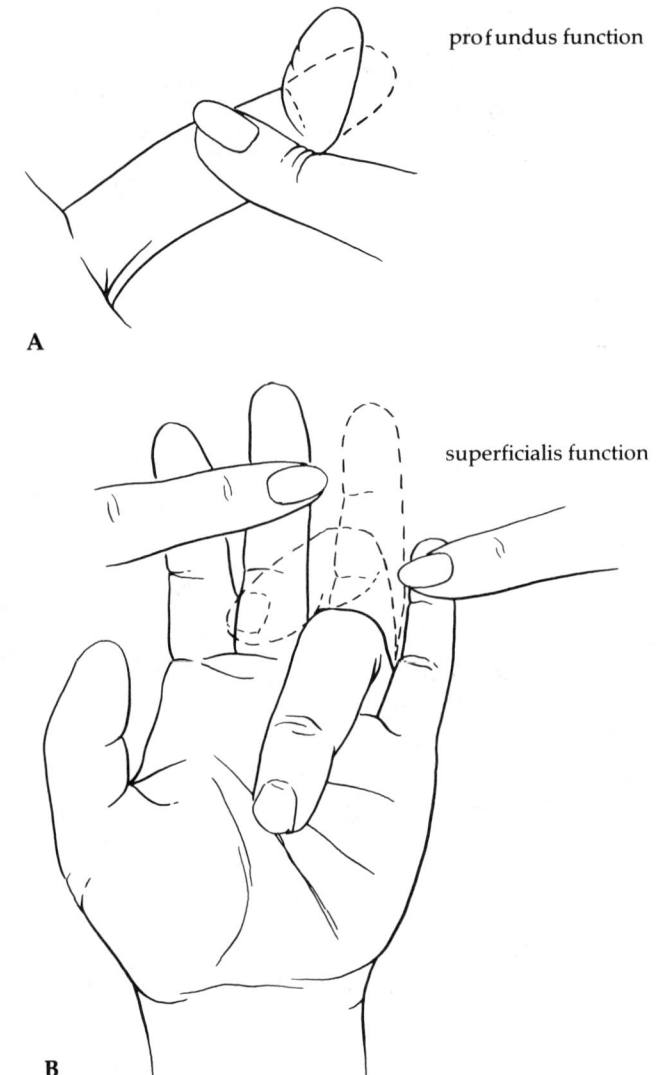

Figure 6-32. Tests of flexor tendon function.
A. If the proximal interphalangeal joint is splinted in extension, active flexion of the distal interphalangeal joint indicates a functioning profundus tendon.
B. The independent superficialis tendon is evaluated by holding adjacent digits in extension. If the patient can flex the PIP joint actively with the distal joint in extension, the superficialis tendon is intact.

    (d) The buttonhole deformity is characterized by flexion at the PIP joint and compensatory hyperextension at the distal interphalangeal (DIP) joint. It is a late sequela of laceration to this central slip and separation of the triangular ligament. The lateral bands fall volar to the axis of rotation of the PIP joint and can no longer assist in extension of the PIP joint.

  c. Intrinsic hand muscles. Limitation of motion of the thumb, particularly inability to abduct the thumb away from the plane of the palm, is most often caused by median nerve injury. However, lacerations over the thenar eminence may transect these muscles. This injury is easily diagnosed by visual inspection of the wound. Inability to abduct or adduct the thumb actively, or to abduct the index finger at the MP joint in the face of small puncture wounds over the thenar eminence or palm, is usually secondary to nerve injury, either median or ulnar.

  d. Pitfalls in tendon examination. A movement may be present or appear to be present in spite of injury to structures normally responsi-

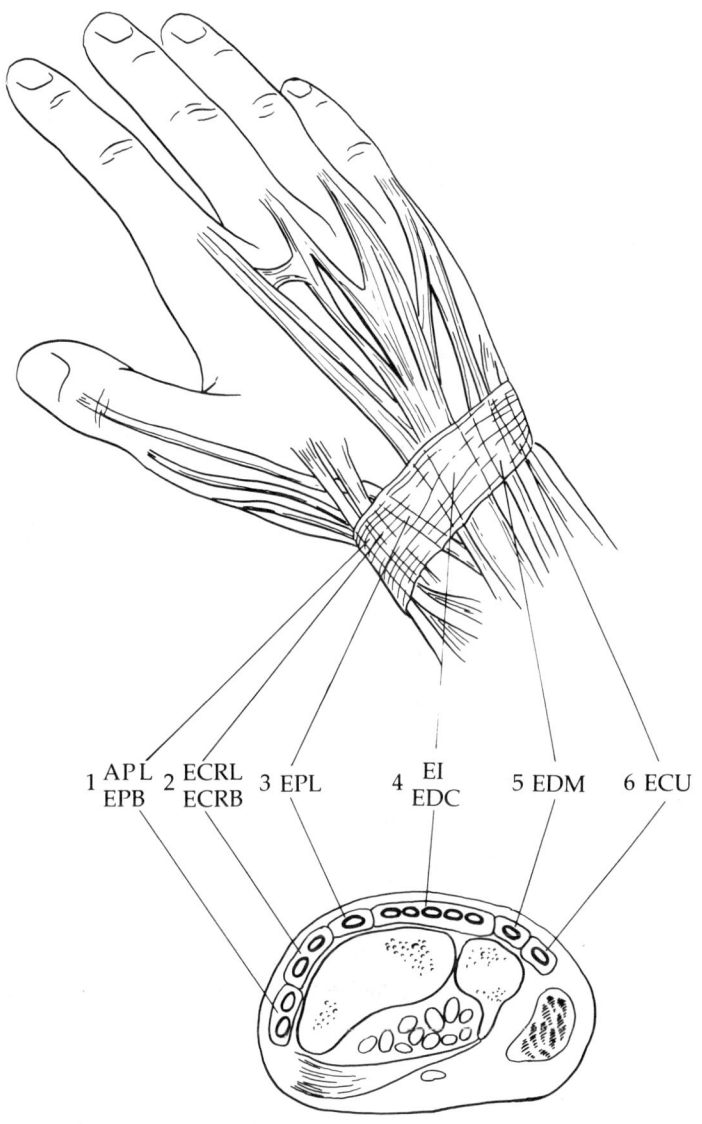

Figure 6-33. The extensor tendons pass through six tunnels in groups, as indicated. APL = abductor pollicis longus; EPB = extensor pollicis brevis; ECRL(B) = extensor carpi radialis longus (brevis); EPL = extensor pollicis longus; EI = extensor indicis; EDC = extensor digitorum communis; EDM = extensor digiti minimi; ECU = extensor carpi ulnaris.

ble for movement. For example, weak extension of the MP joint may occur through intertendinous connections, although the principal extensor slip has been divided.

Transection of the profundus tendon can be overlooked if each digit is not independently tested. The patient can open and close the fist by trapping the injured digit with an adjacent one, thus appearing to have full flexion.

When the long extensor of the thumb is divided, the thumb tip can still be extended through intrinsic muscle contributions to the extensor mechanism. Testing for independent function of the extensor pollicis longus (EPL) requires the patient to demonstrate the ability to extend the entire ray in the so-called hitchhiking position.

Diagnosis of injuries to the central slip mechanism at the PIP joint is difficult, particularly with closed crush injuries. The patient may appear to extend the PIP joint through the intact lateral band. If the

Figure 6-34. Digital extensor anatomy.
A. Over the digit, the extensor mechanism becomes an aponeurosis, or flat sheet, formed by both extrinsic and intrinsic extensor contributions. This system is most vulnerable to injury where important tendon coalescence occurs (e.g., at the central slip and distal insertion). Here, the extensor mechanism is better defined, more tendon-like.
B. The deformity and limitation of extension at the three different sites.

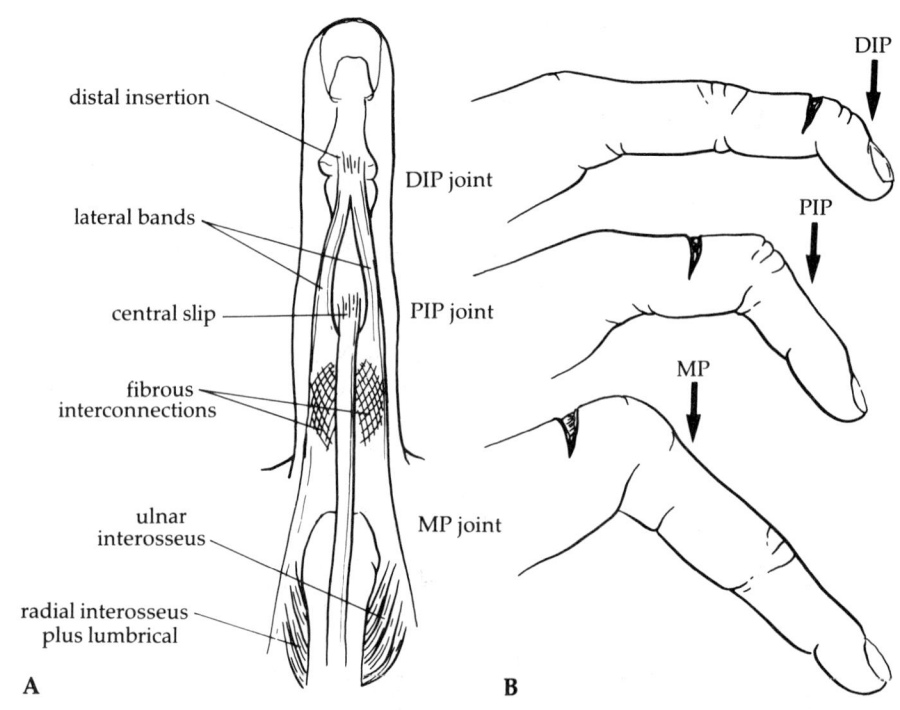

injury is missed and the digit not splinted, any remaining fibers may be disrupted and the lateral bands may fall below the axis of joint rotation and no longer be able to extend the PIP joint. The result is the so-called buttonhole, or boutonniere, injury.

3. Management of tendon transections
   a. Partial transections
      (1) If at least one-fourth of the tendon is in continuity, there is adequate strength without sutures.
      (2) Surgical repair only increases the scar adhesions because of surgical manipulation and sutures.
      (3) One-fourth of a tendon can be adequate for good healing and eventual function if postoperative immobilization or limited protected motion is instituted. For lacerations of approximately one-half of the tendon, the investing paratenon can be tacked together with a 7–0 or 8–0 monofilament nylon suture.
      (4) The surrounding fascia can be partially excised if the cutaneous and fascial lacerations directly overlie the tendon laceration.
      (5) The tendon should be immobilized so that the skin wound does not overlie the tendon wound. When lacerations occur with the finger in flexion, the tendon and sheath lacerations are not overlying each other if the finger is immobilized in extension.
      (6) The length of time for immobilization varies according to the degree of injury. A minimal laceration (less than 25%) may require only the immobilization necessary for good cutaneous healing (7–10 days). A more complete laceration might warrant 2 to 3 weeks of immobilization in association with guarded exercises.
   b. Isolated wrist flexors (Fig. 6-36). Isolated wrist flexor tendons (flexor carpi ulnaris, flexor carpi radialis, and palmaris longus) may be

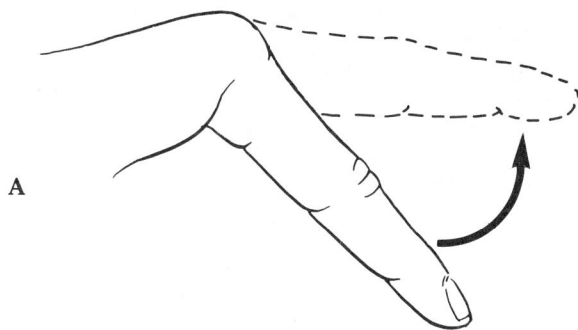
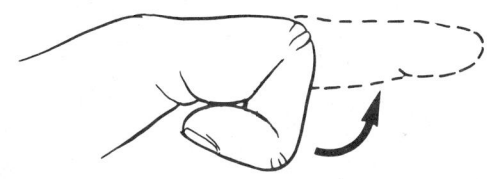

Figure 6-35. Extrinsic and intrinsic extensor systems.
A. The prime function of the extrinsic extensor system (EDC, EI, EDM) is to extend the digit at the MP joint.
B. The intrinsic system cannot extend the digit at the MP joint but is the principal extensor system for the IP joints.

amenable to treatment in the emergency room. These may be injured at the level of the muscle tendon juncture.

An unrepaired isolated wrist flexor will reconstitute itself because of its position within the tendon sheaths and because of its limited excursion. The wrist should be immobilized in slight flexion. This argument may appear to speak against repairing any isolated lacerations of the wrist flexor tendons; however, if both the flexor carpi radialis and the flexor carpi ulnaris are divided, weak wrist flexion may result. Factors such as vocation and age are the primary determinants of the need for repair of divided wrist flexor tendons. In an elderly person, for example, 3 to 4 weeks of wrist immobilization after repair may cause serious and prolonged residual joint stiffness. In a heavy laborer, however, a strong wrist flexor is essential and the risks of immobilization are acceptable.

The method of repair is illustrated in Fig. 6-36. Deeper injuries involving the finger flexors at the wrist should be treated in the operating room because there are often additional injuries to nerves not easily diagnosed without adequate exploration. Following repair, the wrist should be immobilized in 20° to 30° of flexion for about 3 weeks. This is followed by a period of graded exercises.

c. Palmaris longus tendon. This tendon is not essential for wrist function. Therefore, the ends can be debrided so that they are not adjacent to the healing wound. Repair can be done but is not essential. *Be sure the median nerve has not been injured and mistaken for a tendon end!*

d. Extensors in the arm and wrist (Fig. 6-37). Isolated extensor tendon lacerations about the distal forearm or wrist may be repaired in the emergency room. If muscle contraction occurred at the time of tendon division, the tendinous portion of the motor unit may retract within its muscle, making identification difficult through the usually small laceration wound. If tendon ends are readily visible, they

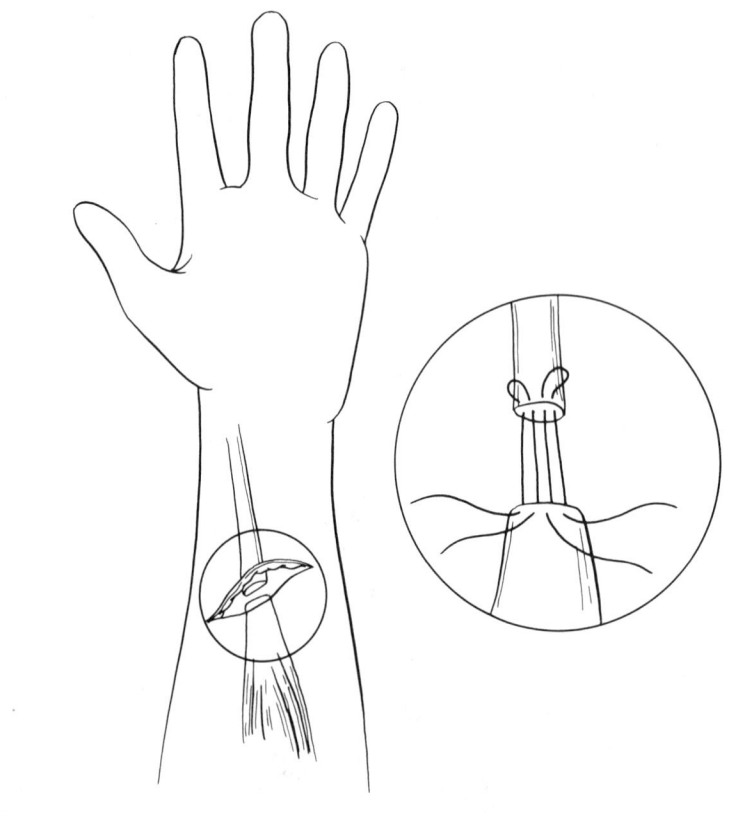

Figure 6-36. The isolated flexor or extensor tendon transection can be reapproximated by any of a number of techniques. Shown here is a mattress technique using a 4–0 nylon or polypropylene suture.

should be sutured. If not, repair should be deferred or performed in the operating room. The method of repair is the same as for wrist flexors, and the postoperative care is also essentially the same, except that the wrist should be splinted in a 30° to 45° extension.

e. Extensors over the dorsum of the hand (Fig. 6-38). Extensor tendons are exceedingly vulnerable to injury over the dorsum of the hand and at the MP joint level. There is minimal subcutaneous tissue for protection and the underlying metacarpal bone acts much like a cutting block. Several anatomic features of the area influence treatment.

Tendon ends do not retract and usually can be retrieved through the wound without undue trauma. The dorsal skin is very thin, however, and tendon sutures may be visible through the skin. Also, the tendon at this level is flattened. This ribbon-like configuration does not lend itself to Bunnell crisscross-type sutures. A useful method for repair of extensor tendons at this level is to place a pullout 4–0 monofilament wire in a continuous, over-and-over fashion. This rolling-type suture holds the tendon in good approximation. If wire sutures are unavailable, other sutures that can be used include horizontal mattress sutures of 4–0 or 5–0 nylon and 4–0 Vicryl or Dexon (Fig. 6-39).

The extensor tendons are small and without the same structural integrity as their flexor counterparts. Immobilization is necessarily

PENETRATING INJURIES AND DEEP TRANSECTIONS

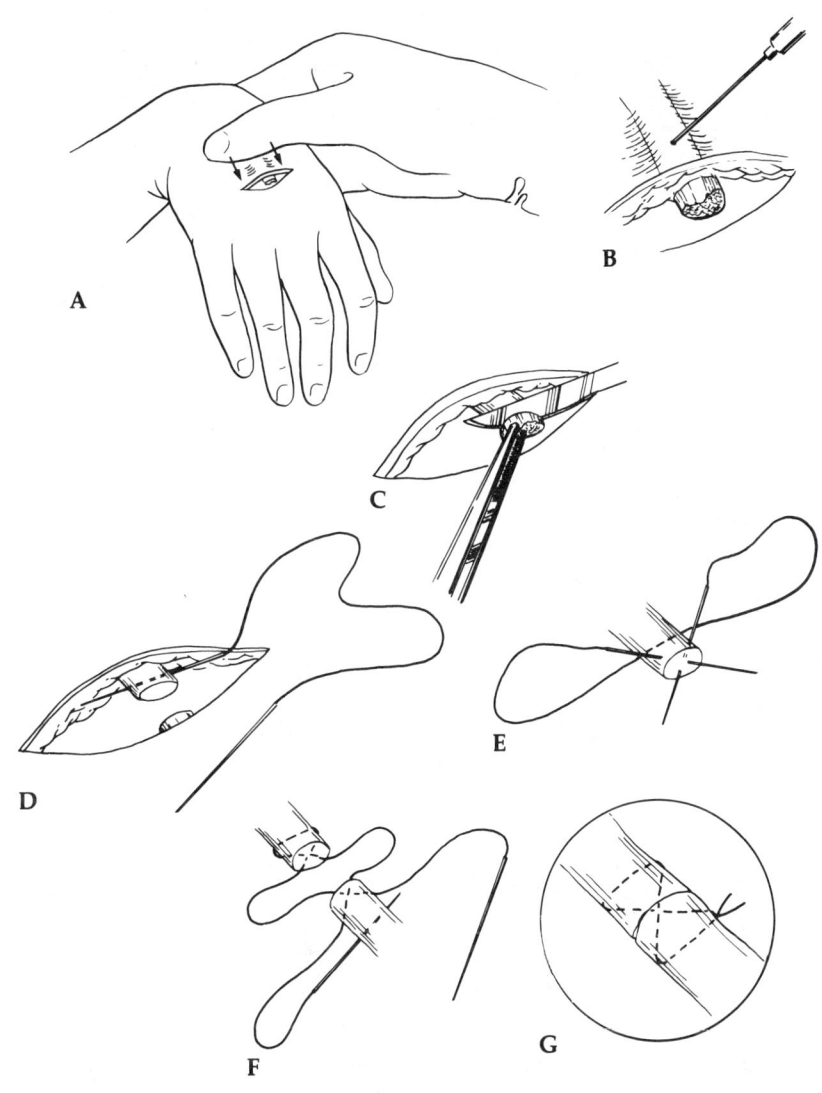

Figure 6-37. Arm and wrist extensors.
A. A useful maneuver for identifying the proximal portion of the tendon is to hold the wrist in full flexion or extension and "milk" the muscle in a distal direction. Look for a collection of blood to identify the tendon sheath.
B. The tendon should be atraumatically grasped with a hook or forceps and gently pulled distally. A #25-gauge 1¼ needle can be passed percutaneously through the skin and the tendon proximal to the laceration to fix it in place.
C. If the tendon has been sharply and cleanly divided, no debridement is necessary. The crushed tendon end should, however, be sharply debrided. This is best accomplished by clamping completely across the damaged portion of the tendon and dividing the tendon close to the edge of the clamp with a sharp new #10 blade in one sweep onto a tongue blade. The wooden blade protects underlying structures and gives a firm cutting surface. A sawing motion usually compromises the integrity of tendon architecture, causing fraying and softening of the freshened tendon end.
D through G. A figure eight or Bunnell crisscross stitch of 4-0 nylon or stainless steel wire is used.

longer—about 5 weeks—to prevent undue stretching of the fibrous tendon union. Immobilization should be with the wrist in extension and fingers in a relaxed functional position, MP joints at 30°, and IP joints *not* immobilized.

  f. Extensors over the digits (Fig. 6-40). Because of the nature of the extensor aponeurosis, complete lacerations over the proximal phalanx are unusual. Smaller wounds may be approximated with fine absorbable sutures and the PIP joint immobilized in full extension until the skin sutures are removed at 10 to 14 days. It is unnecessary to splint the MP joint following repair of this injury.
    (1) Ragged avulsion-type injuries of finger extensors
      (a) If the tendon is bluntly torn rather than sharply lacerated, there are usually a few interdigitating strands of tendon.
      (b) Immobilization of the IP joints in extension for 5 to 6 weeks achieves adequate healing.

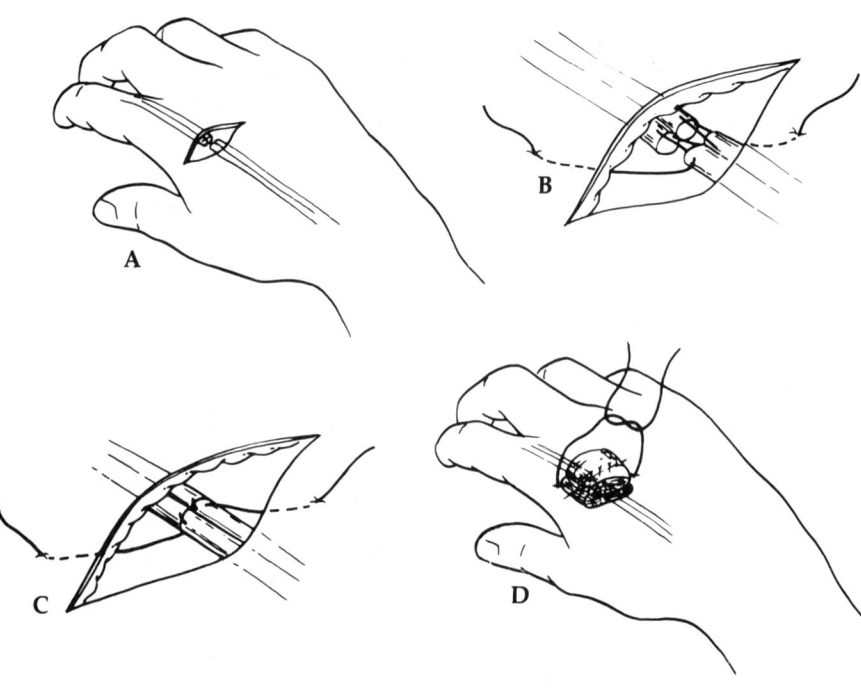

Figure 6-38. Suturing of extensor tendons on the dorsum of the hand.
A. The location of the wound.
B. Place a 4–0 monofilament wire as a rolling over-and-over suture, without kinks or overlaps, so that it will "pull-out" smoothly.
C. Pull the two suture ends to approximate the tendon juncture.
D. Following closure of the skin with 5–0 nylon, tie the wire ends loosely over a bolster, which acts as the initial layer of dressing.

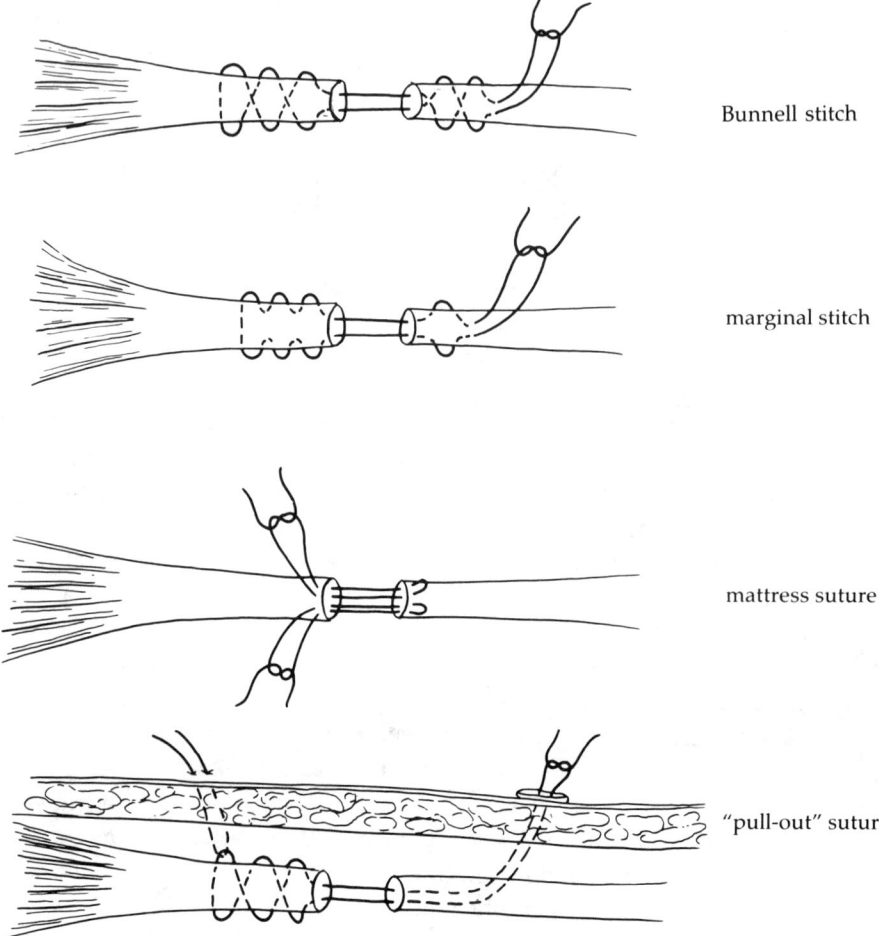

Figure 6-39. Several of the most common techniques for tendon repair.

Bunnell stitch

marginal stitch

mattress suture

"pull-out" suture

(2) Sharp lacerations
  (a) Division of the central slip of the extensor aponeurosis at the PIP joint results in a late deformity termed a *buttonhole deformity* (Fig. 6-40).
  (b) A similar injury may occur at the DIP joint and cause the mallet-finger deformity (Fig. 6-41); it should be treated in the manner described below.

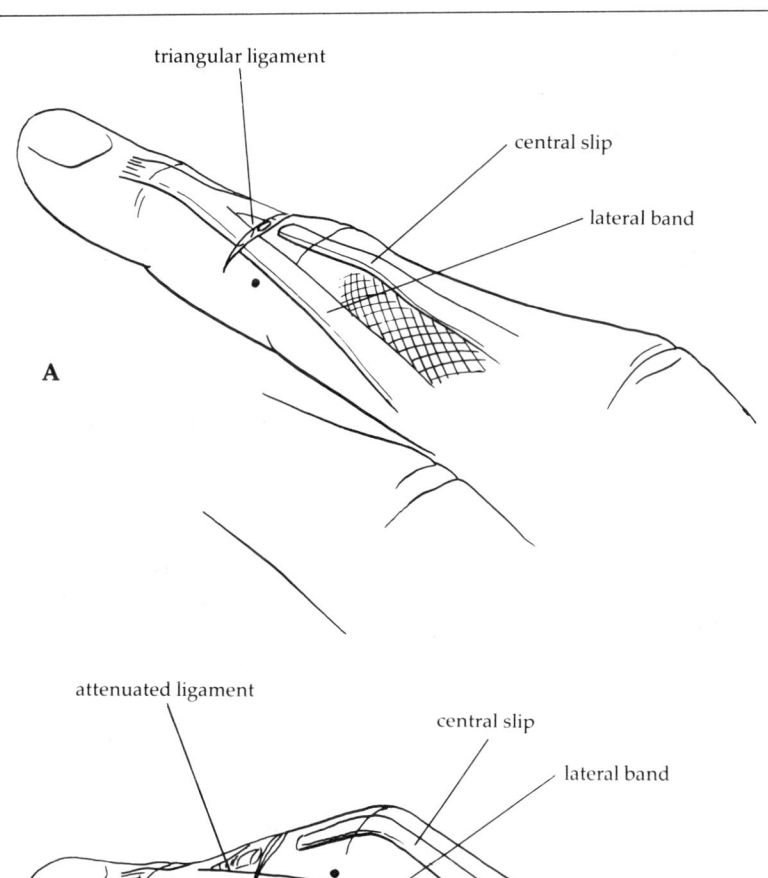
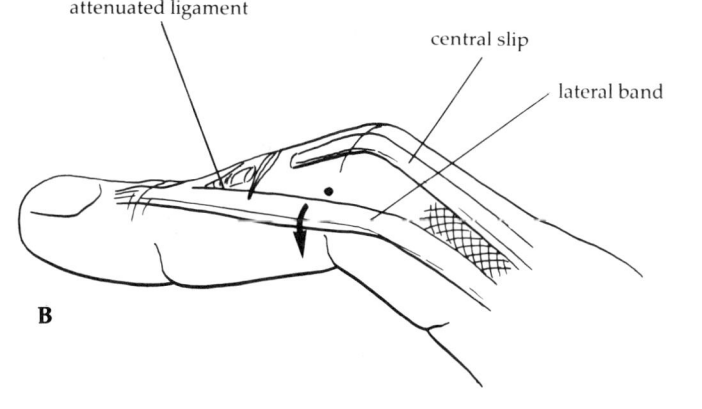

Figure 6-40. The buttonhole injury is the result of transection of the central slip over the proximal interphalangeal joint (A). If uncorrected, over time the lateral bands slide volarly below the axis of the joint, causing PIP flexion and DIP extension (B).

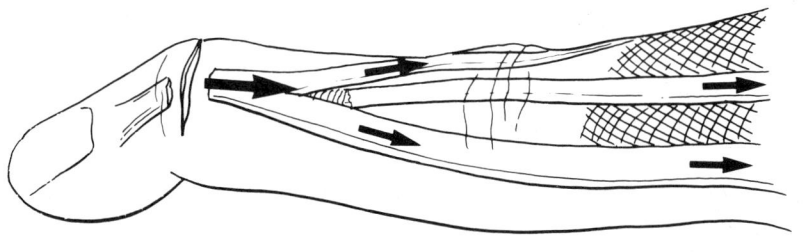

Figure 6-41. The mallet-finger injury, or drop tip, is caused by transection of the distal extensor insertion. The unbalanced pull tends to force the PIP joint into hyperextension, and the now unopposed pull of the FDP forces the DIP into flexion.

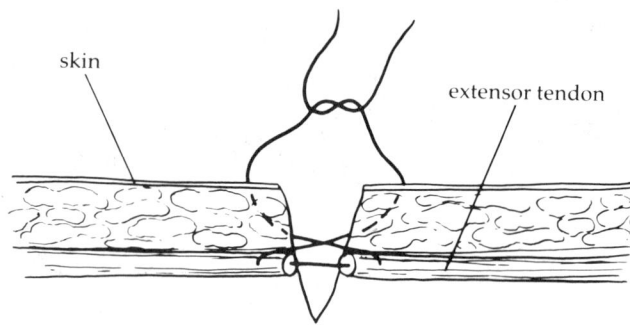

Figure 6-42. Extensor tendons can be simply repaired with figure eight sutures through skin and tendon.

        (3) Treatment (Fig. 6-42). Laceration of the extensor tendons over the digits should be repaired by specialists in the operating room whenever possible but can be repaired in the emergency department by experienced surgeons.
           (a) Technique
              (i) 6–0 clear nylon, simple interrupted or horizontal mattress sutures with the knot inverted
                  OR
              (ii) A figure-eight suture through skin and tendon. A 5–0 nylon is also a useful suture at this site.
           (b) Postoperative care. The PIP is immobilized in almost full extension for 4 weeks to ensure adequate healing. Some MP movement is tolerable. Progressive flexion is then begun.
        Extensor tendon lacerations over the middle phalanx or lacerations dividing the insertion onto the distal phalanx should be similarly sutured. Postrepair, the DIP joint is immobilized in full extension for 5 weeks. It is unnecessary to splint the PIP joint. At 5 weeks, gentle exercises are begun, but the DIP joint should be splinted in full extension between exercise sessions and at night for 2 additional weeks. Night splinting in full PIP extension is sometimes helpful to avoid extensor lag.
    4. *Management of tendon injuries requiring operating-room treatment!*
        a. Multiple flexor tendons in the wrist
           (1) Rationale. Their complex arrangement and location deep within the distal forearm and wrist make repair of multiple tendon lacerations at the wrist difficult even in the best setting. Although these injuries should be cared for in the operating room by a specialist, many factors may delay their definitive care in a definitive setting (e.g., availability of a specialist, availability of operating-room facilities, and presence of other, more life-threatening, conditions.
           (2) Initial care. If definitive care cannot be given within 6 to 8 hours, the wound edge should be debrided, the wound irrigated, the skin carefully closed, and the extremity splinted in a functional position and elevated.
           (3) Delayed care. If definitive treatment is expected but delayed,

prophylactic antibiotics are initiated. If definitive care must be provided secondarily either days or weeks later, prophylactic antibiotics are unnecessary in an uncontaminated wound.

(4) Definitive care. Tendons take priority over nerves in acute injuries at the wrist, because if treatment is delayed beyond several days to weeks, myostatic contracture of the divided muscle-tendon unit occurs to such a degree that subsequent repair at useful length is impossible. Therefore, flexor tendons divided at the wrist must be repaired soon after injury. Although sensation is equally as important or perhaps more important than motion, nerve repair can be performed secondarily, and some authors believe that secondary repair offers better results. In keeping with the "one wound, one scar" concept, tendons repaired in close proximity will probably heal as one mass, restricting their differential motion. Many surgeons suggest that only the deep flexor tendons (flexor pollicis longus and flexor digitorum profundus) be repaired and that the superficialis tendons be resected.

Recently, however, more surgeons have suggested that with careful and accurate approximation of tendons associated with very early motion, some independence of function may be maintained. They state that *in ideal circumstances all lacerated tendons should be repaired*. The key element is the phrase *ideal circumstances*. Every wound is different and should be individually evaluated with many options in the mind of the surgeon, ranging from just closing the skin to immediately repairing all structures. The treatment is dictated by all the factors mentioned earlier.

b. Flexor tendons in the palm and digits. The same management should be followed for flexor tendon wounds in the palm or digits. Here the close arrangement of many essential structures (nerves, vessels, and other tendons) and the complex fascial arrangements of tendon compartments warrant specialized operating-room care. In the finger, tendons move independently of one another in the close confines of a fibro-osseous tunnel. The term *no-man's-land* has been given to that area bounded proximally by the MP joint flexor crease and distally by the flexor digitorum superficialis insertions at the midportion of the middle phalanx. The poor results of primary repair of injured tendons at this level gave impetus to the use of the term. In the finger, lacerations involving both tendons traditionally have been managed secondarily by tendon grafting. Beginning in the early 1970s, several authors reported equal or better results with primary or delayed primary repair in the so-called no-man's-land. These authors continually admonish that this be done only in ideal circumstances and by a skilled specialist. Many point to the necessity of beginning motion early (1–2 days) to maintain gliding of the flexor tendons. Different schemes have evolved, depending on which tendon or tendons are divided and at what level. It bears repeating that flexor tendon repair in the digit is an operating-room procedure. Prompt wound toilet, skin closure, and referral to a specialist constitute quality medical care.

INJURIES TO NERVES
1. Anatomy
   a. Sensory nerves. Sensibility is provided by all three major forearm nerves. The typical sensory distribution of these nerves is indicated in Fig. 6-43. Both the ulnar and median nerves are mixed motor and sensory nerves. The radial nerve is purely sensory in the hand.
   b. Motor nerves
      (1) Extrinsic nerves. All dorsal extrinsic muscles are innervated by the radial nerve (Fig. 6-44). All volar forearm muscles except the ulnar-innervated flexor carpi ulnaris and the ulnar two flexor digitorum profundus muscles are median nerve–innervated (Figs. 6-45 and 6-46).
      (2) Intrinsic nerves. Except for the adductor pollicis and the ulnar half of the flexor pollicis brevis, the thenar muscles are innervated by the median nerve (Fig. 6-46) and the hypothenar muscles by the ulnar nerve (Fig. 6-45).
         (a) The radial two lumbricals are median nerve–innervated.
         (b) All the interosseous muscles and the ulnar two lumbricals are ulnar nerve–innervated.
         (c) The median nerve enters the hand through the carpal tunnel.
         (d) The ulnar nerve enters through a separate, adjacent tunnel.
            Injury to either the ulnar or median nerve diminishes both motor and sensory hand function. Without sensibility, the hand is "blind," and its movements must be guided by the eye. Without adequate motor innervation, its function can only be passive (i.e., a paperweight).
2. Testing of nerve injury
   a. Motor nerves. As mentioned previously, the inability to move a part may be caused by loss of tendon integrity or injury to the motor nerve. The same systematic muscle evaluation usually localizes the site of injury to a motor or mixed sensory and motor nerve (Figs. 6-44, 6-45, and 6-46).
   b. Sensory nerves. Inaccurate testing of sensibility accounts for the most frequent errors in the initial assessment of hand trauma. Most manuals depicting sensory nerve distribution illustrate the average or most frequent pattern. Just as differences occur in handedness, differences occur in sensory patterns. There are areas of specific sensory innervation, however, in which overlap between fibers of different nerves rarely occurs (Fig. 6-47). The following areas should be examined:
      (1) The pulp of the index finger for median nerve function
      (2) The tip of the little finger for ulnar nerve sensory function
      (3) The dorsal first web space for radial nerve function
3. Methods of testing for sensation (Fig. 6-48)
   a. The texture and wetness or dryness of the skin may provide all the necessary information.
      (1) Skin devoid of sensibility feels dry and smooth (silk-like), secondary to loss of sudomotor (sweating) activity.
      (2) Normally innervated skin feels velvety and moist. This knowledge is very helpful in children and unconscious or uncoopera-

PENETRATING INJURIES AND DEEP TRANSECTIONS

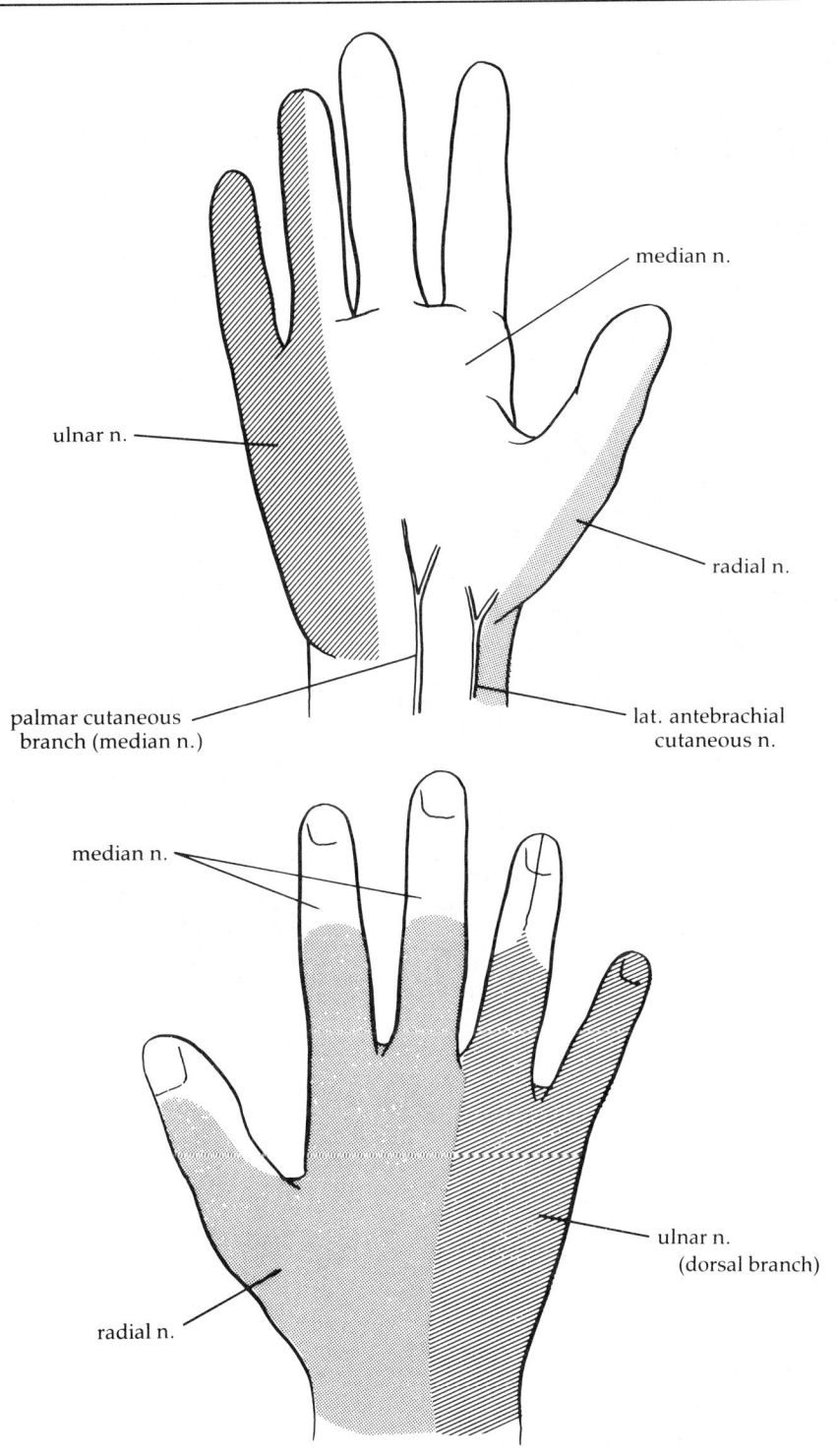

Figure 6-43. Sensory pattern of the hand.

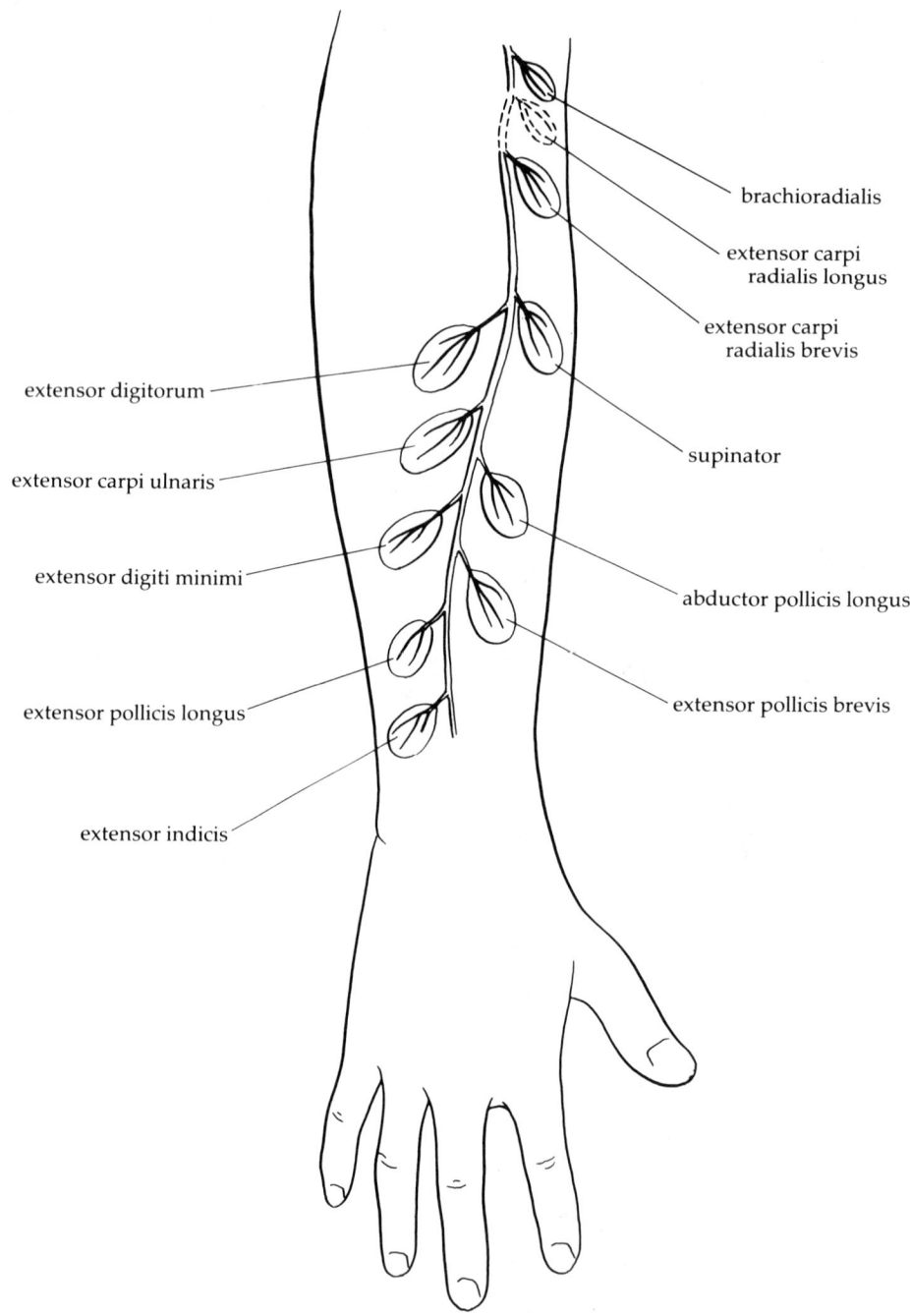

Figure 6-44. Sites of muscle innervation from the radial nerve.

tive patients, because sudomotor activity is severely diminished within minutes following nerve transection.

Sensory testing should begin with nonpainful stimulus testing for the presence of refined sensibility (i.e., two-point discrimination).

b. Two-point discrimination. The most useful test for fine touch is the Weber two-point discrimination test. A bent paper clip is the only instrument necessary. Normally, two-point discrimination varies from 2 to 4 or 5 mm, depending on the finger tested. Comparison with the opposite side is extremely useful.

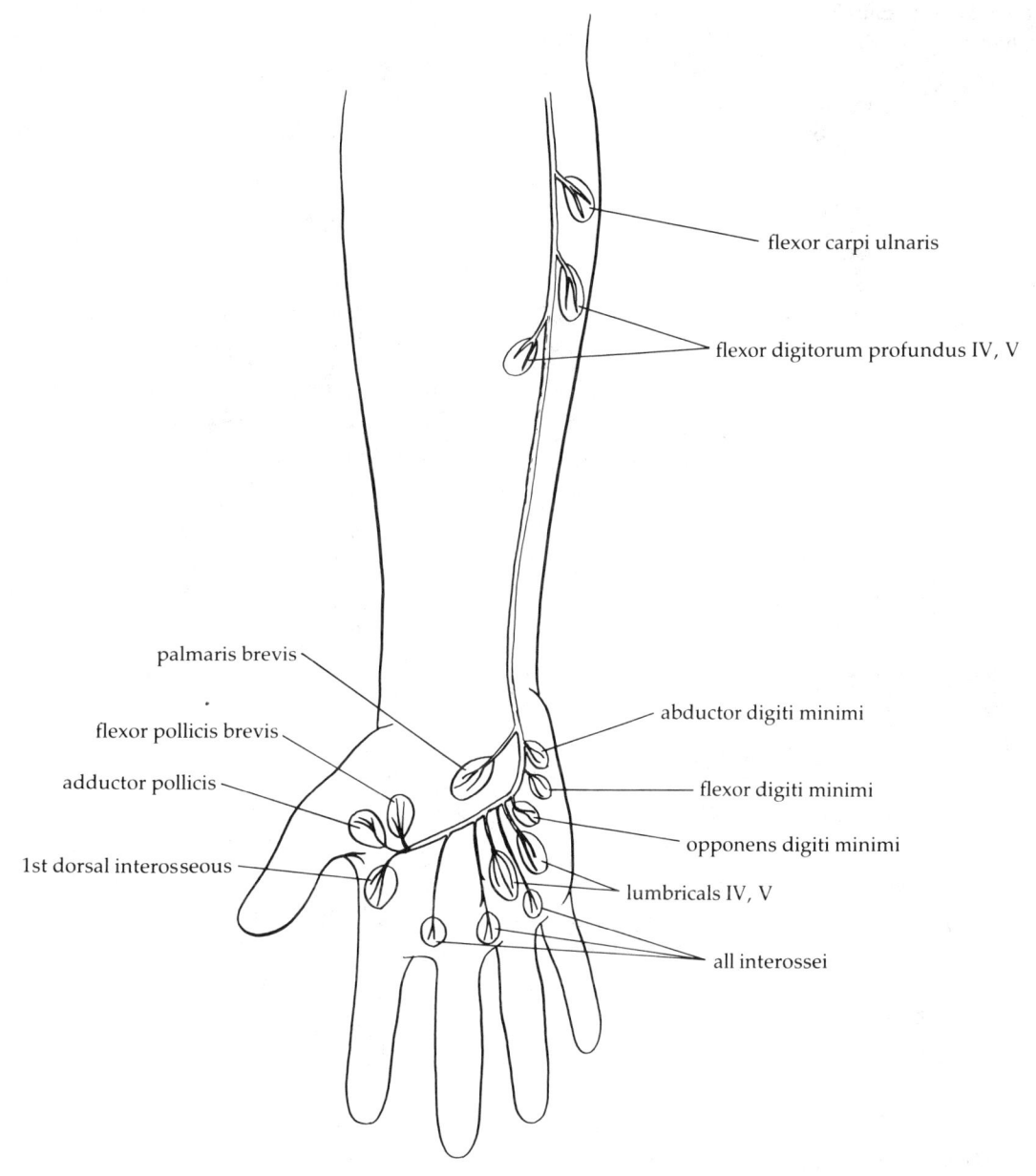

Figure 6-45. Sites of muscle innervation from the ulnar nerve.

Both sides of the digit should be tested separately. Diminished two-point discrimination (greater than 10–12 mm) is evidence of severe nerve injury.

c. Sharp-dull. Sharp-dull discrimination is a less specific test used for determining coarser sensory modalities. An applicator stick sharpened on one end and blunt on the other serves as the testing instrument. The use of a hypodermic needle or safety pin is to be condemned. It is useful to demonstrate sensory testing on oneself, particularly sharp-dull testing, especially to a child, to reinforce that no pain is involved.

4. Difficult diagnostic problems. Partial nerve transections, anatomic variations (nerve crossover patterns), or combination nerve and tendon

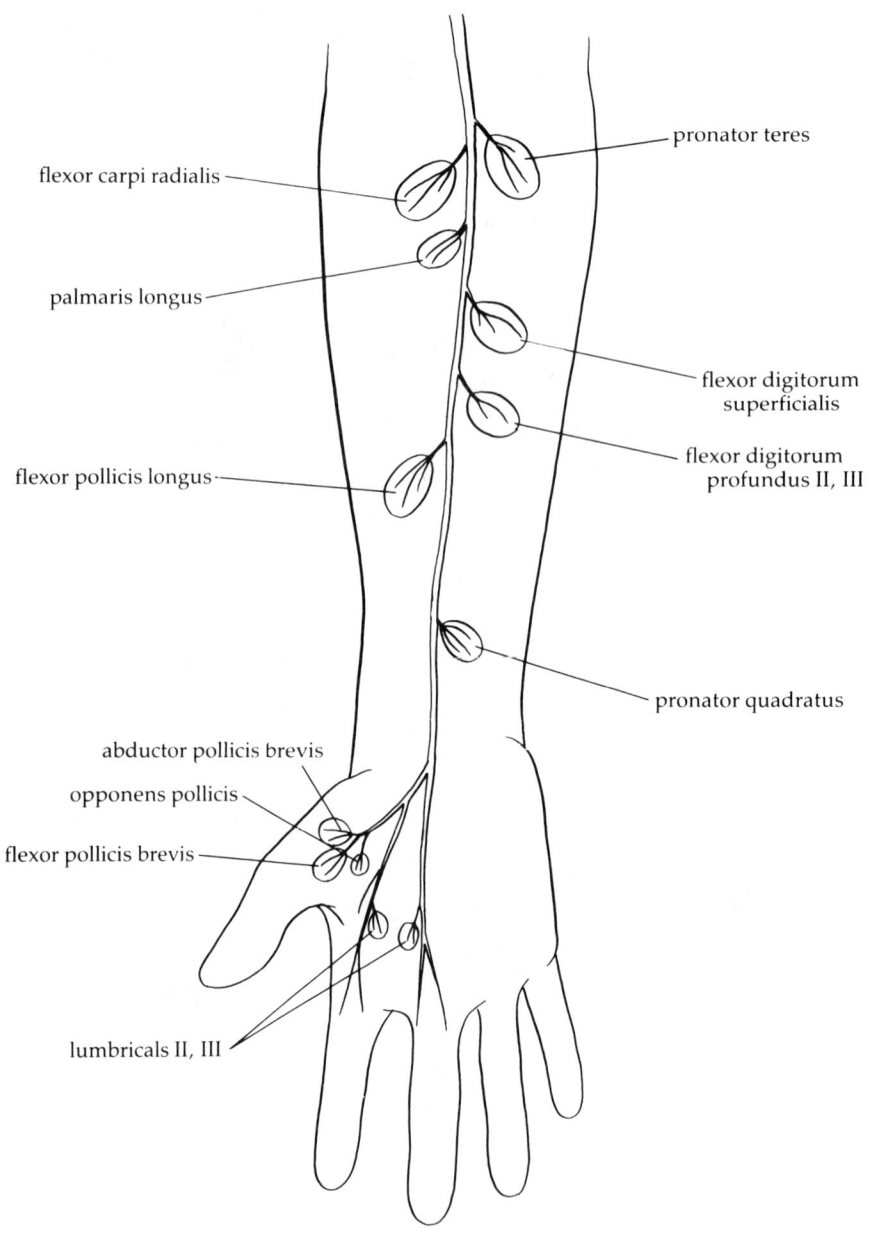

Figure 6-46. Sites of muscle innervation from the median nerve.

injuries provide difficult diagnostic problems. There are, however, criteria to help make these diagnoses.

a. Partial transections. Most peripheral nerves are mixed nerves carrying both motor and sensory fibers. As a general rule, the sensory nerves are more superficial and the motor nerves deeper within the peripheral nerve. Sunderland has mapped out the typical location of the sensory and motor components of most of the peripheral nerves. These maps can be used as a guide for evaluating partial transection of a nerve. It is most common for the superficial part of the nerve to be cut and the deeper part left intact. Thus, there may be a sensory loss, loss of some of the more proximal muscle groups, but retained function of the distal muscle groups. The maps of the ulnar and

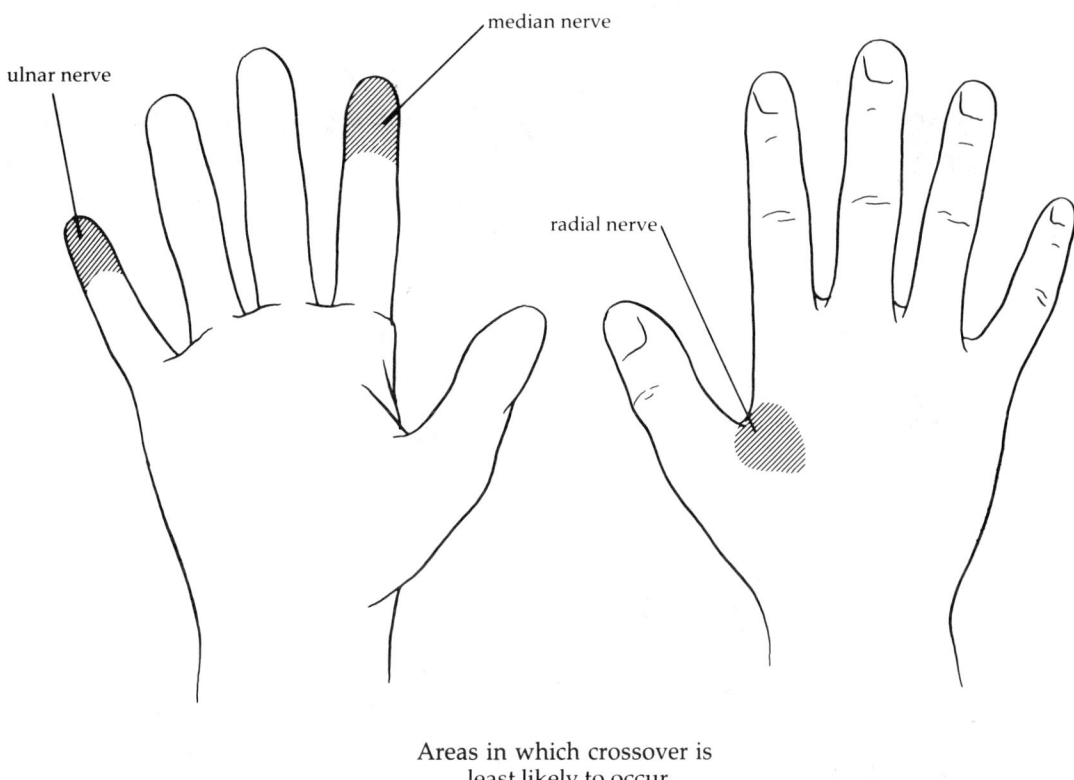

Areas in which crossover is
least likely to occur

Figure 6-47. Areas of sensibility that are the most consistent and not affected by anomalous variations and overlap.

median nerves at the forearm and wrist are given as examples (Fig. 6-49).

b. Crossover patterns and anatomic variations. There are documented instances of crossover of nerve fibers from the ulnar nerve to the median nerve or from the deep interosseous nerve to the median nerve, for example.

One of the most common crossover patterns is the "Martin-Gruber" communication between the median and ulnar nerves, which occurs in 15 percent of limbs. In this pattern the motor fibers to the intrinsic muscles, which normally are in the ulnar nerve, cross over in the midforearm to join the median nerve through a branch of the anterior interosseous nerve.

The diagnosis of these complicated variations and crossovers depends on the physician's awareness that they exist, followed by confirmation by specific nerve blocks. The interpretation of these nerve blocks is relatively complicated and generally is not appropriate for emergency situations.

c. Injuries in children. Nerve injuries in young children are notoriously difficult to diagnose and probably best explored in the operating room under a light general anesthetic, such as ketamine. It may be necessary to admit the young child for observation of the injured part.

5. Types of injuries. For most tissues, functional integrity is synonymous with the reestablishment by wound healing of anatomic integrity with scar. For nerve injuries, however, healing and anatomic continuity are

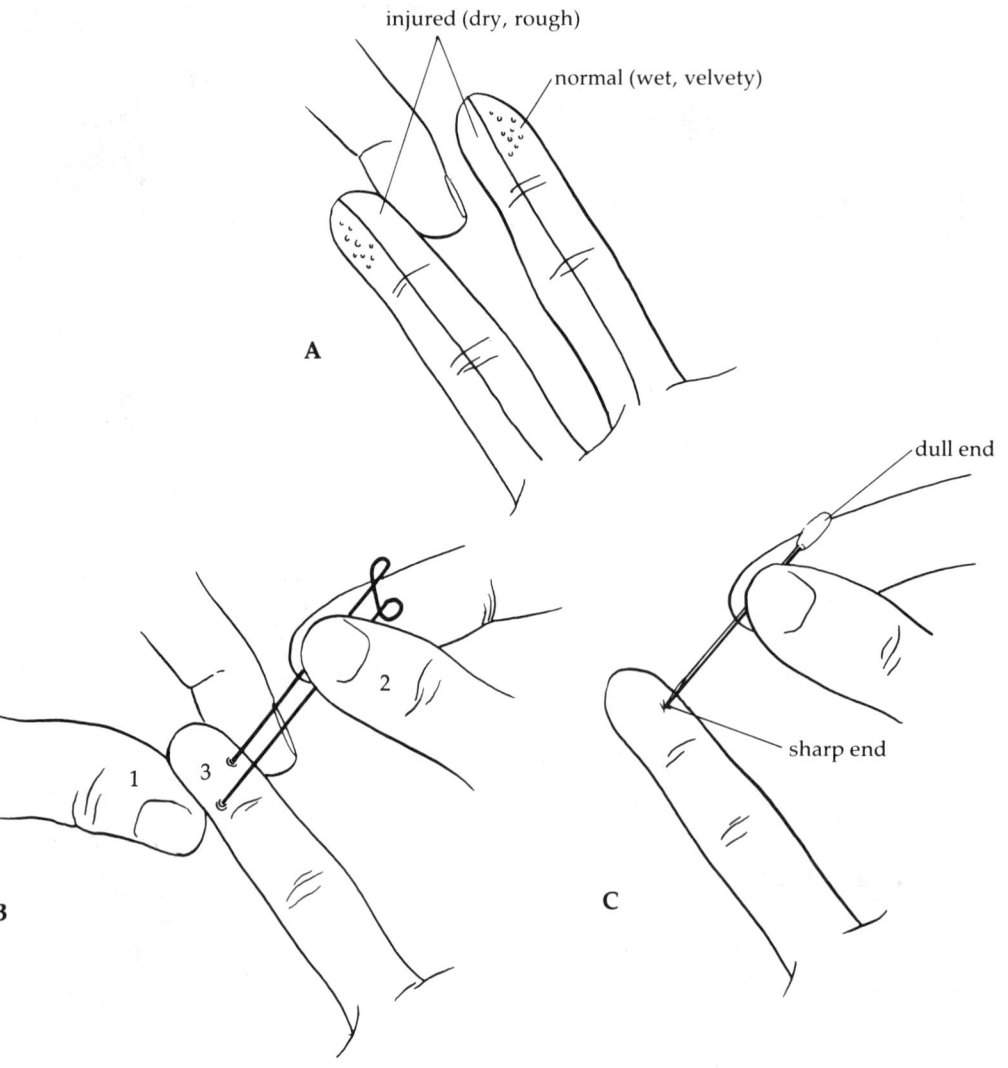

Figure 6-48. Sensory testing.
A. The texture of innervated skin is moist and velvety, and that of non-innervated skin is dry and rough.
B. Two-point discrimination can be tested with a paper clip. Only very light pressure is applied. First, the examiner (1) steadies the patient's finger; then the examiner steadies his or her own hand, holding the bent paper clip (2); the dull points of the instrument barely blanch the skin (3).
C. Sharp-dull discrimination is tested with a cotton-tipped wooden applicator.

much less important than axon regeneration and end-organ reinnervation. Three distinctive types of nerve injuries have been identified, based on the pathology of the injury and, to some extent, on the course and level of recovery (Fig 6-50):

a. *Neurapraxia* refers to the condition of an anatomically intact nerve with a functional (physiologic) inability to repolarize. The myelin sheath and connective tissue remain in continuity. This type of injury is most common with short-term compression, *mild traction, slight ischemia,* or hematoma. Neurapraxia results in a short-term partial or complete interruption of electrical transmission. Dysfunction can last for minutes or days. The most common neurapraxia is compression of the ulnar nerve at the elbow, or "funny bone."

b. *Axonotmesis* refers to a partial anatomic disruption of a nerve caused by death or division of the axons only. The external neural connective tissue sheaths remain intact. This type of injury is most commonly caused by localized prolonged compression and crush injuries. Regeneration of axons and spontaneous occurrence require weeks or months, depending on the site.

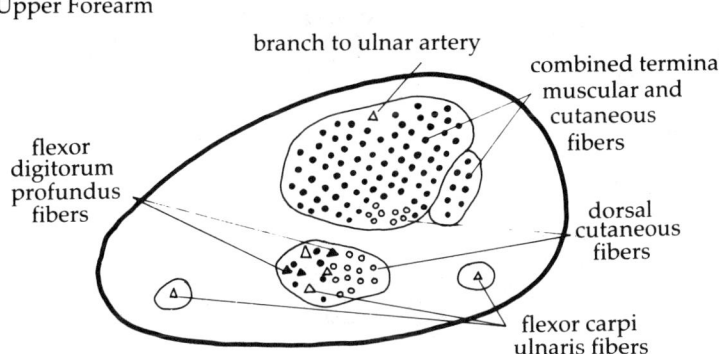
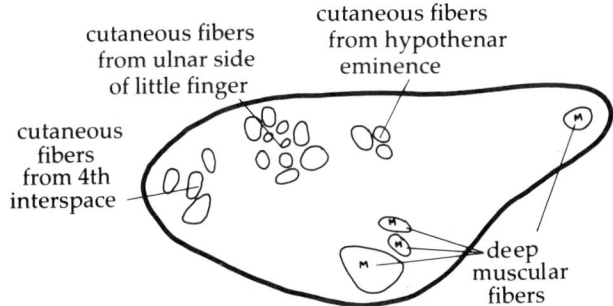
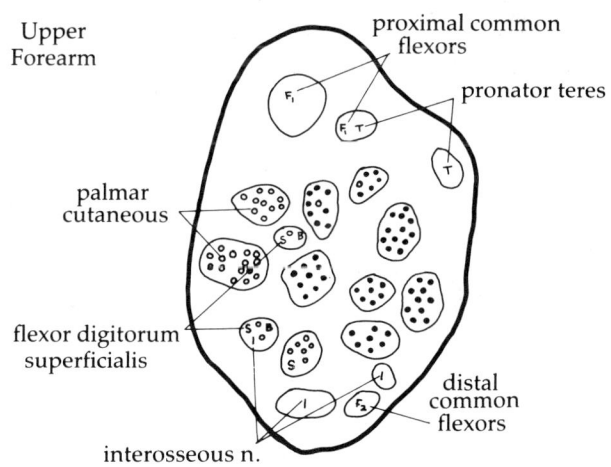
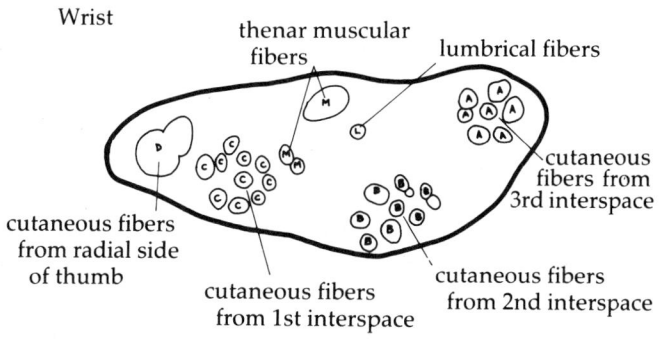

Figure 6-49. Cross-sectional maps of the ulnar and median nerves at forearm and wrist. They can be used for distinguishing partial nerve transections from combined nerve and tendon injuries.

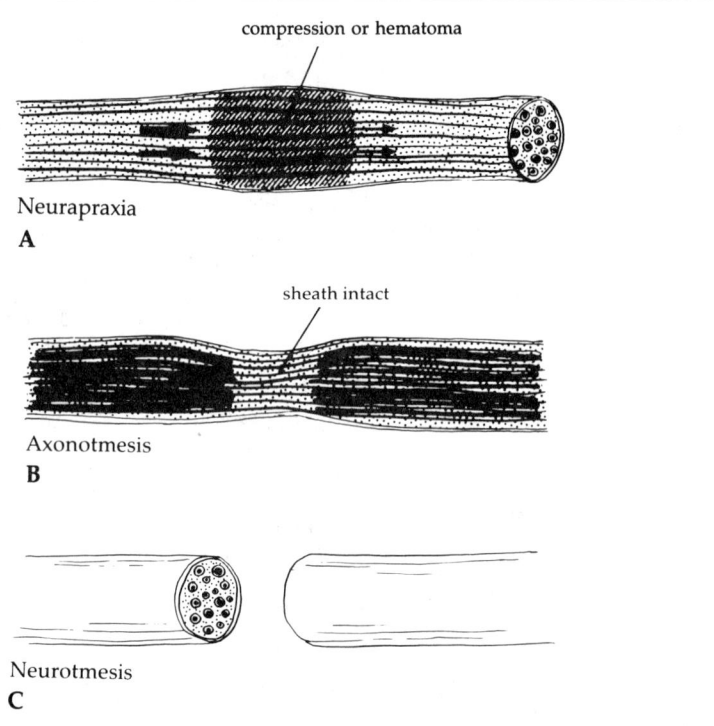

Figure 6-50. Types of nerve injury.
A. *Neurapraxia* is a dysfunction of electrical transmission caused by internal ischemia or herniation. All structures are anatomically intact.
B. *Axonotmesis* is a partial discontinuity caused by death of axons from pressure, with intact sheaths, perineurium, and epineurium.
C. *Neurotmesis* is a complete anatomic discontinuity.

    c. *Neurotmesis* is the complete physical disruption of the entire nerve (all axons and connective tissue). This type of injury usually occurs with lacerations or major avulsions.

    From the point of view of wound repair, only neurotmesis, or complete transection of the peripheral nerve, requires surgical intervention. Neurapraxia almost always results in spontaneous return of function within minutes to days, and axonotmesis may result in spontaneous recovery in days to weeks or months. In severe injuries, however, particularly of the proximal nerves, return of function may not occur, with either axonotmesis or neurotmesis.

6. Nerve repair and regeneration (Fig. 6-51)
    a. Repair. A lacerated nerve, surgically repaired, heals by collagen scar formation between the fibrous supporting tissues (the epineurium and perineurium) of the nerves. However, regenerative continuity between proximal and distal axons does not necessarily occur coincident with surgical repair. A scar may create a physically strong repair site but block axon regeneration across the repair site.
        (1) Choice of surgical facility. Most peripheral nerve injuries should be repaired in the operating room, with anesthesia, tourniquet, and magnification. Single injuries to sensory nerves can be treated in the emergency department by epineurial repair, usually with local anesthesia, loupe magnification, and 8-0 or 7-0 suture. Even these relatively small and seemingly functionally unimportant sensory branches can cause considerable discomfort because of neuromas if they are not adequately repaired.
            (a) Emergency department. Nerves that may be repaired in the emergency department with ideal conditions are:

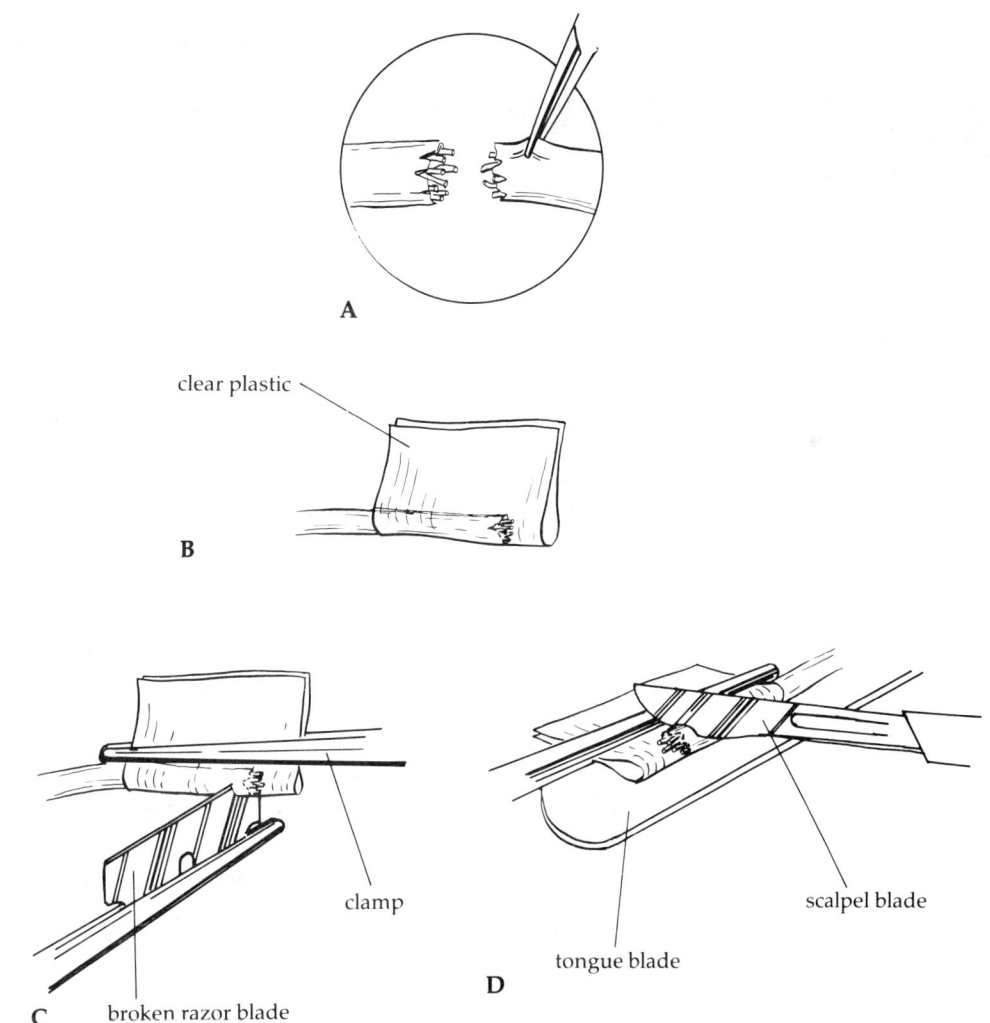

Figure 6-51. Debridement of ragged nerve ends (A) can be achieved by fixation of the nerve in clear plastic wrap (B) and straight clamp (C). The nerve is cut with either a razor or scalpel blade, with or without a tongue blade (D).

      (i) Cutaneous branches of the arm and forearm
      (ii) Dorsal sensory branches of the radial nerve
   (b) Operating room. Nerves to be repaired in the operating room include:
      (i) Digital nerves because of their critical functional importance
      (ii) Deep motor nerves
      (iii) Median and ulnar nerve transections at or proximal to the wrist

(2) **Localization of cut ends** (Fig. 6-52). A thorough understanding of the regional anatomy and careful observation are required for this task. Branches can retract beyond the margins of the wound because of a rubber band–like action if cut while under tension.

(3) **Debridement** (Fig. 6-51). Ragged nerve ends must be debrided for contusions or avulsion ruptures, but debridement is not required for sharp transections.

Debridement of severe injuries may result in a large gap between nerve ends. If so, the repair requires an interposition

Figure 6-52. Nerve ends are accurately aligned by identifying superficial vessels, size and position of individual fascicles, or obliquity of cut. The initial epineurial sutures are placed using these landmarks as guides.

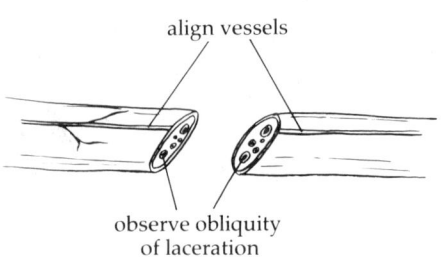
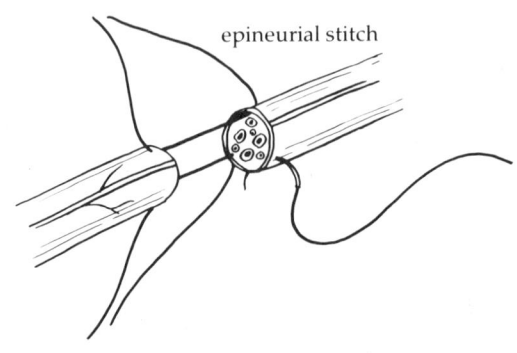

nerve graft, and the patient should be referred for specialty care in the operating room.

(4) Accurate alignment (Fig. 6-52). Matching of fascicles is of great importance with large mixed motor and sensory nerves (ulnar, median) but is of less importance in small, pure nerves, such as the facial nerve (motor) or digital nerve (sensory). Proper rotation is achieved by identifying the longitudinal blood vessels and matching the obliquities of the cut nerve ends and fascicles according to size and position.

(5) Epineurial or perineurial placement. Perhaps the major controversy in this area is whether the perineurial (fascicular) or epineurial placement should be used. However, for the small, pure motor or sensory nerves repaired in the emergency department this controversy is academic. Simple approximation of the epineurium is the only practical alternative (Fig. 6-53). This is achieved by placing sutures such as 8–0 or 10–0 nylon in the surrounding epineurium rather than into the nerve itself.

The question of fascicular perineurial repair for larger mixed nerves such as the median or ulnar nerve is more complex. However, these repairs should be done in the operating room by a specialist (Fig. 6-54).

(6) Splinting. Postoperative immobilization without tension for 7 to 14 days, followed by gradual reactivation, is required.

The events occurring after a repair of a peripheral nerve can be considered in three distinct phases: degeneration, regeneration, and reinnervation of muscle end-plates and sensory organs. However, there is overlap of the events in this sequence.

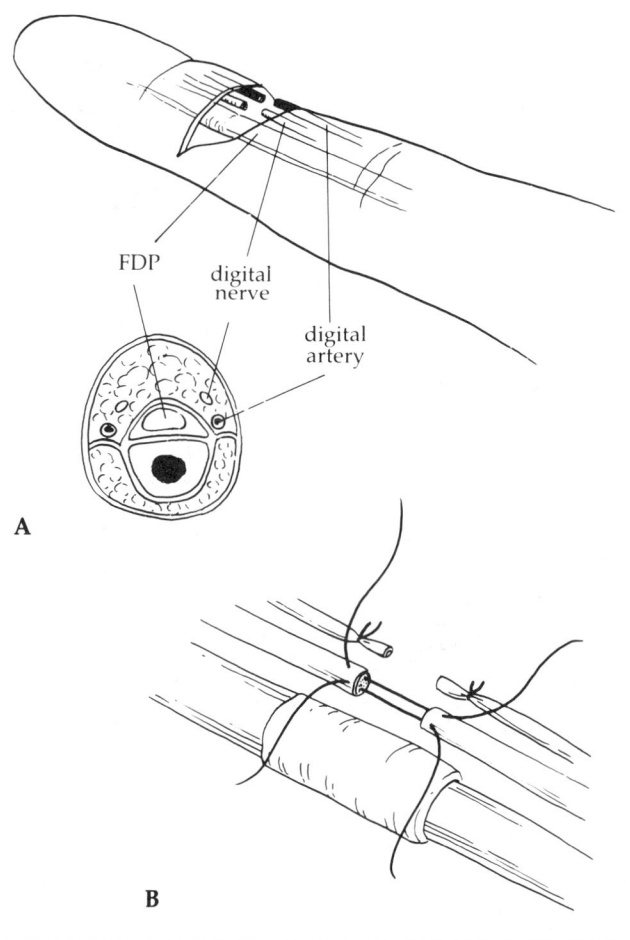

Figure 6-53. Epineural placement.
A. The digital nerve is slightly volar and medial (toward the tendon) to the artery. When only one neurovascular bunch has been lacerated, the artery may be ligated.
B. When both neurovascular bundles are divided, digital arteries should be repaired. Repair the nerve with 8–0 nylon.

(1) Degeneration
  (a) Distal axon. The degenerative process takes approximately 2 or 3 weeks. The distal axon undergoes "Wallerian degeneration," which is disintegration of the distal axon myelin sheath and proliferation of new cords of Schwann cells. The Schwann cells have two functions: phagocytosis of axonal and myelinic debris and sprouting of new cords of Schwann cells to provide a conduit down which regenerating axons can grow.
  (b) Cell body. Ribonucleic acids (RNA) in the cytoplasm begin to increase from the fourth day in preparation for migration down microglobules within the axon. If the cellular insult is excessive, and particularly, if there are very proximal nerve injuries, the nerve cell body will die.
  (c) Proximal axon. The proximal axon undergoes degeneration to the level of the first or second node of Ranvier (1–2 mm).
  The Schwann cells proliferate and assume a phagocytic role. The amount of proximal degeneration and Schwann cell response is proportional to the severity of the injury.
(2) Regeneration. After 2 weeks, the degenerative processes are completed and the regenerating axons must cross the gap from

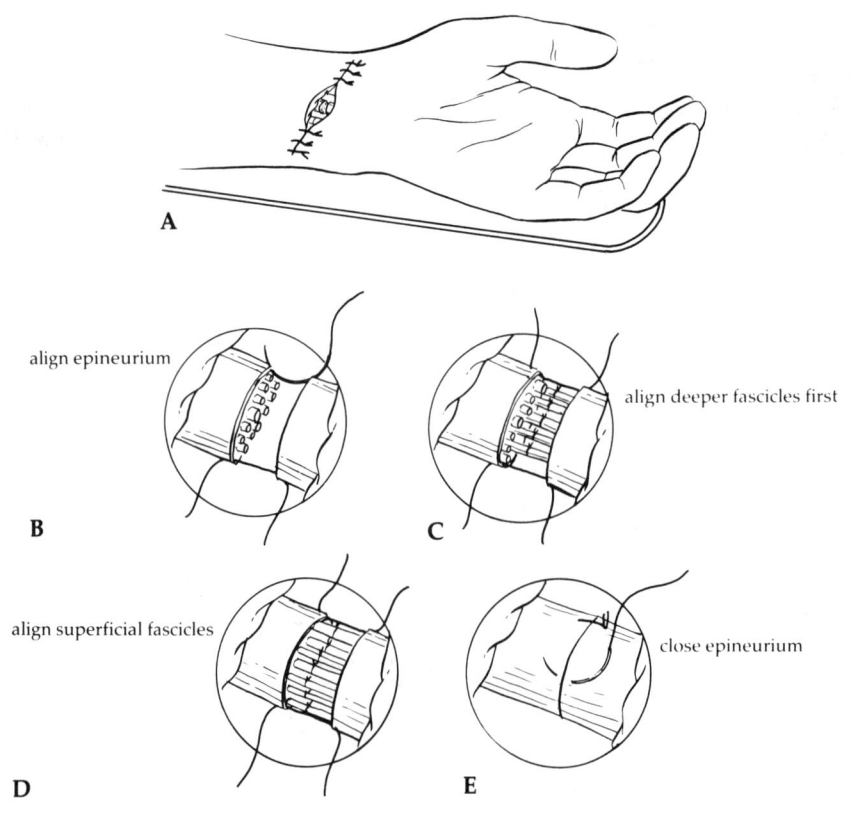

Figure 6-54. Perineurial repair of larger, mixed nerves.
A. Close other structures, including tendons and lateral skin; splint the hand.
B. Align the nerve and close the posterior epineurium with a 6–0 or 7–0 nylon suture to take tension off the repair.
C. Repair matched fascicles with two 10–0 nylon sutures; begin posteriorly.
D. Progress anteriorly to close fascicles.
E. Repair anterior epineurium.

proximal to distal. Excessive scar or separation of the ends caused by tension can prevent axons from crossing.

The rate of regeneration is related to the type of injury, location, and whether it is a motor or sensory fiber. The rates from time of injury until functional maturation as determined by electromyographic impulses in previously denervated muscle are approximately (1) ½ mm per day in the more distal extremities, (2) 1 mm per day in the leg or forearm, and (3) as rapid as 3 mm per day in the upper arm and thigh. Perineurial cells also grow into the distal nerve.

(a) Fibrin clot. Normally, a fibrin clot interposes between the surgically approximated nerve ends.

(b) Tension alignment. Tension from nerve retraction causes the fibrin strands to form a series of linear bridges across the gap. Tension from sutures can alter fibrin orientation.

(c) Axon migration. Axons use the fibrin alignment for directional guidance across the gap to the distal side. After the axons enter the distal nerve, they use the Schwann cords for guidance.

(3) Reinnervation. Sensory organs and motor end-plates do not degenerate and thus can be reinnervated. The functional maturation related to muscle reinnervation is a relatively slow process. The time for physical regeneration of nerve axons represents only 10 to 30 percent of the total time from injury to return of

normal muscle function, whereas the functional maturation of the muscle represents 70 to 90 percent of the total elapsed time.

(a) Muscle end-plates. The muscles and peripheral axons are metabolically dependent on the nerve cell body. After nerve sectioning, muscle fibers shrink and muscle spindles begin to atrophy. The synaptic distance between the termination of the nerve and the motor end-plate widens. This sequence of events in muscle atrophy begins as early as 3 to 4 months after injury, but viable muscle may survive 5 or 10 years. However, any degree of denervation atrophy is harmful to future reinnervation because the thickened muscle sheath blocks end-plate formation. It has been estimated that 1 percent of motor function is lost for every week of denervation after the initial 3-week metabolic delay.

The return of muscle function is better in the more proximal muscles than in the distal muscles. The reasons for this are that (1) the bundles are more compact, (2) the rate of axon growth in the proximal extremities is more rapid, (3) there is less denervation atrophy and muscle fibrosis because axons reach the end-plates more rapidly; proximally located muscles function more by gross, simultaneous contraction and less by finely controlled movements than do intrinsic muscles.

(b) Sensory end-organs. The sensory end-organs are less dependent on axon innervation for their own survival. The return of sensory function is considerably more rapid than motor return. There is also a differential in the rate of return of specific sensory modalities. The order of functional return is as follows: deep sensation (proprioception), paresthesias (e.g., Tinel's sign), light touch (e.g., with a cotton-tipped applicator), pain (e.g., pinprick), and stereognosis (e.g., two-point discrimination and object identification).

7. CLOSED AND BLUNT INJURIES

GENERAL PRINCIPLES

Mechanisms

Blunt injuries are characterized by major damage to skin, underlying soft tissue, and skeletal support, with or without skin disruption. Blunt injuries can be caused by direct rapid *impact* from another object, sustained *compression* between nonyielding objects, or *torque* and stretch (Fig. 7-1).

Each type of injury subjects different tissues to specific types of damage. Thus, an accurate history of how the injury occurred provides a clue to the most likely type of tissue damage. Diagnosis and treatment of specific tissue injuries are discussed later in this chapter, according to anatomic site and wound condition.

IMPACT

Impact injuries are caused by forceful or high-velocity physical contact between the body and another object. The force of a moving object, such as a car, ball, fist, or stone, can be duplicated by the movement of the person toward an immobile object, such as the ground, wall, or car interior.

Regardless of the mechanism, the high energy of direct impact is likely to cause disruption of deep tissues. Fractures, dislocations, hematomas, and ruptured viscera are most likely to occur; skin disruption may or may not occur.

COMPRESSION AND CRUSH

Compression injury is caused by physical forces applied over a longer period of time. The predominant effect of prolonged compression is tissue death from reduced vascular perfusion. Ischemia may result from relatively low compression forces of 25 to 40 mm for 2 to 3 hours. Ischemia initiates the processes of inflammation and repair.

Ischemia may perpetuate itself even if the compressive force is removed. Injured capillaries leak intravascular fluids; the resultant edema in a closed fascial compartment may cause ischemia, release of vasoactive substances from injured cells, and additional inflammation and ischemia. A vicious cycle is initiated and perpetuated until cell death occurs; thus, release of compartment pressure is an essential part of treatment.

Examples of compression injury include transient ulnar nerve palsies (Saturday night palsy), Volkmann's flexor compartment syndrome, and decubitus ulcers.

TORQUE (SHEAR, DISLOCATION, STRETCH)

A force can occur at an angle, causing shearing, stretching, or dislocation of the tissue. With a shearing injury, the skin is separated from the underlying fascia. Blood vessels are ruptured and nerves are stretched, causing hematomas and nerve dysfunctions. The washing machine wringer injury is a typical example. Rotational forces applied to tissue may cause spiral fractures in long bones, sprains, or dislocations at joints. Stretch and rotation cause ligament sprains, "pulled muscles," torn ligaments, and ruptured tendons.

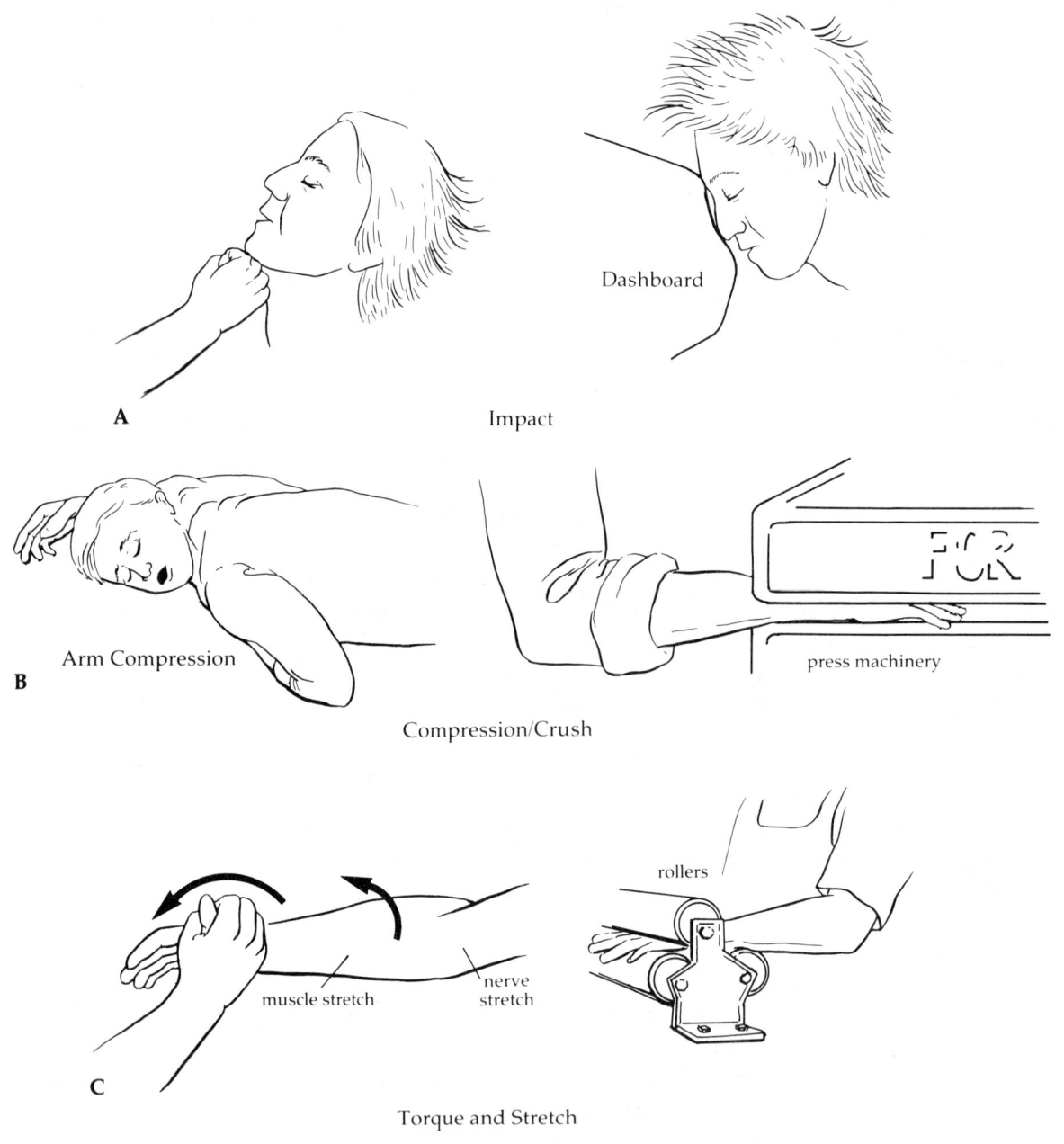

Figure 7-1. Mechanisms of blunt trauma.
A. Impact injuries cause fractures, dislocations, and hematomas.
B. Crush injuries cause ischemia of skin, muscle, and nerves.
C. Torque injuries cause dislocations, sprains, and skin separation.

Tissue Damage

Regardless of the mechanism of trauma, there is variation in severity of tissue response. Any or all of these tissue responses can occur: anatomic discontinuity, direct traumatic cellular death, indirect cellular death from ischemia or toxins, and physiologic dysfunction without cellular death.

ANATOMIC DISRUPTION (COMPLETE OR PARTIAL)
Rupture is caused by physical force that is greater than the tissue (collagen and cellular) can tolerate. The mechanism through which the force is applied partially determines which tissues are injured. Examples of tissue

disruption include fractures; sprains; avulsions; dislocations; and ruptures of muscle, tendon, nerve, bone, cartilage, fat, vessels, or ducts.

NECROSIS (CELL DEATH)

High-energy impact or prolonged compression can cause a localized cellular death at the site of contact. This primarily affects the skin and muscular compartments and is caused by direct and immediate damage to the cells.

ISCHEMIA

This is an important aspect of closed injuries because the surgeon has the opportunity to intercede to prevent additional ischemia and eventual delayed necrosis or infection.

Most secondary tissue damage is caused by vascular compromise from edema, hematoma, intravascular thrombosis, and ischemic devascularization. Additional damage can be caused by infection. Elevation, decompression, debridement, drainage, and antibiotics can be used to limit the damage.

DYSFUNCTION (PHYSIOLOGIC)

Minimal injury from partial circulatory compromise, pressure, edema, inflammation, or impact can result in temporary dysfunction without cell death. Function can return minutes, days, or weeks after injury. The following categories of tissue response are used for nerve injuries:

1. *Neurapraxia* is a temporary, physiologic tissue dysfunction caused by pressure or circulatory compromise. *Saturday night palsy* is an ulnar nerve compression at the elbow with functional loss that lasts minutes or days. A similar insult to the radial nerve in the axilla can result from incorrect use of crutches and is termed *crutch palsy*.
2. *Axonotmesis* involves an indirect or direct death of the nerve axon with continuity of myelin sheath maintained; nerve regrowth and functional return may occur many weeks later.
3. *Neurotmesis* is the complete disruption of all components of the nerve.

After categorizing tissue response in this way, it is important to distinguish a temporary dysfunction from permanent damage so that appropriate therapy can be defined.

SPECIFIC ANATOMIC SITES

Cutaneous Injury

Cutaneous blunt injuries have a spectrum of clinical presentation related to the severity and mechanism of injury. Impact usually causes erythema, ecchymosis, or hematoma, but can result in necrosis with severe impact if the skin ruptures.

Compression usually causes edema or transient ischemia but can cause severe damage with necrosis. The "decubitus" pressure injury results in necrosis of the subcutaneous tissue and muscle as well as the dermis.

Shearing injuries usually result in skin blisters or subcutaneous hematomas but can be associated with skin avulsion. The diagnosis and treatment of cutaneous injuries follow.

ERYTHEMA

Minimal impact or compression to skin can cause vasodilation of the dermal vascular arcade. This is probably caused by release of vasoactive amines.

1. Diagnosis
   a. Erythema and local heat occur without severe swelling or pain.
   b. There is no systemic temperature elevation.
   c. Persistent erythema (after 36 hours) suggests underlying injury, particularly muscle and fat necrosis.
2. Treatment. Immobilization, elevation, and avoidance of additional injury for 24 to 36 hours are required.

EDEMA

There is transudation of protein-rich fluid into the extravascular tissues, although the capillary remains intact.

1. Diagnosis
   a. Edematous skin "pits" with pressure and/or has the dimpled appearance of an orange skin (termed *peau d'orange*).
   b. Paresthesias, pallor, and stiffness are characteristic.

2. Treatment
   a. *Elevation* is the most important aspect of treatment.
   b. *Cool packs* cause local vasoconstriction, which minimizes additional swelling and reduces pain but does *not* reduce established edema. Thus, cooling should be used for the first 12 to 24 hours after injury for comfort and prevention of edema.

      Avoid direct application of ice because this can freeze tissue, causing cellular death. Chemical cool packs or ice wrapped in a plastic bag is used if the wound is to be kept dry. A cloth soaked in ice water or direct immersion in cool water can be used if a wet environment is needed.
   c. *Light compression dressings* can be used, but care must be taken to avoid excessive tightness. Incorrect application or excessive compression itself can cause edema and ischemia.

      The pressure must be checked frequently to determine if progressive edema has occurred in spite of treatment. Additional edema results in a relatively tightened compression dressing. The method for applying a compression dressing is shown in Figs. 8-17 to 8-28.

BLISTERS

Blisters can be caused by shearing, compression, or burns. Proteinaceous fluid accumulates at the basement membrane epidermal-dermal junction.

1. Diagnosis. The clinical appearance of a blister is of an elevated dome of fluid-filled skin.

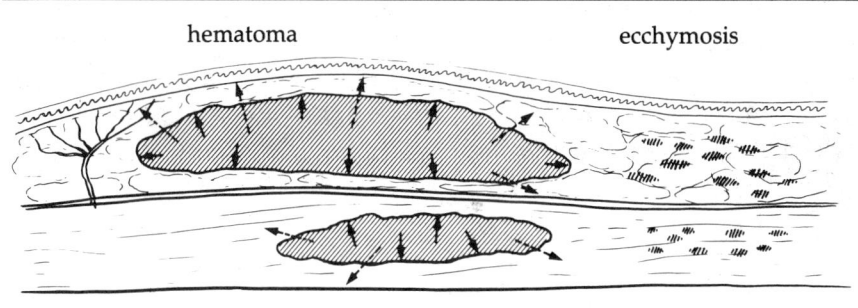

Figure 7-2. A localized hematoma is most likely to occur in distensible tissues such as fat, muscle, or fascia, whereas a diffuse ecchymosis is seen in dermis or minimally traumatized soft tissue. Hematomas cause additional damage by direct pressure and release of toxins.

2. Treatment
   a. Leave blister intact; do not aspirate or remove the skin cover.
   b. Cover with a nonadherent protective dressing for 3 to 5 days and avoid pressure or shearing.
   c. Blister fluid can be aspirated or the blister "unroofed" after 5 days.

ECCHYMOSIS (BRUISE, CONTUSION)
An ecchymosis is an area of interstitial blood caused by rupture of small vessels and capillaries. The extravascular blood is a diffuse extravasation within the tissue, whereas a hematoma is a localized collection (Fig. 7-2). The occurrence of an ecchymosis or hematoma is related to the anatomic site, whether there is a potential space for blood collection, and whether a large vessel or small capillaries are ruptured.

1. Diagnosis
   a. Initial red-blue discoloration with slight swelling
   b. No fluctuance
2. Treatment (similar to that for blister)
   a. Elevation and immobilization
   b. Cooling for 12 to 24 hours
   c. Warm packs after 12 hours

HEMATOMA
A hematoma is a localized collection of blood that forms a clot between or in fascia, muscle, fat, or distensible soft tissue (Fig. 7-2).

1. Diagnosis
   a. Signs and symptoms. A hematoma is suspected when there is:
      (1) Localized swelling
      (2) Pain
      (3) Red-blue discoloration
      (4) Fluctuance
   b. Needle aspiration. The distinction between a hematoma and a large interstitial ecchymosis can sometimes be made by needle aspiration. A #14 to 18 needle is passed through anesthetized skin into the area and slowly withdrawn with continuous negative pressure. If a

liquefied or fresh hematoma is encountered, blood may be aspirated. Aspiration not only confirms the diagnosis, but also may be therapeutic. In most cases, however, the blood has clotted and cannot be aspirated; therefore, *failure to withdraw blood does not exclude the presence of a clotted hematoma.*

2. Treatment. Treatment may be symptomatic to relieve discomfort, or the situation may require immediate drainage of the hematoma through either a surgical incision or delayed aspiration-drainage following liquefaction. Treatment is determined, in part, by the anatomic area and the volume of hematoma. It is most important to avoid the secondary complications of untreated hematomas: ischemic necrosis, disabling pain or dysfunction, metaplasia that can form scar, bursa, or ectopic ossification, and prolonged cosmetic disfigurement. The indications for drainage are as follows:

   a. High risk of necrosis. Large cutaneous hematomas can cause secondary necrosis of initially viable overlying skin through occlusion of venous flow and release of toxins. Risk of secondary necrosis is related to several factors (Fig. 7-3).

      (1) Type of skin. Tight nonexpandable skin carries a high risk. Examples of this include *digital palmar and plantar skin,* with underlying fascial aponeurosis, *pretibial skin,* scalp, and other sites in which the skin is relatively fixed to underlying tissue and strongly dependent for vascular supply on muscular perforators that may be occluded or compressed by the hematoma.

      Skin that is distensible is found on the face, ventral aspect of the trunk, proximal extremity, and dorsum of hands and feet.

      Thus, a small hematoma can exert great pressure on a nondistensible site, such as the palm or finger pad, and a large hematoma can accumulate relatively unnoticed and with minimal risk to the skin of the abdomen or upper extremity.

      (2) Severity of injury to overlying tissue. If the soft tissue overlying the hematoma is bruised and questionably viable, greater consideration should be given to hematoma drainage.

      (3) Anatomic area (see Fig. 7-3)

         (a) Blood supply. The type of blood supply to the skin and distensibility of the skin influence the risk of necrosis.

         There are two patterns of vascular distribution: axial direct cutaneous and perforating musculocutaneous. In the axial direct cutaneous pattern, there is a large central artery that passes through mobile soft fascia and radiates parallel to the skin surface. The small axial vessels running parallel to the skin are less likely to be injured. Areas of axial blood supply include the scalp and face, chest, and groin.

         Skin with a perforating blood supply has many small blood vessels emerging from the underlying muscle perpendicularly into the skin. These vessels are more likely to be severed by the original injury and may be more susceptible to compression. Areas supplied by musculocutaneous perforators include the extremities, hands and feet, back, and buttock regions. Many areas have overlapping sources of blood supply.

CLOSED AND BLUNT INJURIES 255

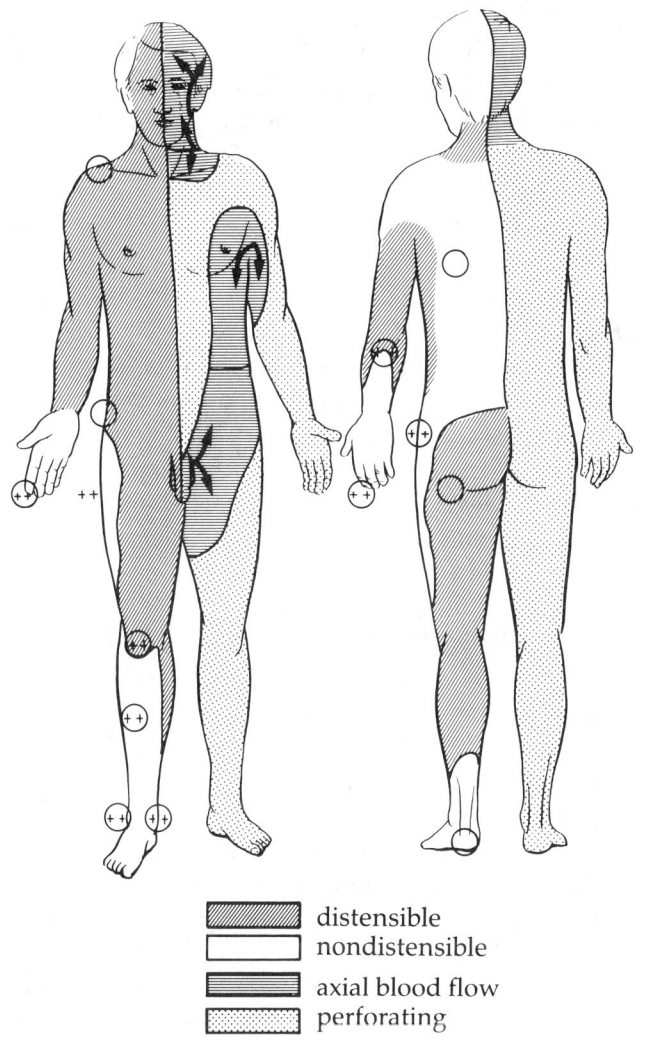

Figure 7-3. Skin characteristics that affect formation of hematomas. Highest risk of necrosis from hematoma is in areas of less distensible skin; areas of perforating blood supply; the lower extremity, in general; and bony prominences.

▨ distensible
☐ nondistensible
▤ axial blood flow
▦ perforating

(b) Bony prominences (see Fig. 7-3). There is a higher risk of tissue necrosis over bony prominences because of greater susceptibility to injury and greater pressure against the tissue. Areas of particular susceptibility include the pretibial, prepatellar, malleolar, and subungual regions.

The evaluation for skin ischemia and need for hematoma removal depends ultimately on a cumulative clinical assessment, including mechanism of injury, volume of hematoma, anatomic site, and associated tissue damage; other diagnostic clues are the rapidity of capillary blanching and refill and results of the fluorescein dye test.

(4) Fluorescein dye test. This test is becoming more widely used and better understood as an adjunct to clinical evaluation for skin necrosis. Fluorescein seems to be the best available vital dye; although others such as Evans blue dye have been used, they are somewhat more toxic and allergenic. Moreover, fluorescein can be identified using the Wood's ultraviolet light and is easily identified except in very dark-skinned people.

The test is usually used intraoperatively with the patient under general anesthesia so that the rare allergic reaction can be more easily managed. However, fluorescein is used with the awake patient if adequate precautions are taken against major allergic reactions. The awake patient may experience transient nausea and/or vomiting. The usual adult dose is 2 vials (500 mg/vial) injected slowly over 4 to 5 minutes through an indwelling venous catheter. Vascularized areas are characterized by multiple pinpoint sites of yellow fluorescein that occur 5 to 10 minutes after infusion. These can be seen by direct visualization or with the ultraviolet light and remain for 24 to 48 hours.

    (a) Positive test. The presence of stippled fluorescein indicates adequate vascularization of the traumatized area (at the time of the test). Subsequent skin death can occur from the progression of the hematoma, infection, or additional trauma.

    (b) Negative test. The absence of fluorescein is highly suggestive of severe skin ischemia and eventual complete or partial skin necrosis; however, some nonfluorescent areas may survive.

Because injecting an inadequate dose, not waiting long enough between injections of the drug and examination with the Wood's U-V lamp, or local vasoconstriction contribute to false negative readings, the negative fluorescein test must be interpreted in conjunction with all other clinical signs. It can be helpful in deciding when to incise and drain hematomas that are causing pressure on damaged skin.

The test also can be used in combination with clinical judgment as the indication for skin *excision* for open, untidy lacerations and skin ruptures, as well as hematomas that require debridement.

b. Disabling pain and dysfunction. Very large hematomas and small hematomas at specific locations require drainage for relief of pain or dysfunction. Pain is a signal of tissue ischemia (muscle, skin) or nerve compression.

    (1) Subungual hematomas of the digits can cause great pain because of pressure between nonexpansible nails and bone. Bone necrosis can occur.

    (2) Hematomas of joints (hemarthrosis) are most likely to cause pain and dysfunction because of nonexpansibility of the joint space. Hemarthroses are very common following trauma to individuals affected with hemophilia. Excessive joint pressure can cause cartilage necrosis and arthritis.

c. Secondary scarring and metaplasia (formation of bursa, ossification). A hematoma usually liquefies and is slowly absorbed, resulting in return to the original tissue contour. However, for poorly understood reasons, some hematomas are not resorbed but undergo ossification, chondrification, or formation of a bursa. Thus, large hematomas at critical functional or cosmetic areas should be drained. This includes *periarticular hematomas*, to avoid joint limitation, and *perichondrial hematomas* of the ear and nasal septum, which are susceptible to replacement by scar and cartilage. The end result of an

untreated hematoma at these sites may be "cauliflower" ear, septal deviation, nasal obstruction, or even cartilage necrosis.
   d. Open wound. A hematoma is an ideal culture medium. A hematoma in the drainage pathway of a more distal open wound is susceptible to infection. Bacteria in any open wound can gain hematogenous access to the hematoma. Any hematoma in continuity with an open wound should be drained.

Facial Injury

Blunt trauma to the face causes skin and soft tissue trauma and unique ocular and periorbital injuries and facial fractures.

OCULAR AND PERIORBITAL INJURY

Blunt injuries of the globe and periorbital structures can be overlooked easily because globe injuries may be detectable only by intraocular ophthalmoscopy. Although this examination is difficult because of pain, lid edema, and lack of patient cooperation, a thorough screening examination must be performed. Very few ocular injuries should be treated in the emergency room or by the nonspecialist. *The emphasis should be on recognition, protective dressing, and referral to a specialist.* Many of the penetrating injuries are described in Chapter 6; only blunt injuries are described here.

The eye is partially protected against injuries by the surrounding orbit, fat, and lids. The orbital rims, zygoma, and nose protrude anterior to the globe and afford a bony barrier. The globe is suspended in periorbital fat, which acts as a cushion against blunt injuries. The lids close by reflex action, thus offering a screening protection. In spite of these protections, globe injuries are often encountered. An approach to diagnosis follows.

1. Pain control. Pain can be temporarily controlled for examination with topical anesthetics, such as tetracaine or proparacaine. Anesthetics should not be used for continuous therapy without consultation with an ophthalmologist.
2. Visual acuity testing. Each eye is tested independently using the Snellen acuity chart, and depth perception is tested. If the chart is not available, testing can be achieved by having the patient read from a book and count fingers. If the patient notes decreased vision, an initial evaluation for the cause of blurring should be made, but in most cases, an ophthalmologist should also be consulted.

    Be sure that the decreased vision is not caused by a refractive error or ointments applied to the wound.

    Causes of loss of visual acuity from trauma include acute glaucoma; bleeding into anterior chamber; conjunctival edema; corneal abrasions; traumatic iritis; retinal detachment; optic nerve transection; retinal artery occlusion; and ruptured anterior chamber, posterior chamber, or lens (Fig. 7-4).
3. Conjunctiva. Trauma can cause symptoms of grittiness, burning, pain, loss of visual acuity, and blurring. A visual inspection of the conjunctival surface of the globe and the sulci can provide a basis for diagnosis (Fig. 7-5). Free-floating foreign material should be removed immediately

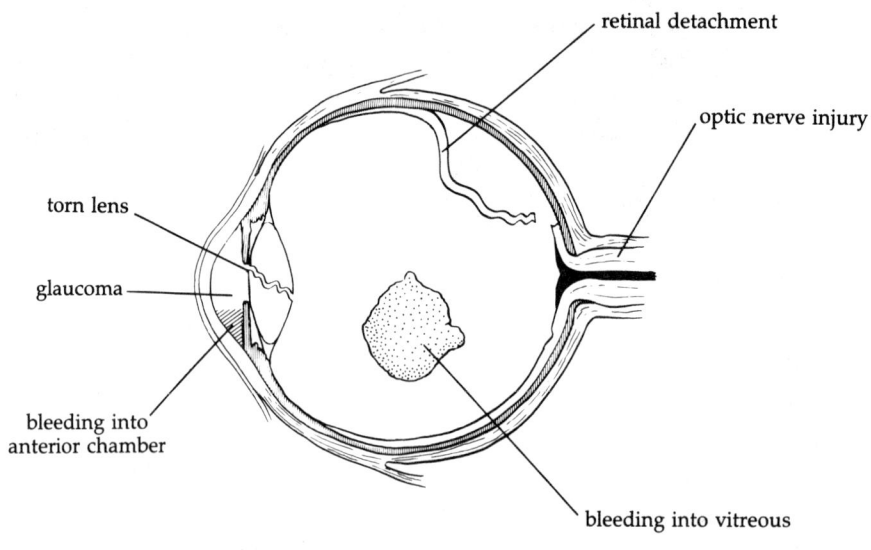

Figure 7-4. Some causes of loss of visual acuity. These conditions may be accompanied by eye pain or redness.

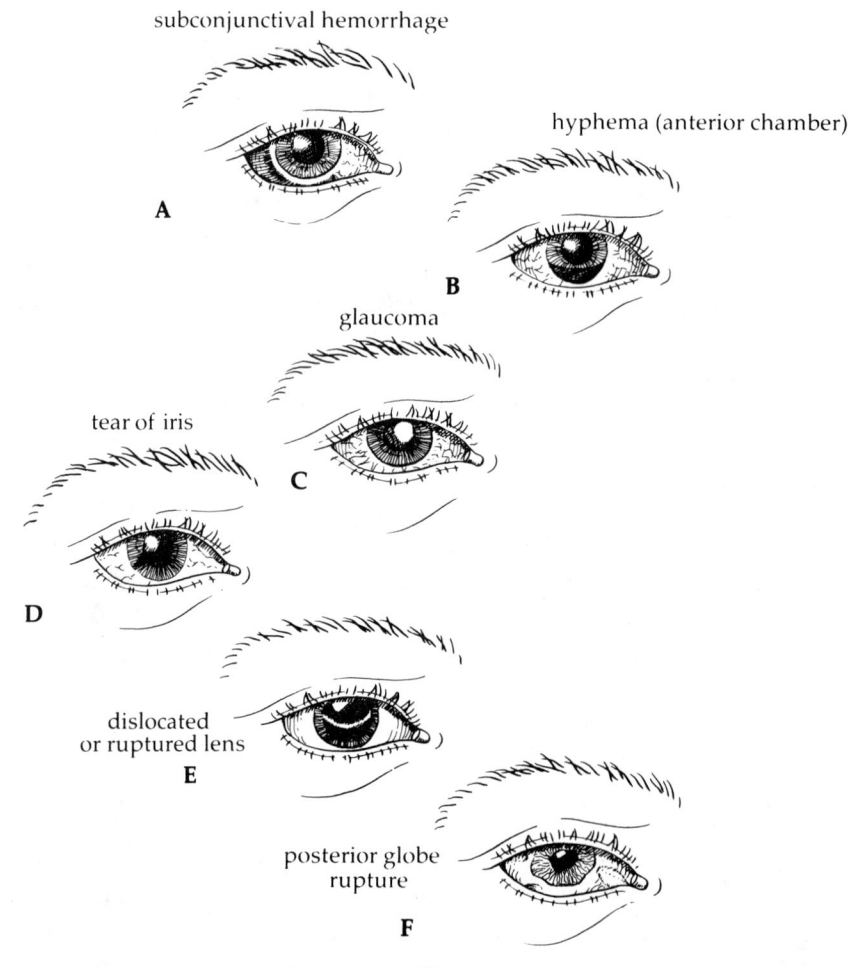

Figure 7-5. Typical appearance of the eye with various injuries.
A. In subconjunctival hemorrhage, there are irregular patches of blood that do not extend to the iris.
B. An injury to the anterior chamber can show a dependent accumulation of blood and surface contour irregularities (hyphema).
C. Acute glaucoma. An acute obstruction of the anterior chamber may be seen in isolation or in association with hyphema. Vessels may be dilated (dilated pupil and eye pain), or the conjunctiva may extend to the iris.
D. A tear of the iris is seen as an irregular contour and often has associated hyphema.
E. Lens rupture has an irregular light reflection.
F. Posterior chamber rupture presents with irregular buckling of the globe.

with a moist cotton-tipped applicator or sponge pledget or with irrigation with saline solution using a bulb or needle syringe. Examine the upper lid by eversion. Small foreign bodies in the conjunctiva or sclera should be removed whenever encountered. Large foreign bodies that may perforate into the anterior or posterior chambers should not be removed because of possible leakage of vitreous or aqueous. If a large foreign body is encountered, it should be left in place and the eye protected against additional damage with eye pads placed over both eyes until an ophthalmologist is consulted.

A red eye may be a sign of numerous conditions, including acute glaucoma, iritis, conjunctivitis from abrasion or foreign body, or conjunctival hemorrhage.

Subconjunctival hemorrhage is perhaps the most common and least severe of these conditions. Subconjunctival hemorrhage may vary from petechiae to large extravasations. A diffuse hemorrhage appearing hours after injury suggests an orbital fracture, whereas a localized hemorrhage usually indicates contusion to the eye. The conjunctiva is firmly attached to the lids and loosely attached to the globe, and blood migrates toward but stops short of the limbus.

Don't forget to ask about and *look for a contact lens!* A contact lens may be difficult to identify if dislodged into the upper lid sulcus. Contact lenses are the most common cause of eye pain from corneal abrasion. The symptoms include conjunctivitis, epiphora, and blepharospasm (see Figs. 7-4 and 7-5).

4. Removal of contact lens. First, ask the patient to remove the lens. If the patient is unable to do so, proceed with removal.

   One of the most common problems is eye pain and redness caused by contact lens dislocation. Corneal abrasions may also occur. It is essential to remove the contact lens (Figs. 7-6 and 7-7) and treat corneal abrasions, if present.

   Care must be taken when removing the lens because a dry suction can occur and lead to avulsion of the corneal conjunctiva.

5. Upper lid levator muscle. Careful observation of the lid may show that a portion of it does not elevate completely. It may be difficult to distinguish between ptosis caused by muscle injury and that caused by edema.

6. Extraocular muscles. Limitation of globe movement commonly occurs because of muscle contusion, and rarely, because of nerve injury or muscle entrapment in orbital-floor fractures.

   a. Limited upward gaze—orbital-floor fracture (Fig. 7-8). Limitation of upward movement of one eye with associated diplopia is commonly caused by either a fracture of the orbital floor with entrapment of the inferior rectus muscle in the orbital bones or muscle contusion. The differentiation between an inferior rectus entrapment and muscle contusion or nerve injury can be made by additional testing and examination, including:

      (1) Forced duction test (Fig. 7-9). This is usually done in the operating room with the patient anesthetized but can be done on a sedated patient with topical anesthesia.

      (2) Water's facial x-ray. Look for depression or "teardrop" of maxillary roof.

Figure 7-6. Removal of hard contact lenses.
A. If possible, the lens should be irrigated and the contact slid off the cornea and onto the bulbar conjunctiva to avoid accidental avulsion of corneal conjunctiva.
B. If the lens cannot be slid off, it should be gently "rocked" off the cornea by pressing on the edge to break the suction effect.

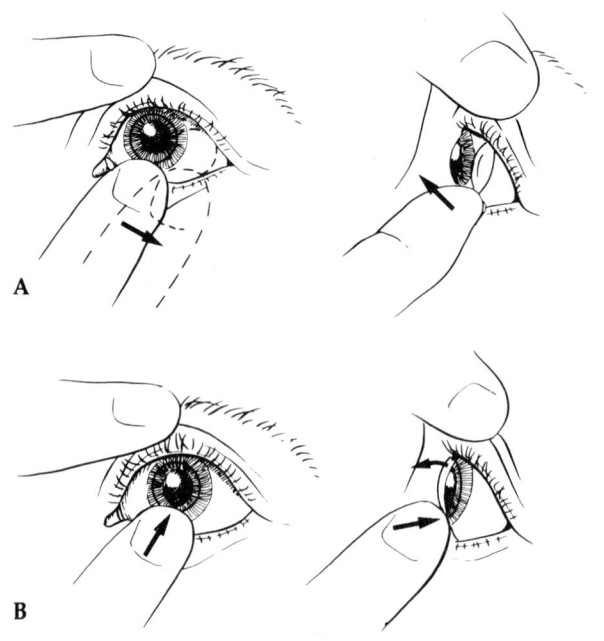

Figure 7-7. Removal of soft contact lenses. The soft contact lens can be removed by pinching the lateral edges of the lens, causing it to buckle.

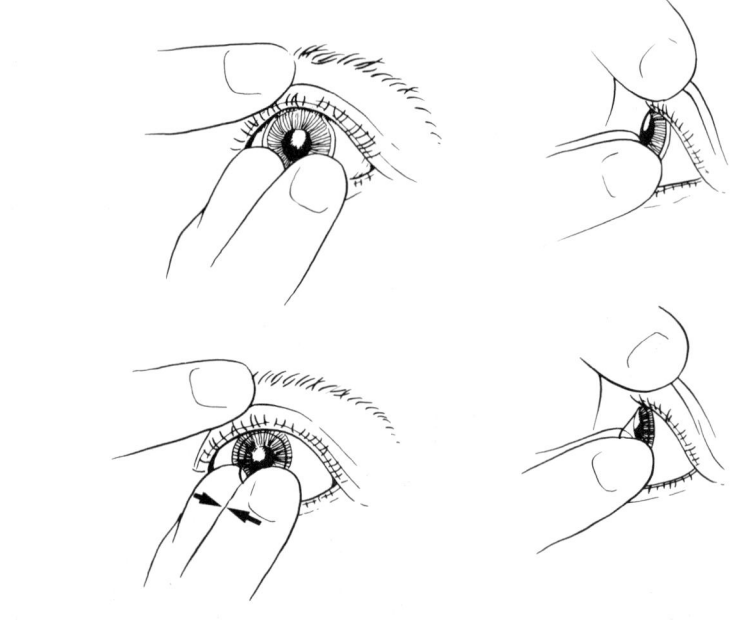

(3) Physical evidence of fractures, including palpable or visible deformities, or infraorbital nerve anesthesia.

Ultimately, the diagnosis may require surgical exploration. Ninety percent of patients with diplopia have transient muscle contusion, and normal vision returns in 3 to 7 days. Orbital-floor exploration can be delayed for 7 to 10 days.

b. Limited gaze in multiple fields. Limitation of motion in several fields of muscle movement is most likely caused by a hematoma of the

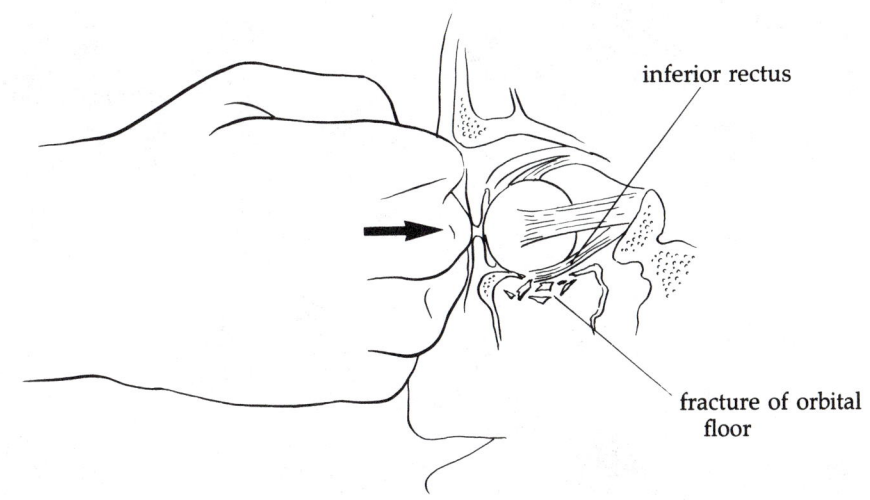

Figure 7-8. Limitation of ocular movement can occur from entrapment of the inferior rectus muscle in the bones of the orbital floor. If only the inferior rectus is entrapped, other muscles function normally.

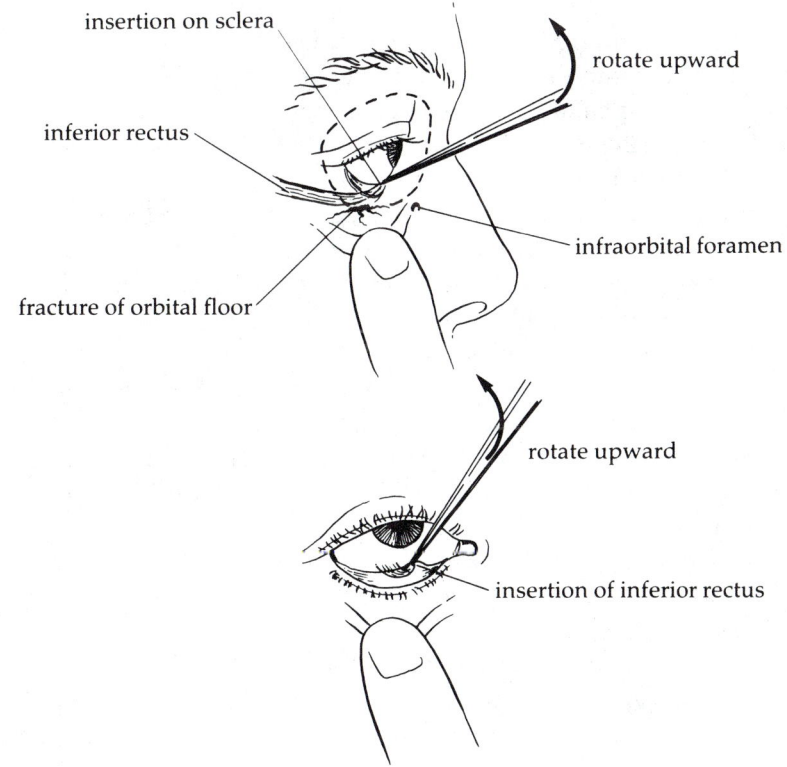

Figure 7-9. Forced duction test to identify inferior rectus muscle entrapment. Grasp the insertion site of the inferior rectus on the globe with forceps and rotate upward to assess range of motion and resistance to pull. Compare this side to the normal uninjured side.

retroorbital fat pad and muscle but may be caused by a fracture through the superior orbital fissure, with associated injury to cranial nerves III, IV, and VI.

7. Pupils. The injured globe may show either a constricted or a dilated pupil depending on the site and nature of injury. A preexisting anisocoria (unequal pupil size) can be misleading.

A miotic (constricted) pupil is a sign either of irritation to the third cranial nerve as a result of intracranial compression or the presence of Horner's syndrome.

Figure 7-10. Anatomy of nasolacrimal apparatus. Key sites are the canaliculi under the orbicularis muscles, the ampulla behind the canthal tendon, the nasolacrimal duct penetrating the nasal bone (fenestra), and the duct exiting beneath the inferior turbinate.

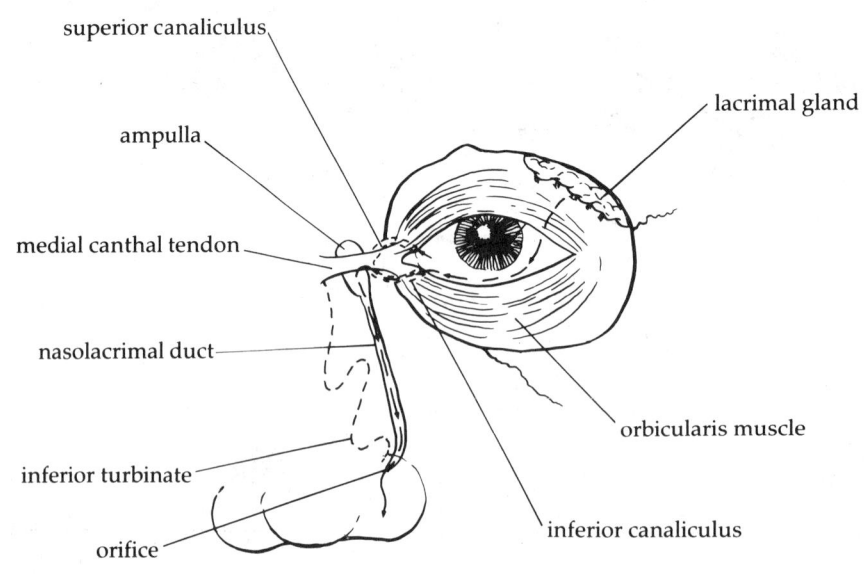

A mydriatic (dilated) pupil is more common with direct ocular injury but can also occur with a total third nerve intracranial paresis.

8. Nasolacrimal apparatus. Injury to the lacrimal apparatus commonly occurs from fractures of the frontal and nasal bones. Early repair is far more likely to achieve patency and function than is secondary repair; thus considerable detail is given to diagnosis of this problem.
   a. Anatomy (Fig. 7-10)
      (1) Tears are formed by the lacrimal gland in the superior lateral region of the orbit.
      (2) Secretions accumulate in the fornices, and blinking distributes tears over the globe and propagates tears medially toward the paired superior and inferior lacrimal puncta.
      (3) The great majority (80–90%) of tears are drained through the lower punctum, but the superior punctum can drain all of the basal secretions.
      (4) The puncta open into the upper and lower lacrimal canaliculi, which pass into the lacrimal sac (the sac is behind the medial canthal tendon).
      (5) The lacrimal sac then passes through a bony window into the nasal cavity as the nasolacrimal duct. The nasolacrimal duct courses inferiorly along the lateral wall of the nasal cavity to empty just below the inferior nasal turbinate.
   b. Testing for nasolacrimal obstruction
      (1) *Observation.* The transected or obstructed system is sometimes identifiable by direct visualization. The lacrimal sac lies behind the medial canthal tendon. If there is severe fracture of the frontonasal area, there is presumptive evidence of lacrimal sac injury.
      (2) *Dye passage test* (Fig. 7-11). A colored dye, such as fluorescein, is placed in the lower lid fornix. Fluorescein is the preferred test dye because the Wood's ultraviolet lamp can be used to identify fluorescein if there has been severe associated bleeding that might otherwise obscure the color of another dye.

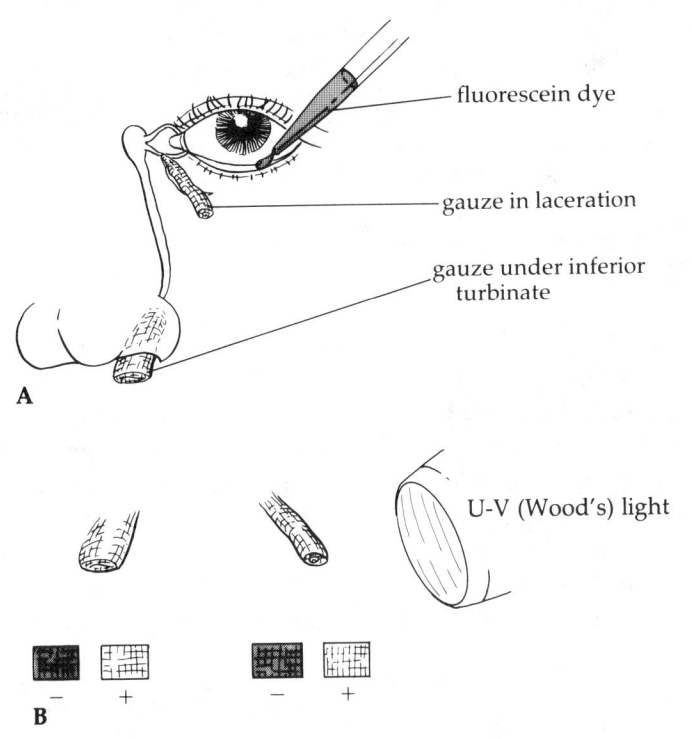

Figure 7-11. Fluorescein dye test.
A. The test examines for dye passage into lacerations and under the nasal turbinates. Several minutes after installation of the dye, the gauze is removed and examined with an ultraviolet Wood's light.
B. The interpretation of this test is described in the text.

A 2 × 2 gauze pad is placed in the nasal cavity on the side of the injury directly underneath the inferior nasal turbinate. A small gauze pad is also placed in any laceration near the canaliculi. Additional fluid ("artificial tears" or 0.2 N saline) is placed in the conjunctival sulcus.

Failure to identify fluorescein on the intranasal pack after 20 to 30 minutes is presumptive evidence of lacrimal apparatus obstruction by a fracture but may only indicate edema of the duct lining.

This test does not determine the level of obstruction; moreover, the presence of dye in the nose pad does not exclude transection of one of the canaliculi and patency of the other. Presence of dye in a laceration at the injury site indicates a transection of the canaliculus or ampulla.

If the dye tests suggest lacrimal injury, the patient should be referred to an ophthalmologist or plastic surgeon for repair in the operating room.

(3) *Malleable lacrimal probes* are used to test the patency of the lacrimal drainage system. Although this test ordinarily is performed by the ophthalmologic consultant, with experience it can be done successfully by the emergency physician. Each of the canaliculi is individually tested for patency. Extreme care must be taken not to force the probe into a false passage or the tissues will be damaged additionally. Details of this technique are described in Figs. 6-19 and 6-20.

(4) *Dacryocystograms* are rarely used for emergency diagnosis because the diagnosis can be made by other methods; however, if

there are equivocal results, it may be justifiable to do an emergency dacryocystogram. The dacryocystogram is most helpful for diagnosis of the level of obstruction of the nasolacrimal duct associated with naso-orbital fractures, rather than for laceration of the canaliculi. The procedure requires cannulation of both canaliculi and injection with a radiopaque contrast material such as iodized oil (Lipiodol). Radiographs indicate the level of obstruction or disruption.

FRACTURE OF THE FACIAL SKELETON

Most fractures of facial bones can be evaluated in a leisurely manner with the objectives of identifying the fracture sites and referring for treatment. The exceptions are severe bleeding, usually from a maxillary fracture; airway obstruction, usually from mandibular fractures; and acute blindness, associated with orbital fractures. The acute treatment of these problems is discussed in relation to the fracture site.

The diagnosis of a facial fracture can usually be made on physical examination and confirmed radiologically (standard and tomographic x-ray, CT scan).

1. Diagnostic examination
   a. Deformity. Observe and palpate for malposition of fractured bones. Be aware that extensive swelling may disguise deformity.
   b. Swelling and ecchymosis. Hemorrhage and edema may disguise deformity but also can be signs of underlying fractures.
   c. Malocclusion. The normal occlusal relations usually are altered by fractures of the facial skeleton. The patient may tell you that his or her teeth do not fit properly. Checking dental records may be very helpful.
   d. Pain and tenderness. The fracture site may be tender to palpation.
   e. Instability. Facial bones may be quite mobile.
   f. Muscle spasm. Temporalis, masseter, and suprahyoid muscles may be in spasm. This is manifested as local pain and causes malocclusion.
   g. Bleeding. Intraoral bleeding occurs with compound fractures of the mandible and maxilla.
   h. Sensory loss. Anesthesia or hypoesthesia of the face and teeth may occur because of compression or transection of sensory nerves that pass through bony foramina.
   i. X-rays. The initial x-ray screening examinations should be appropriate for the suspected fractured site (Tables 7-1 and 7-2).
2. Periorbital fractures. Fractures involving the orbital walls are often associated with other fractures of the nose, zygoma, or maxilla, but they may occur independently.

   The areas of fracture can best be described as fronto-orbital (superior), naso-orbital (medial), maxillo-orbital (inferior), and zygomatico-orbital (lateral). All these fractures require consultation and operative reduction. The following are guides to diagnosis.

Table 7-1. Initial x-ray screening for facial fractures

Facial bone	Suggested routine x-ray projections
Mandible	
Coronoid processes, ascending ramus, and body	Lateral and oblique of mandible
Symphysis, body, and ascending rami	Posterioanterior of mandible
Condyle and subcondyle	Modified Towne's view (anteroposterior of mandible)
Anterior mandible	Dental occlusal view of anterior of mandible
Maxilla	Stereo Water's view; PA and lateral facial view
Zygomatic arch	Stereo Water's view; submental—vertex
Nasal bone	Lateral view of nose, superoinferior nasal view
Orbit	Stereo Water's view

Table 7-2. Special x-rays for facial fracture

Facial bone	X-ray
Mandibular condyle	Tomograms of the temporomandibular joint with the mouth open and closed; Panorex
Maxilla (orbital floor)	Tomograms of the orbital bones (AP and/or lateral)
Orbit	CT scan (computerized tomography)
Zygomatic arch	Trispiral tomography
Dental alveolar	Dental x-rays; Panorex (or orthopantogram)

  a. *Fronto-orbital* (supraorbital) *fractures* involve the superior orbital rim and frontal sinuses (Fig. 7-12). The signs and symptoms of these fractures include:

    (1) *Depression* of frontal bone and superior orbital rim

    (2) *Proptosis* of the globe, which occurs because the orbital roof is usually depressed and thus reduces the volume of the bony orbit

    (3) *Diplopia*, which may occur because of damage to cranial nerves III, IV, and VI as they pass through the supraorbital fissure

    (4) *Ptosis* of upper lid, usually caused by edema, but possibly indicative of displacement of levator insertion

    (5) *Supraorbital anesthesia,* caused by compression or transection of supraorbital or supratrochlear nerve

    (6) *Blindness,* caused by compression of the optic nerve at the foramen

    (7) *Meningitis* (late), a serious infection caused by extension of frontal fracture lines into the cranial vault

    (8) *Frontal mucocele and sinusitis,* late complications caused by obstruction of the frontal sinus

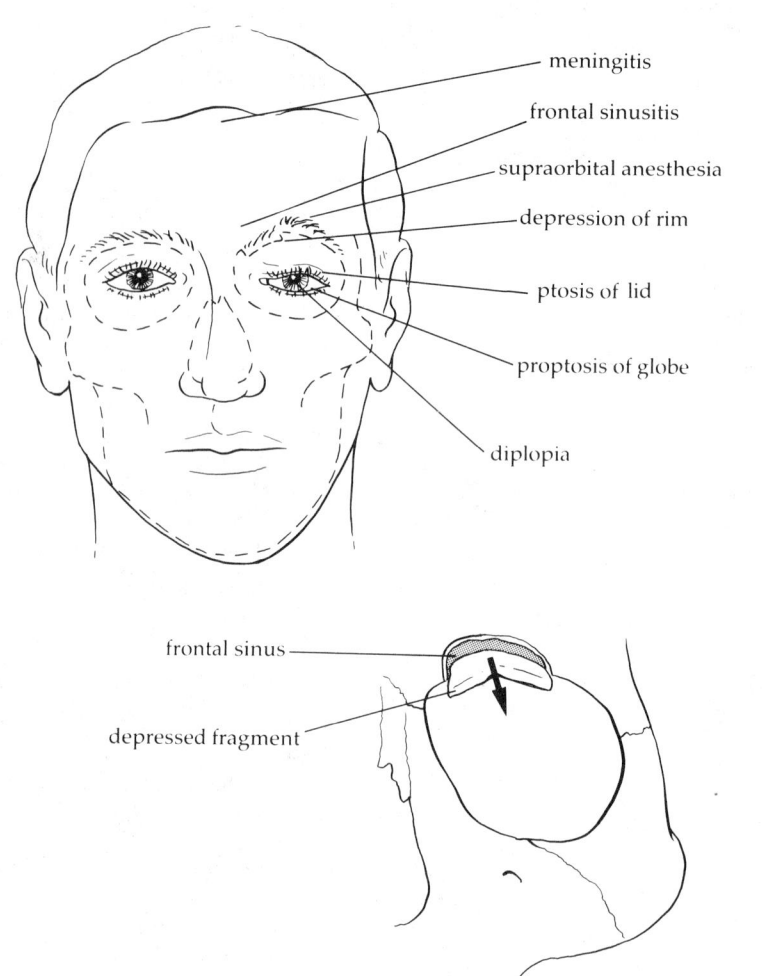

Figure 7-12. Signs and symptoms of supraorbital fractures. These include depression or impaction of the orbital rim and frontal sinus.

    b. *Naso-orbital fractures* commonly occur as part of complex fractures of the midface (Fig. 7-13). The signs and symptoms include:
        (1) *Epicanthal fold*—an apparent web across the medial lid.
        (2) *Telecanthus*—increased distance between the canthi, caused by distraction of the lacrimal bone by the pull of the orbicularis muscle on the medial canthal tendon
        (3) *Depressed nasal bridge*—flattened nasal bridge, caused by crushing of nasal dorsum
        (4) *Early exophthalmos*—caused by hemorrhage and edema of the orbital contents
        (5) *Late enophthalmos*—caused by fractures of the eggshell thin medial wall, which allow displacement of orbital fat into the ethmoidal or sphenoidal sinus. The relatively increased orbital cavity size allows sinking inward of the globe.
    c. *Infraorbital fractures* are relatively common and associated with maxillary, nasoorbital, and zygomatic fractures (Fig. 7-14). The signs and symptoms include:
        (1) *Infraorbital nerve anesthesia.* The nerve is often contused or compressed, causing anesthesia of the medial cheek, upper lip, and lateral nose.

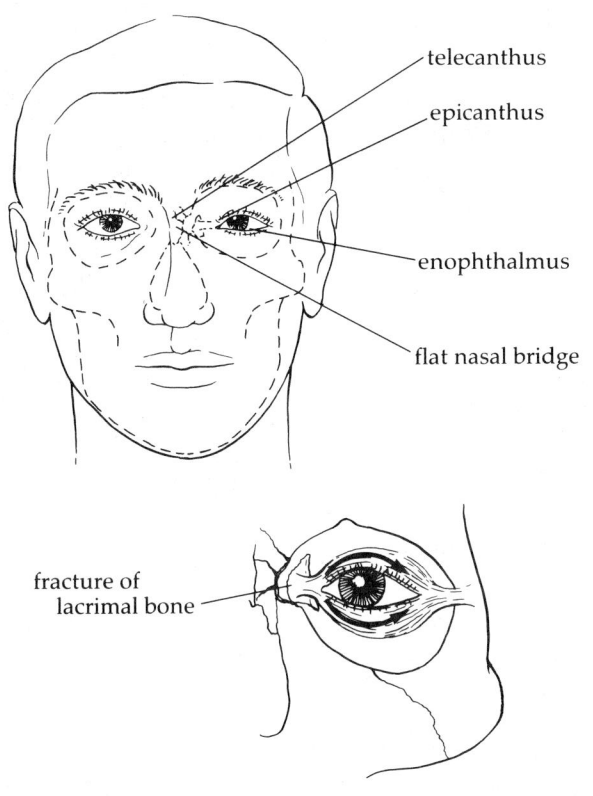

Figure 7-13. Signs and symptoms of naso-orbital fractures. These include depression of nasal bones, fractures into ethmoidal and sphenoidal sinuses, and displacement of the medial canthal tendon insertion.

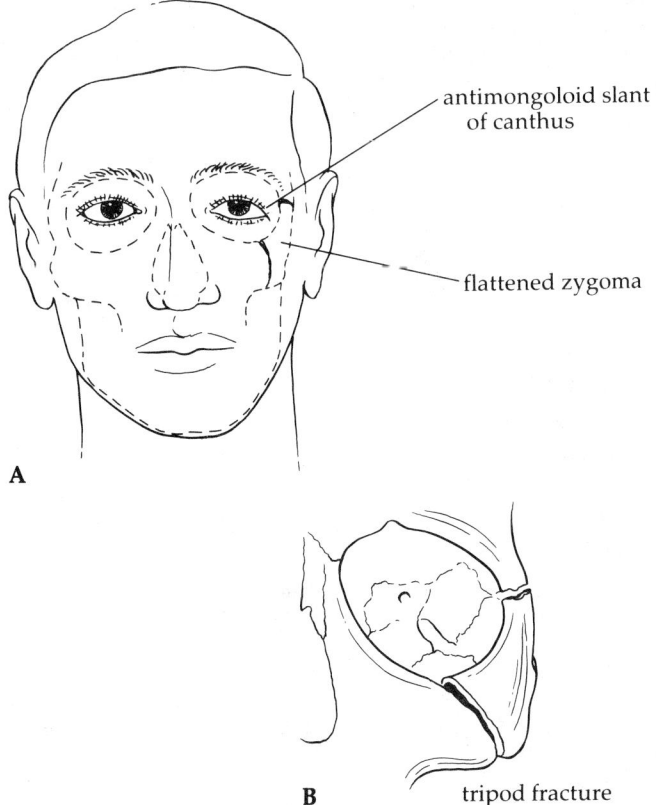

Figure 7-14. Signs and symptoms of infraorbital fractures.
A. Depression of zygoma and attached canthal tendon.
B. Tripod fracture. Not seen is the third element of this fracture, the zygomatic temporal fracture.

(2) *Diplopia.* This may be caused by entrapment of the inferior rectus (this is described under "blowout" fractures of the orbital floor).
(3) *Early exophthalmos.* Initial hematoma and swelling cause apparent exophthalmus.
(4) *Late enophthalmos.* Displacement of orbital contents into the maxillary sinus and scar contracture of periorbital ligaments and intraorbital contents lead to enophthalmos. Enophthalmos is characterized by the presence of *lid ptosis* and *abnormally deep supratarsal sulcus.*
  d. *Lateral orbit—zygomatic arch fractures* have also been called tripod fractures because of concomitant fracture through zygomaticofrontal and zygomaticotemporal areas (see Fig. 7-14). The signs and symptoms include:
   (1) *Depression of lateral canthus* (antimongoloid slant). The lateral canthus is attached to the zygoma and most commonly is displaced inferiorly.
   (2) *Flattened cheekbone*
   (3) *Infraorbital fracture,* with all the symptoms and signs related to fracture at that site
3. Nasal trauma (fractures and bleeding)
  a. Bleeding
   (1) Common sites of bleeding include the septum and the lateral nasal wall and mucosa. Bleeding from the septum is usually related to minor trauma. Bleeding from the anterior septum (Kiesselbach's area) is most common in younger patients, whereas bleeding that is posterior from the sphenopalatine or posterior ethmoidal artery is more common in older patients. Bleeding from the lateral nasal wall and mucosa is usually caused by nasal bone fractures.
   (2) Diagnosis. Examine the patient in a sitting position using a hand mirror, nasal speculum, and suction. As clots are suctioned, the nasal mucosa can be sprayed or packed with a topical anesthetic agent such as 1% Xylocaine with epinephrine or a 4% cocaine solution (be cautious of dosage), which provides local vasoconstriction as well as anesthesia. Obtain blood, if necessary, for typing and cross-matching.
  b. Intranasal anesthesia
   (1) Anatomy (Fig. 7-15)
    (a) The anterior and posterior ethmoidal nerves exit through the cribriform plate at the dome of the nasal vestibule.
    (b) The sphenopalatine nerve exits from the posterior region of the middle turbinate.
    (c) The posterior nasal vestibule is supplied by the branches from the greater palatine nerve, lesser palatine nerve, vagus nerve, and glossopharyngeal nerve.
   (2) Method of anesthesia (Fig. 7-16). A 4% or 10% cocaine solution spray or cotton pledgets moistened with the solution and placed against the anterior ethmoidal and sphenopalatine sensory nerves achieves regional block.

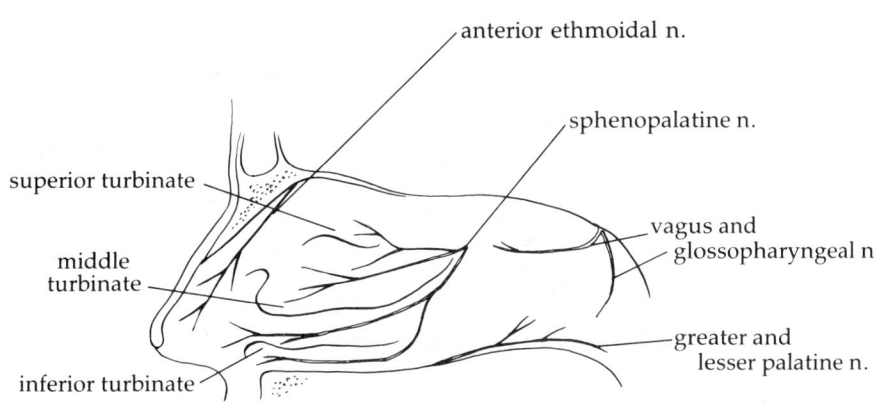

Figure 7-15. Sensory nerve supply to the nasal cavity and nasopharyngeal cavity. The sensory distribution is overlapping.

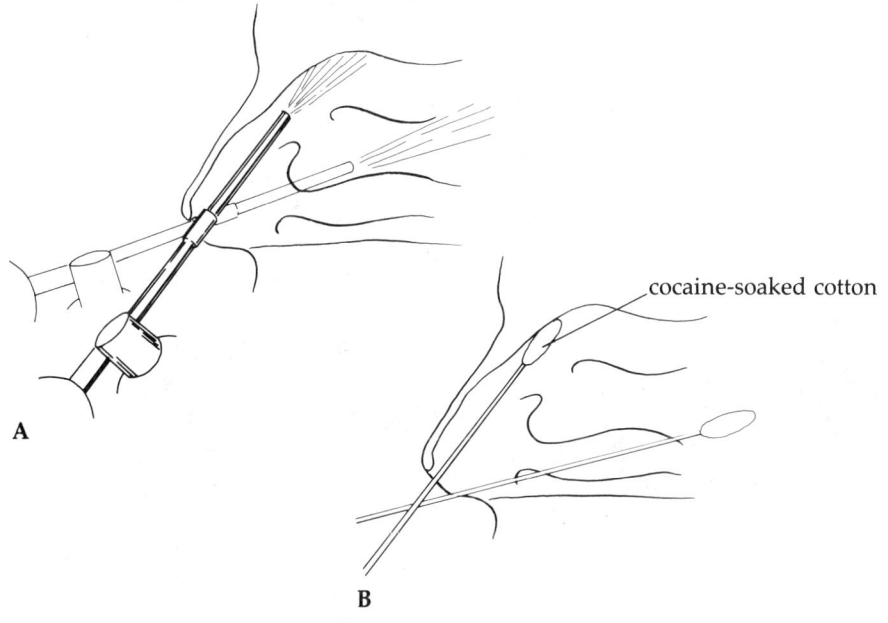

Figure 7-16. Intranasal anesthesia.
A. Spray the septum and vestibule. Additional spray is required for posterior bleeding; ask the patient to inhale deeply through the nose and simultaneously spray into the far posterior.
B. Carefully place cocaine-dampened cotton applicators at the site of the anterior ethmoidal and sphenopalatine nerves.

(a) Intranasal anesthesia in the posterior nose and nasopharyngeal area is achieved by a spray of hexylcaine (Cyclaine) or other topical anesthetic spray.

(b) A cotton pledget is soaked with a 4% or 10% cocaine solution. Remember that the toxic dose of cocaine is 250 mg (2.5 ml of 10% solution or 6 ml of 4% solution). Because it is difficult to assess the actual amount of cocaine, it is preferable to use a considerably smaller amount by wringing free the excess cocaine from each pledget.

Extreme care must be taken to stay within the safe limits of cocaine usage. The first pledget is inserted into the dome of the nasal cavity against the cribriform plate just above the superior turbinate.

(c) The second pledget is inserted under the middle turbinate.

Figure 7-17. Bleeding from the anterior septum usually can be controlled by pressure against the ala.

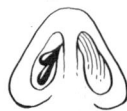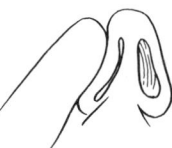

        (d) Additional topical anesthesia can be obtained by packing the posterior nasal cavity with ¼-inch or ½-inch gauze packing soaked with 4% Xylocaine or cocaine.
   c. Treatment of intranasal bleeding
     (1) Initial steps
        (a) Posttrauma nasal bleeding may be controlled by head elevation; the patient should be face down to avoid swallowing blood and to make it easier to estimate the severity of bleeding.
        (b) Direct pressure is attempted next.
        (c) Topical anesthesia with cocaine may also reduce bleeding by its vasoconstrictive effect. This is done before anterior packing.
        (d) The anterior pack is placed (Fig. 7-18).
     (2) Anterior septal bleeding
        (a) First, attempt direct pressure against the septum by pushing the ala of the nose on the side of the bleeding against the septum (Fig. 7-17). Pressure is maintained for 5 to 10 minutes.
        (b) Use an anterior pack (see Fig. 7-18). Anterior nasal packs are rarely required for spontaneous epistaxis but are commonly used for traumatic anterior bleeding. The cotton gauze pack can be impregnated with an antibiotic ointment. This limits adherence of the clot against the gauze and reduces bacterial odor. The pack is left in place for 12 to 24 hours.
        (c) Posterior bleeding (Fig. 7-19). Posterior packs are difficult to position and not particularly effective. Operative intervention may be required if packing and blood replacement seem inadequate.
   d. Nasal fractures without bleeding. Minor nasal fractures can be reduced in the emergency department. Diagnosis is based almost exclusively on clinical examination for deformity. X-rays are of limited value. The procedure is as follows:
     (1) Obtain anesthesia as described in the previous section.
     (2) Elevate the nasal fragment using a blunt flat instrument (scalpel handle, clamp, or Asche forceps).
     (3) Pack the nasal vestibule with antibiotic ointment–impregnated gauze (as for bleeding).
     (4) Apply a nasal splint.
     (5) Packing for a splint should be left in place for 5 to 7 days.
4. Maxillary fractures. Occasionally maxillary fractures are associated with massive hemorrhage from torn venous plexuses or branches to the internal maxillary artery. If there is a probable maxillary fracture, im-

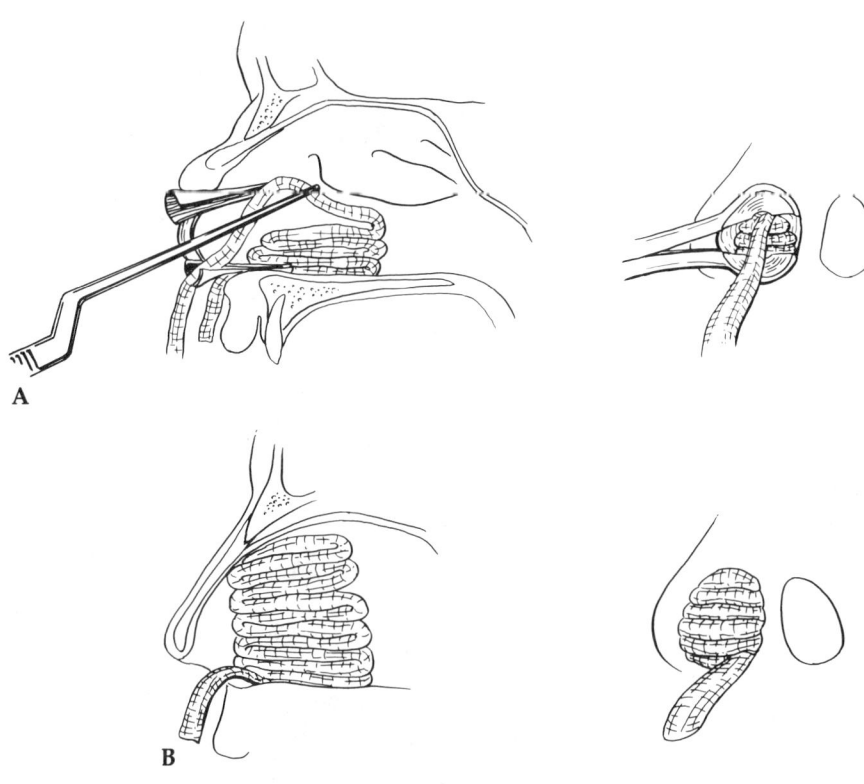

Figure 7-18. Anterior packing.
A. Packing should extend slightly posterior to the observed bleeding site.
B. Final packing should compact the vestibule snugly.

mediate compression of the fracture line is required. Grasp the anterior maxilla and push upward toward the base of the skull. This compresses the fractured bone ends, thus diminishing bleeding (Fig. 7-20).

Maxillary fractures are not treated in the emergency department but require referral for evaluation and surgery. Thus the emphasis is on diagnosis and referral for consultation.

Maxillary fractures can be subdivided conveniently into anatomic areas: periorbital, nasal, zygoma, and maxillary Le Fort I, II, and III. These can occur in isolation or any combination.

Maxillary fractures have been classified according to the most common sites of fracture (Fig. 7-21): Le Fort I—transverse; Le Fort II—pyramidal, through the orbit; and Le Fort III—craniofacial disjunction.

The diagnosis of maxillary fracture is suggested by the following signs and symptoms:
a. Malocclusion. Inability to achieve normal occlusion is often a result of maxillary fracture.
b. Facial flattening and elongation. Separation of the maxilla from the upper face or cranium causes displacement of the axilla in a posterior and inferior direction.
c. Associated fractures of the orbit. These are described earlier in this chapter.
5. Mandibular fractures (Fig. 7-22). Mandibular fractures almost always require consultation and operating-room reduction. The primary responsibility of the emergency physician is to treat acute associated injuries, airway obstruction, and bleeding. Minor injuries such as tem-

Figure 7-19. Posterior packing.
A. Pass a balloon catheter into the nose on the side of the bleeding.
B. Inflate the catheter with 10 to 15 cc of air. Gently pull the catheter forward until it fits firmly in the choanae.
C. Insert a nasal pack snugly against the catheter balloon, particularly in the region of the posterior ethmoidal and sphenopalatine arteries. Tape the catheter in place. The balloon should be deflated every 30 to 60 minutes to avoid ischemic pressure and necrosis at the contact area.

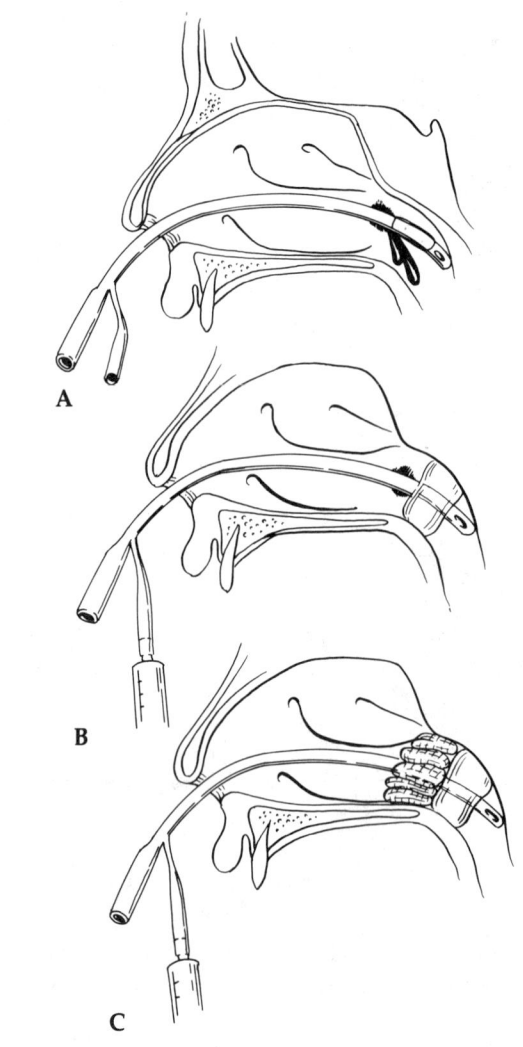

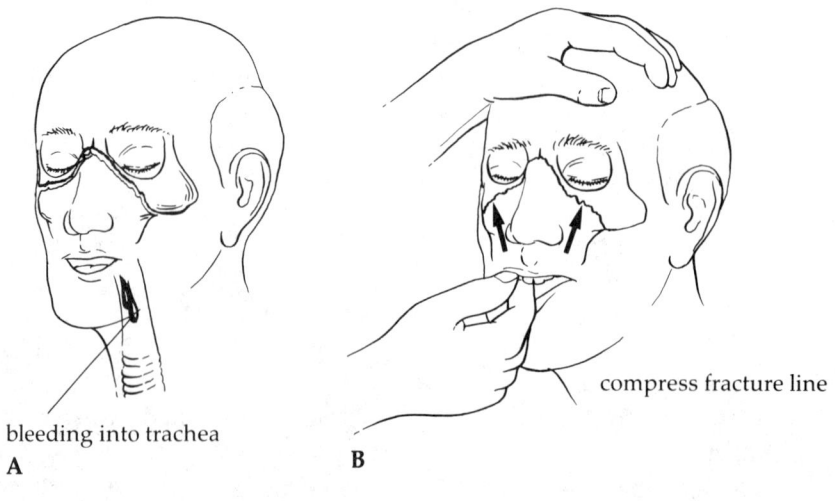

Figure 7-20. Massive maxillary bleeding may compromise the airway (A). Reduction of the fracture by compression of the maxilla against the frontal orbital skeleton helps achieve hemostasis (B).

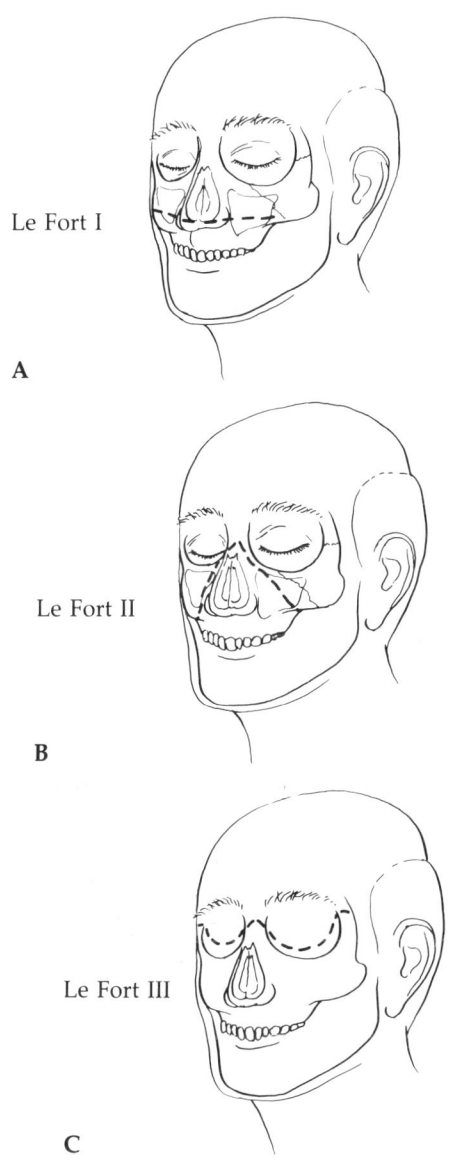

Figure 7-21. Le Fort fractures.
A. The Le Fort I fracture (transverse) passes across the nasal vestibule and sinuses.
B. The Le Fort II fracture (pyramidal) passes through the maxillary sinus, orbital floor, medial wall, and superior nasal cavity.
C. The Le Fort III fracture (craniofacial disjunction) passes behind the sinus, across the orbital floor, and high across the ethmoidals and frontozygomatic junction.

poromandibular dislocation and alveolar fractures may be treated in the emergency department as described in the following two sections.

Airway obstruction is related to tongue injuries and posterior displacement of the mandible. Prone positions and tongue traction may be required to establish an airway.

6. Temporomandibular joint. Limitation of opening or closing the mouth is usually noted immediately after facial trauma, but it can develop weeks or months after a closed injury. Usually this is caused by damage to the temporomandibular (T-M) joint, but it may be related to muscle injury or spasm.
   a. Inability to close mouth
      (1) Diagnosis. T-M joint dislocation can occur with or without associated mandibular and condylar fractures, although forceful impact that causes T-M joint dislocation is also likely to cause a

Figure 7-22. Mandibular fractures may involve any part of the body (symphysis, horizontal ramus, condyle). The signs and symptoms are primarily those of pain, malocclusion, and mental nerve hypesthesia.

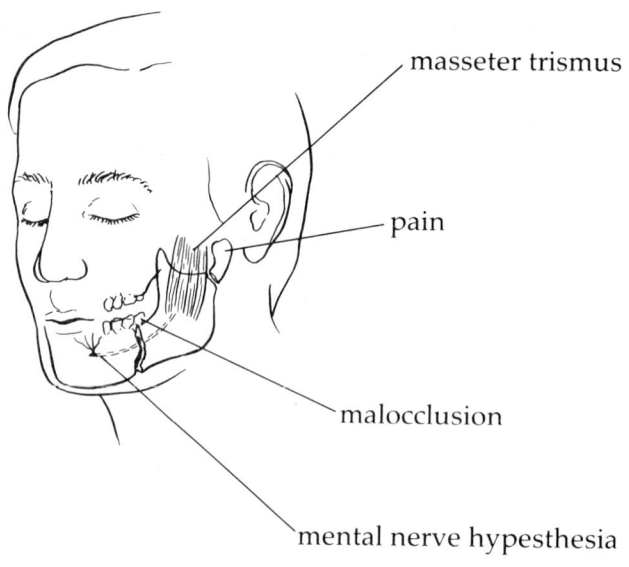

fracture. Isolated T-M joint dislocation can occur nontraumatically as a result of opening the mouth too widely. Diagnosis is made clinically but can be confirmed by T-M joint x-ray.
(2) Treatment. The condylar head should be relocated into the temporal fossa (Fig. 7-23).
   (a) Prereduction and postreduction x-rays. X-rays should be obtained to determine if there is an associated fracture.
   (b) Muscle relaxation (see Fig. 7-23). Relocation of the T-M joint is usually prevented by spasm of the masseter muscle; therefore, relief of muscle spasm is essential. This is best achieved with local anesthetic blocks but may also require systemic muscle relaxants.
      (i) Injection of 2 to 5 ml of Xylocaine or other local anesthetic into the masseter (and sometimes temporalis) muscle usually provides rapid and safe relaxation.
      (ii) IV muscle relaxants, such as diazepam (Valium, 5–10 mg), should be given very slowly with careful monitoring.
   (c) Manual manipulation. The mandible is grasped and the posterior teeth forced downward and anteriorly so that the condyle slides around the prominence superiorly and posteriorly and then into the fossa. Failure to achieve reduction may be caused by persistent muscle spasm or soft tissue interposition.
   (d) Postreduction immobilization. A Barton bandage or maxillomandibular interdental wires should be used and maintained for 7 to 10 days to allow scar formation of ligaments and prevent recurrent dislocation. A liquid diet is necessary during that interval. Careful mouth opening is necessary for 3 to 4 weeks.

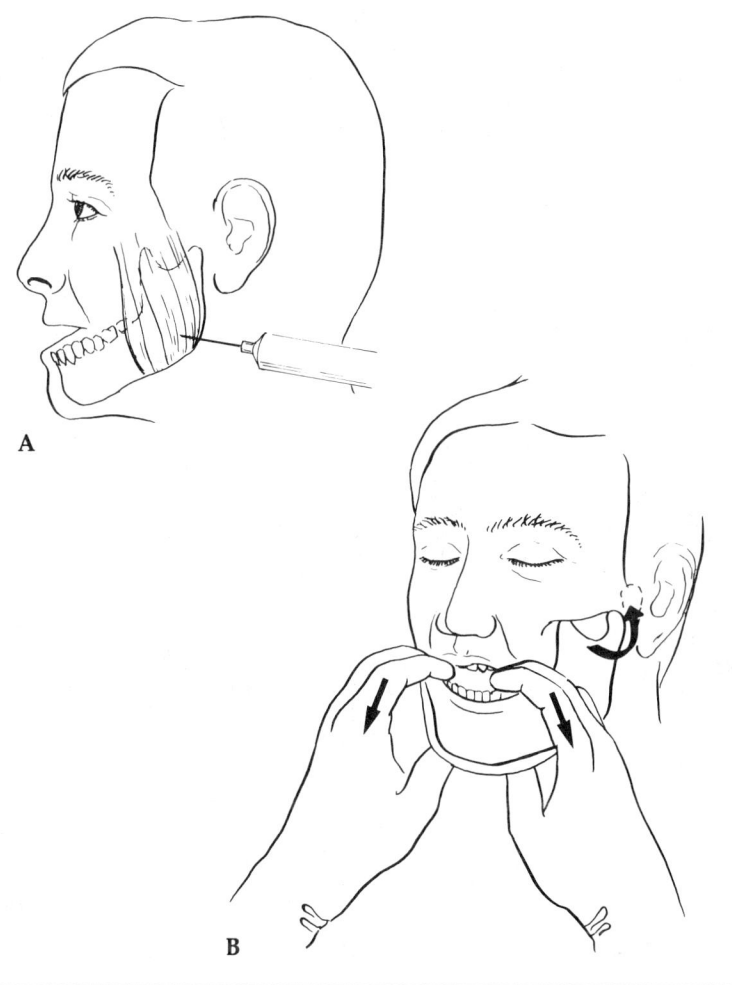

Figure 7-23. Dislocated condyle.
A. The dislocated condyle sits anteriorly on the prominence and is held in that position by muscle spasm. Injection of Xylocaine directly into the temporomandibular joint or the masseter muscle relieves the spasm and may result in spontaneous relocation.
B. The dislocated condyle can be reduced by forceful downward movement of the fingers on the posterior teeth. Once the condyle slips below the prominence, it will move posteriorly and upward into the fossa.

b. Inability to open mouth. Trismus may be caused by (1) masseter or temporalis spasm or fibrosis, (2) condylar head fractures or perforation through the joint meniscus, or (3) zygomatic arch fracture.

    (1) Diagnosis. Trismus is usually the immediate result of direct impact to the side of the face or jaw; however, trismus can occur several days or weeks after injury.

        Infectious tetanus (*Clostridium welchii*) must be ruled out; other unusual causes of trismus may be psychogenic and neuro-epileptic in origin. This discussion is limited to immediate post-traumatic trismus.

        (a) X-rays. Before attempting forceful opening or closure of the jaw, x-rays of the T-M joint, condyle, zygomatic arch, and mandible should be taken.

        (b) Examination. Palpate for spasm of muscle and fractures.

        (c) Use diagnostic (and therapeutic) test injection with local anesthetic agents.

    (2) Treatment

        (a) *Masseter spasm* is caused by muscle tears and hematomas or fractures of the underlying mandible. Spasm without frac-

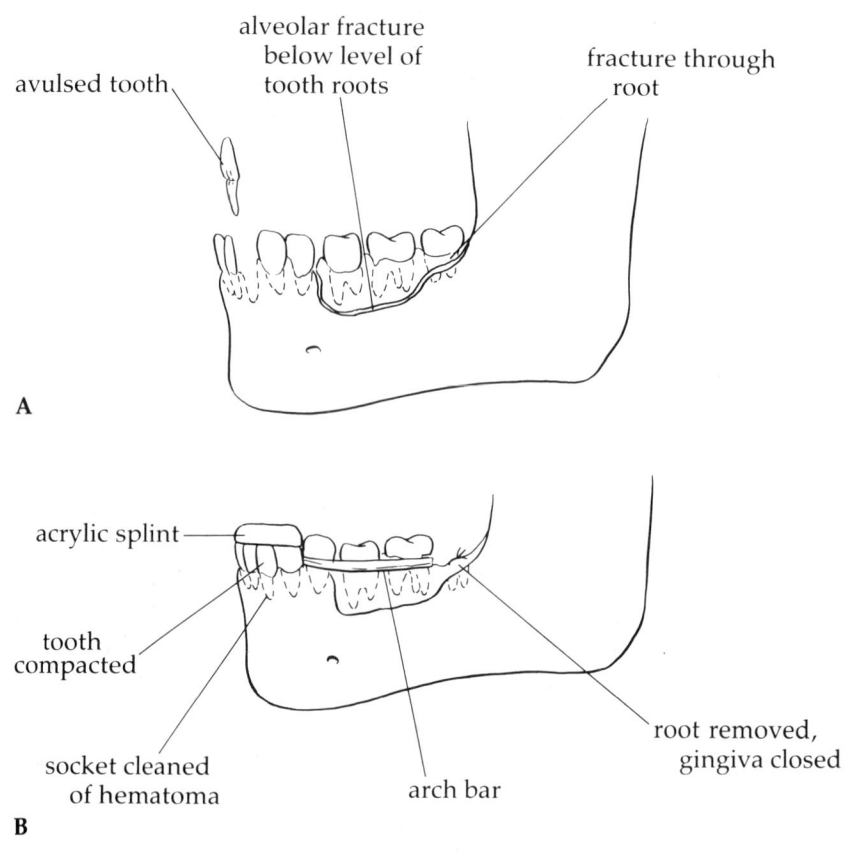

Figure 7-24. Alveolar injury may avulse a tooth, fracture below tooth roots, or fracture through the root (A). The recommended management for these various types of dentoalveolar injuries is illustrated (B).

ture is treated by intramuscular injections of Xylocaine and systemic muscle relaxants.

Because of a propensity to late fibrosis, a postoperative program of careful, full-range mouth opening should be instituted.

(b) *Condylar head fracture or perforation* injuries are diagnosed by x-rays, and treatment should be determined by specialists.

(c) *Zygomatic arch fracture.* A depressed zygomatic arch can cause mechanical limitation of the temporalis and may result in muscle necrosis and secondary fibrosis. Immediate reduction by a specialist in the operating room should be arranged.

7. Dentoalveolar fractures (Fig. 7-24). Some fractures across the alveolar ridge and tooth can be treated in the emergency department. Dental consultation and x-ray should be obtained if available.

   a. Alveolar fractures. Fractures across the alveolar ridge should be confirmed with x-ray. Incomplete fractures need to have the ridge repositioned and teeth stabilized with an arch bar, splint, or interdental wires. Complicated fractures need to have tooth roots removed or root canals performed. These procedures are better performed in the operating room by a specialist or dental surgeon. Antibiotics should be given for all dentoalveolar fractures.

   b. Tooth avulsions without fractured basal bone. As a temporary mea-

CLOSED AND BLUNT INJURIES

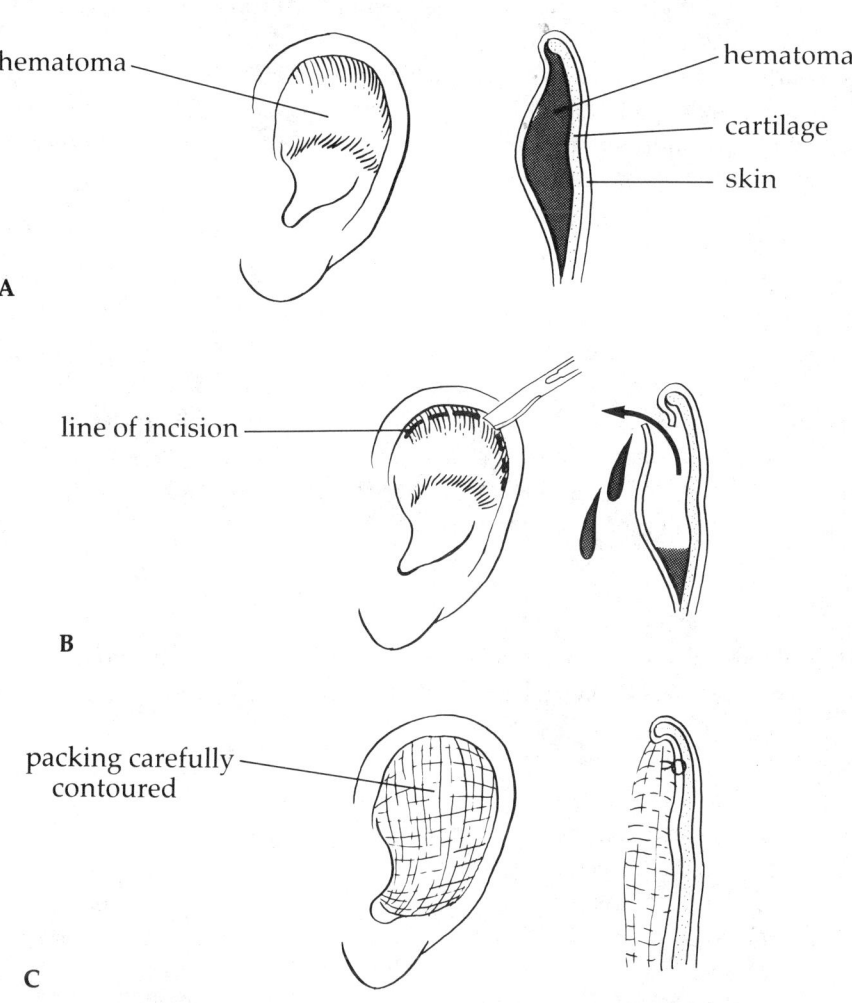

Figure 7-25. Cartilage hematomas of ear and septum.
A. Appearance is of a swollen blue bulge.
B. An incision is made in a conveniently located and hidden site, and the hematoma is evacuated.
C. Packing is placed.

sure until dental consultation is obtained, avulsed teeth are treated as follows:

(1) The sockets are cleaned and *all hematoma removed*.
(2) The tooth is firmly pressed into the socket.
(3) A splint is placed over the occlusal surface of the avulsed tooth and uninjured adjacent tooth.
(4) A liquid diet and antibiotics are given.

CARTILAGE INJURY

1. Perichondrial hematoma (Fig. 7-25). Hematomas under perichondrium can cause distortion by scar, neocartilage formation, or pressure necrosis. This can occur on the ear or nasal septum. Untreated ear hematomas lead to "cauliflower ear," and septal hematomas lead to septal deviation or perforation.
   a. Diagnosis. A tense or fluctuant blue swelling with minimal pain usually indicates a subperichondrial hematoma.
   b. Treatment
      (1) Incision and drainage of blood with thorough irrigation and hemostasis.

(2) Contoured packing to flatten perichondrium and skin against the cartilage.
2. Cartilage fractures or avulsions from bone. The major concern is avoidance of bacterial chondritis. Thus, external manipulation of the skin with packs and splints is the best treatment. Opening of wounds and suture repositioning should be avoided!

NECK INJURY

Blunt trauma to the neck can cause severe injury from (1) crush of the airway, causing acute respiratory obstruction and aphonia; (2) cervical spine fractures and dislocation, causing quadriplegia and acute respiratory paralysis; and (3) carotid injury, causing acute cerebral insufficiency.

In Chapter 6, discussions of penetrating injuries to the neck emphasize the importance of operating-room exploration. With blunt injuries, the emphasis is on emergency prophylaxis to prevent airway obstruction and cervical injury.

1. Etiology. Blunt trauma most commonly occurs from automobile accidents but also is seen with assaults, strangulation, and bicycle and skimobile accidents.
2. Diagnosis
    a. Symptoms
        (1) Airway compromise—stridor, dyspnea
        (2) Muffled voice or aphonia
        (3) Hemoptysis
        (4) Neck pain
        (5) Dysphagia
        (6) Drooling
    b. Signs
        (1) Loss of neck contour (absence of Adam's apple)
        (2) Bruising of neck skin
        (3) Subcutaneous emphysema and crepitus
        (4) Neck tenderness and muscle spasm
    c. Radiologic evidence (the PA and lateral chest x-ray or CT scan may lead to diagnosis of minor trauma)
        (1) Subcutaneous emphysema
        (2) Distortion of esophagus or pharynx by hematoma
        (3) Dislocation and fracture of larynx or cervical spine
3. Treatment. Treatment is directed toward airway maintenance and cervical stabilization until consultation can be obtained.
    a. Careful observation. Because rapid development of airway symptoms can occur, close monitoring (particularly if x-rays are being obtained) is mandatory.
    b. Endotracheal intubation. This is the primary method if competent, well-trained physicians are available, and if cervical-spine injury has been reasonably excluded as a possible problem.
    c. Tracheostomy
    d. Referral for surgical exploration and repair

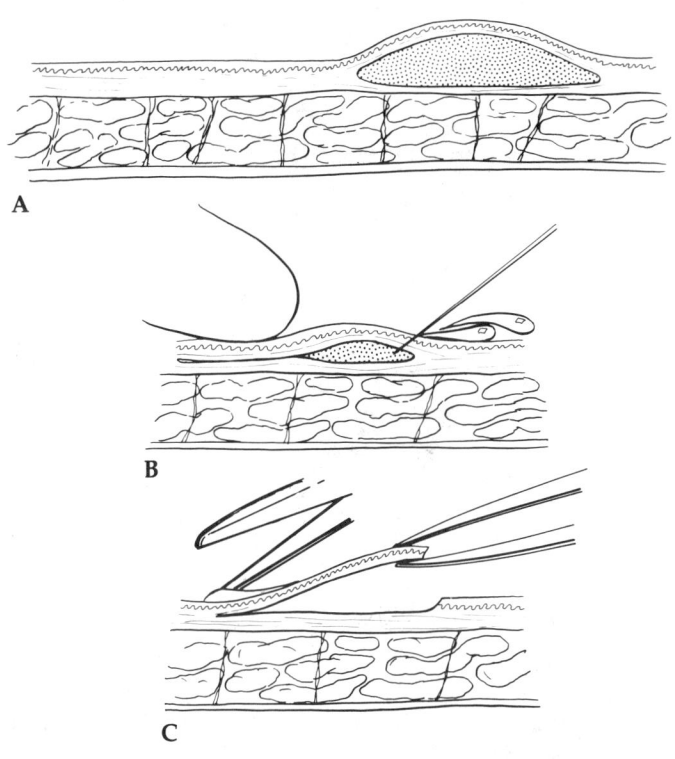

Figure 7-26. Friction blister.
A. Leave blister intact for 3 to 5 days, unless it becomes infected. Unroof the blister if infected. The blister is at the epidermal-dermal junction.
B. At 3 to 5 days, the fluid can be removed by needle puncture, the roof of the blister is compressed flat against the base.
C. After 1 week, the dry blister can be removed.

Injuries of the Extremities

SKIN, SUBCUTANEOUS TISSUE, AND NAIL

1. Palmar skin. The palmar skin is reinforced by a thick keratin layer with many ridges that increase surface contact and enhance grip. The palmar skin is firmly attached to the bony skeleton by vertical bands of the palmar aponeurosis, with fat compartments in between. This anatomy prevents shearing, maximizes stability, and provides a cushion. Common injuries include:
   a. Blisters (Fig. 7-26). Because of skin stability and the hand-grasp function, friction blisters are quite common. Treatment is the same as described for blisters in other cutaneous areas.
   b. Fingertip and palmar hematomas. Because of the tight, unyielding skin and abundant nerve supply, palmar and fingertip or pulp hematomas can be very painful and jeopardize vascular flow.
      (1) Diagnosis
         (a) Pain, usually extreme
         (b) Ecchymosis and localized swelling; frequently, hard swelling
         (c) Hypoesthesia
         (d) X-ray to rule out an associated fracture
      (2) Treatment (Fig. 7-27)
         (a) Elevation and cold pack may be satisfactory treatment for most small, nonpainful hematomas.
         (b) Drainage. If symptoms of pain persist or ischemic necrosis seems likely, drainage is performed directly over the hematoma. The incision is performed parallel to the palmar crease

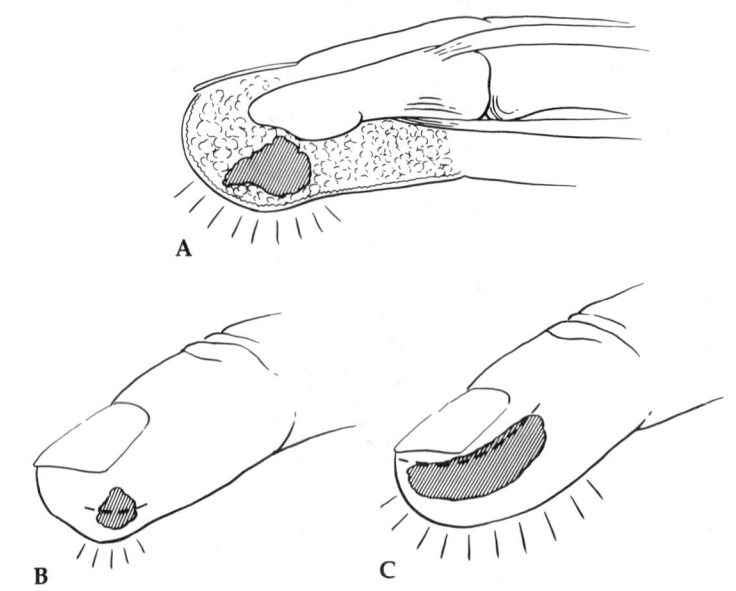

Figure 7-27. Alternate sites for drainage of pulp hematomas.
A. A hematoma within the confined pulp space usually causes great pain and tenderness.
B. Drainage is directly over hematoma for small superficial collections, particularly if hematoma has caused skin softening and is "pointing."
C. A midaxial "fishmouth" incision is used for extensive deep hematomas. This avoids a large scar on the tactile surface but is not as direct a path for drainage.

or longitudinally in the digit. The incision may be relatively small and of a size just sufficient to allow the hematoma to be expressed.

If the hematoma has been present for some time or is associated with a great deal of subcutaneous or pulp edema, the incision should be extended to serve as a relaxing incision.

Some surgeons advocate a lateral midaxial incision at the distal fingertip pulp to avoid a scar on the tactile surface.

A rubber drain or packing for 24 hours may improve drainage.

The incision should not be closed with sutures but allowed to close by secondary intention.

    (i) A sterile dressing is applied, followed by a splint to rest involved tissues.
    (ii) Elevation is essential.
    (iii) Antibiotics may be required.

2. Dorsal and upper extremity skin
   a. Prefibrotic hematoma. The dorsal skin is thin and stretches with motion of the hand; however, there is only sufficient skin to allow full flexion of the fingers, as evidenced by the blanched knuckles of the clenched fist. The dorsal skin has a loose areolar attachment to the underlying structures and is readily avulsed. Although hematomas do occur, they are unlikely to cause severe pain or lead to skin necrosis. On occasion, a dorsal hematoma may lead to the development of a firm fibrotic mass that restricts joint and tendon motion. This condition is termed Secretan's "hard dorsal edema."
      (1) Diagnosis. The precursor of this unusual condition is usually marked dorsal swelling that is seemingly out of proportion to the nature of the injury. Typical patients are said to be middle-aged women, especially those classified as "sympathetic overreac-

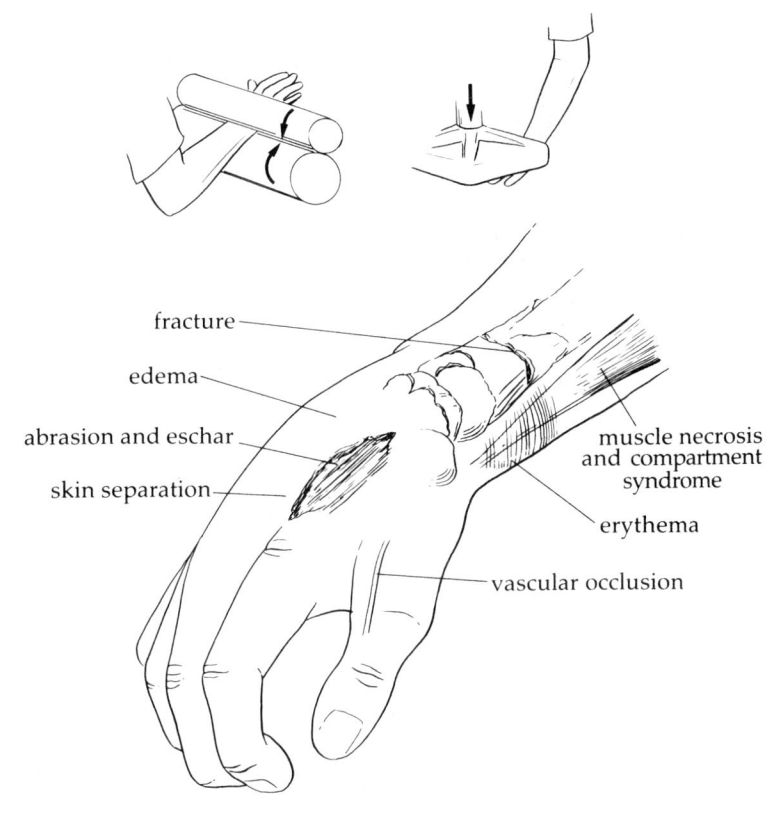

Figure 7-28. A roller, a press, or compression from any heavy object can cause extensive injuries.

tors." An x-ray is necessary to rule out an underlying fracture or dislocation.
- (2) Treatment
  - (a) Any palpable collection of blood (hematoma) should be aspirated.
  - (b) A compressive hand dressing should be applied, followed by a volar or dorsal plaster splint (not circular cast) that maintains the hand and wrist in a position of function (wrist slightly extended, MP joints flexed at least 70°).
  - (c) The hand should be examined after 48 hours to check for reaccumulation of blood.
  - (d) Vigorous physical therapy with active exercise is begun when initial discomfort is past.
  - (e) Occasionally other modalities are necessary, such as a rapidly tapering course of corticosteroids or chemical stellate ganglion blockage.
- b. Wringer and crush injury (Fig. 7-28). The system of diagnosis and management described here, especially splinting in a functional position, is used for any crush injury to the hand.
  - (1) Mechanism. The most common problems are avulsion injuries and closed "wringer" or "roller" injuries. These injuries combine many of the elements of vascular damage, shearing of skin from underlying fascia, and fractures.
    - (a) Initial compression in the rollers causes cellular damage to endothelium (and other cells).

(b) Subsequent torque and shearing disrupt vessels, devascularize overlying skin, and cause a hematoma.

(c) Finally, there is a skin burn caused by friction.

The most severe injuries result from industrial rollers, especially heated rollers, from which severe burn injury may complicate the crush injury. Full-thickness necrosis must be managed as a burn wound is, with proper recipient-site care and eventual skin grafting. There is some risk of ischemic contractures with this condition. These injuries should be managed by specialists, as they can be deceptive, with a benign initial appearance.

(2) Diagnosis

(a) Often there is only erythema and some slightly abraded areas.

(b) Soon edema develops, and skin areas initially thought healthy may demarcate because of ischemic devascularization. The combined effect of direct cellular injury, vascular thrombosis, hematoma, devascularization, and ischemia usually is skin necrosis.

(c) Nerve compression, arterial damage, muscle necrosis, and fractures also may occur.

(d) Thus, a careful examination repeated at frequent (every 2–3 hours) intervals is required. The examination should include vascular status (pulse and color), nerve status, sensibility and movement, and evaluation of muscle compartments (see p. 284).

(3) Treatment

(a) X-rays are imperative to rule out forearm or hand fractures.

(b) Skin abrasions, avulsions, or eschar should be covered with nonadherent sterile dressings.

(c) Muscle compartment compromise must be treated.

(d) The arm is splinted with the elbow slightly flexed and the wrist and hand in a functional position.

(e) Continuous elevation is required for 48 to 72 hours. This is done in the hospital unless the family is exceedingly reliable.

(f) Dressing change in 24 to 48 hours discloses suspicious areas of full-thickness necrosis of skin. Consultation for probable excision and skin grafting should be obtained.

(g) When no full-thickness skin losses are apparent, the arm should be splinted again until the edema has resolved; after that, the patient may be allowed to use the extremity.

(h) Large doses of steroids may be beneficial, but their efficacy has not been proved.

(i) Persistent skin erythema may be a sign of underlying muscle necrosis.

3. Nails—subungual hematoma (Fig. 7-29). This specialized skin appendage is both decorative and functional. It amplifies afferent stimuli because of the rich nerve supply to the nail bed. It supports the soft tissues of the distal phalanx and allows a firmer "digging-in" grasp. The anatomic relation to the distal phalanx and soft tissues is diagrammed in Fig. 7-29. The most common closed nail injury is the subungual hematoma.

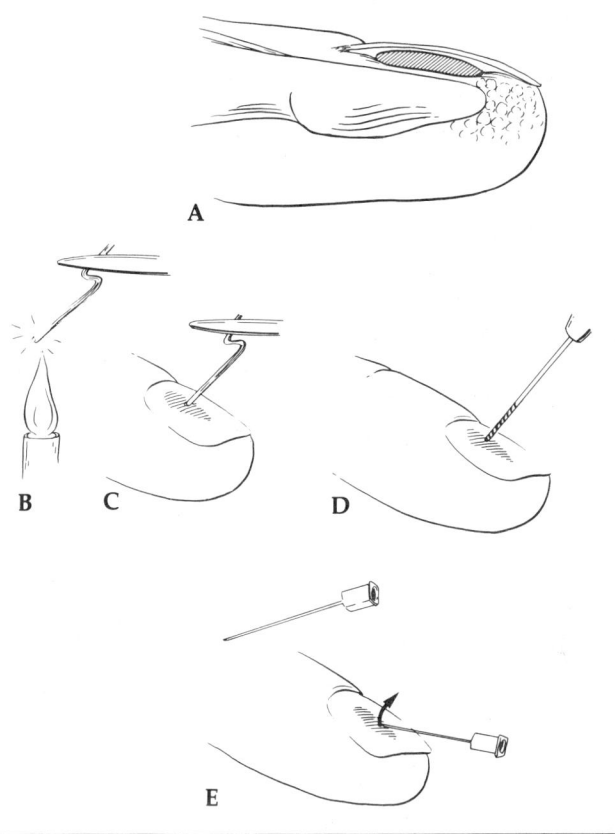

Figure 7-29. Draining a subungual hematoma.
A. The hematoma has elevated the nail plate over the matrix.
B. A paper clip is heated until it is "red hot."
C. Heat from the clip is immediately dissipated by the blood under pressure through the hole in the nail. Pain relief is rapid. Occasionally more than one hole needs to be created to provide complete decompression.
D. The trephine or drill can be used but with minimal pressure. Pressure causes pain.
E. A needle can be used to pick away overlying nail by lightly contacting the needle point and elevating or "flicking" small nail fragments. Do not push the needle inward.

a. Diagnosis and mechanism. The fingertips are frequently crushed by doors, hammers, or other heavy objects without avulsion or laceration of the skin. The result may be a painful collection of blood under the nail. A subungual hematoma can be exquisitely painful; if it is not released, the pressure may cause damage to the nail bed or underlying bony phalanx.

b. Treatment
   (1) An associated fracture of the tuft of the distal phalanx should be suspected and an x-ray obtained.
   (2) The intact overlying nail should be opened to allow evacuation of the hematoma. It can be trephined with a small drill, perforated with the tip of a heated paper clip, or picked away with a sterile, stout needle. Other, more severe crush injuries may partially avulse the nail. If the nail is not lost, it provides a good splint for the nail bed. These injuries are painful because of their tendency toward excessive swelling. Splinting of the injured finger, elevation, and analgesics are necessary.

MUSCLE AND MUSCLE COMPARTMENTS

Closed injury to muscle is usually manifested as either a tear (strain or rupture), bleeding (hematoma or contusion), or edema. Regardless of the basic injury, the major emergency consideration is avoiding the development of compartmental compression syndrome or treating a compartmental compression syndrome if one exists. Even a minor injury with secondary edema can have serious consequences. The second consideration is to diagnose and repair ruptures.

1. Muscle hematoma and compartment syndromes
   a. Mechanism. Many muscle groups are tightly invested by dense fascia and bone. A hematoma in muscle may require drainage if the volume of blood and the edema from injury cause pressure within the compartment.

   Prolonged compression or direct impact may cause edema without hematoma. Muscles swell and compartmental pressure rises; venous outflow is occluded, which causes additional edema; finally, arterial inflow can be occluded. The release of vasoactive substances caused by ischemia can compound the ischemic cycle. Eventually, necrosis of the muscle and accompanying vessels and nerves occurs.

   The best known of these conditions is the so-called acute Volkmann's ischemia of the forearm flexors. Other compartments susceptible to compression are the lumbrical-interossoeus of the hand, rectus abdominis, medial tibial, and anterolateral tibial of the leg.
   b. Diagnostic signs and symptoms
      (1) Pain. Persistent, progressively worsening pain is reported, usually described as a deep ache.
      (2) Muscle group dysfunction. Weakness or complete paralysis of the muscles in the compartment can progress rapidly. The muscle groups offer resistance to passive stretching, and this may cause increased pain.
      (3) Distal nerve dysfunction. Nerve trunks passing through the compartment develop an initial neuropraxia because of ischemia. This usually starts as tingling and progresses to numbness in the affected sensory nerves. Motor nerve paralysis can also occur but is slower to develop than sensory changes.
      (4) Progressive diminution of distal pulse
      (5) Intracompartmental pressure recordings. This involves a new technique that is highly diagnostic but not generally available.
   c. Systemic manifestations
      (1) Myoglobinuria and acute tubular necrosis. Muscle crush can cause release of myoglobin and resultant renal dysfunction. This should be assessed in all muscle crush syndromes by obtaining urinary myoglobin levels.
      (2) Bleeding and shock. Extensive bleeding and hypotensive shock can occur in large muscles (thigh, abdomen). Two or three liters of blood can be lost into thigh muscles without obvious signs of localized bleeding.
      (3) Fat or thrombotic embolism (phlebothrombosis). Fat or thrombotic embolism can occur after severe crush injury. Cardiopulmonary signs and symptoms should be assessed. Phlebothrombosis (traumatic, noninfectious thrombophlebitis) frequently occurs after major leg or pelvic trauma, and the signs may be similar to those of a compartment syndrome. *The diagnosis for the more common areas is described below.*

d. Syndromes
  (1) Forearm flexors syndrome (Volkmann's ischemic contracture). Originally described as an occasional complication of supracondylar humeral fracture, this pathologic condition has been identified as a potential sequela to a number of closed injuries in the arm or hand, including wringer or compression injury to the forearm and prolonged immobilization of the arm following drug overdose. Intraarterial drug injections may cause arterial spasms sufficient to compromise circulation.

  The structures within the forearm muscle compartments include the wrist and digital flexors, the median and ulnar nerve, and the radial and ulnar artery. Volkmann's four *P*s—pain, pulselessness, paralysis, and paresthesia—are infrequently seen together. Early diagnostic evidence is based on the findings of:
  (a) *Paresthesia.* Median nerve sensory dysfunction to the hand
  (b) *Dysfunction* of median nerve–innervated thumb intrinsics
  (c) *Pain* in forearm with wrist or digital extension, which may be the earliest sign of impending ischemia
  (d) *Pulselessness.* Loss of radial and/or ulnar pulse
  (e) *Tenseness and swelling* of forearm

  (2) Intrinsic muscle compression syndrome. This condition commonly follows crush injuries to the hand, burns, other accidents, intraarterial injections, and prolonged compression. An unconscious patient, such as a victim of stroke or drug or alcohol overdose, may cause this syndrome by lying on the hand.

  This compartment contains the lumbricals, interosseous muscles, and median nerve. The thumb intrinsics and nerves may be separately involved.
  (a) Early diagnostic signs
    (i) Hand pain
    (ii) "Intrinsic plus" hand posture (MP flexion, DIP extension), caused by spasm of intrinsic muscles
    (iii) Pain and resistance to passive extension of MP joint, which may be the earliest sign of impending ischemia
  (b) Later manifestations
    (i) Intrinsics are paralyzed, and the hand assumes the "intrinsic minus," or "clawhand," posture.
    (ii) Resistance to passive finger and thumb extension
    (iii) Erythema and edema of overlying skin without signs of infection

  (3) Anterior tibial syndrome (extensor compartment). This syndrome occurs most commonly with crush injuries of the lower leg. The compartment contains the extensor hallucis longus, extensor digitorum longus, and peroneus muscle, and the deep branch of the peroneal nerve. The signs include:
  (a) Anterolateral leg pain with passive plantar flexion
  (b) Inability to extend the foot or toes
  (c) Paresthesia in peroneal distribution

  (4) Medial tibial syndrome (flexor compartment). This is the very common jogger's injury, "shin splints," but also occurs rarely

from acute trauma. This compartment contains the flexor digitorum longus, tibialis posterior, and flexor hallucis longus muscle, and the posterior tibial artery and nerve. The signs include:
- (a) Anteromedial leg pain with passive foot extension (dorsiflexion)
- (b) Inability to flex the foot (against gravity)
- (c) Loss of posterior tibial pulse
- (d) Paresthesia of posterior tibial nerve

e. Treatment. The treatment for all compartments is essentially the same and is determined by the severity of compression.
  (1) Early minor syndromes. A minimal early compartment syndrome can be treated conservatively with:
   - (a) Elevation
   - (b) Diuretics, such as furosemide (Lasix, 10–40 mg IM) or mannitol
   - (c) Cortisone (prednisone, 40 mg IM)
   - (d) Urinalysis and monitoring for myoglobinuria
   - (e) Frequent reassessment for local circulatory or neurologic changes and pain
  (2) Early, severe syndromes and nonresponsive or progressive syndromes. The treatment is the same as for mild syndromes, but in addition, surgical decompression is required.
   - (a) Fasciotomy. If the symptoms are severe, an immediate decompressive fasciotomy should be performed. The appropriate consultant should be called and preparations made for operating-room surgery.
   - (b) Reduction of fractures. Supracondylar and other fractures may cause direct vascular obstruction by kinking of compartment vessels or by compression from the hematoma.

2. Muscle tears (strain, rupture). These injuries are most commonly caused by a sudden or restricted movement with spontaneous muscle tear. They are less likely to occur from direct impact.
  a. Diagnosis. The mechanism of injury allows some estimation of the relative severity of injury to muscles. The following are signs and symptoms of muscle tear:
   (1) Tenderness to palpation
   (2) Pain
   (3) Resistance to passive stretch
   (4) Muscle spasm
   (5) Deformity—bulges proximally and distally, concavity at the rupture site
   (6) Ecchymosis of skin
  b. Treatment
   (1) Symptomatic mediation—analgesics, antiinflammatory agents
   (2) Rest
   (3) Heat
   (4) Splinting
   (5) Muscle relaxants

Once symptoms diminish, progressive exercises generally lead to rapid recovery. The same recommendations are made for simple sprains in which joint stability is not compromised. Surgical repair of muscle rupture (as opposed to tendon rupture) is not essential. Attempts to repair muscle usually fail because sutures pulled through muscle and closure of fascia create a "dead space" that is susceptible to infection after surgical incision exposes the wound. Because distracted muscle ends are pulled into close approximation by scar contraction, little disability occurs. Professional athletes or people interested in maximal functional return may require surgical repair of the fascia.

TENDONS

The recognition of acute closed tendon rupture requires a high index of suspicion. Tendon disruption is much more likely to occur at the *insertion* onto bone or at the muscle-tendon juncture than along the tendon proper.

Any muscle-tendon unit may rupture secondary to excessive force, or especially, to excessive force that is rapidly applied; only the most common of these ruptures is discussed here (Fig. 7-30).

1. Ruptures
   a. Finger extensors. Rupture of the finger extensors occurs most commonly at the distal phalangeal insertion and may or may not be accompanied by a fracture of the distal phalanx. If the injury is closed, the usual history is a strike on the tip of the extended finger by a ball or other object. So common is this history that the condition is termed *baseball* or *mallet finger*.
      (1) Signs of finger extensor rupture include:
         (a) Inability to extend the distal phalanx actively
         (b) Mallet-finger posture (dropped tip)
         (c) Small avulsion fracture from the site of tendon insertion
      (2) Treatment. When there is *no associated fracture*, the finger can be continuously splinted for 5 to 6 weeks in minimal hyperextension, followed by 2 to 3 weeks of night splinting. Results with primary surgical repair are not significantly better than results with conservative closed positioning.
   b. Flexor digitorum profundus. This is a common rupture injury, especially among football players.
      (1) Signs and symptoms. The ring finger is most commonly affected by:
         (a) Pain in the digit
         (b) Swelling along the course of the tendon sheath
         (c) Inability to flex the terminal phalanx actively
      (2) Treatment. Referral to a hand specialist for *operative reinsertion* of the affected tendon is required. Frequently, the tendon retracts into the palm, making retrieval more difficult.
   c. Plantaris tendon. The plantaris tendon ruptures spontaneously in association with vigorous activity such as running and jumping. The patient often states that the pain felt like being shot in the calf and he may hear a "pop." The calf pain may mimic that of thrombophlebitis, but the history of activity and the acute onset delineate this condition. No functional loss can be demonstrated.
      Treatment involves use of elastic wraps, elevation, and mild pain medications.
   d. Achilles tendon (gastrocnemius). This tendon may rupture at the

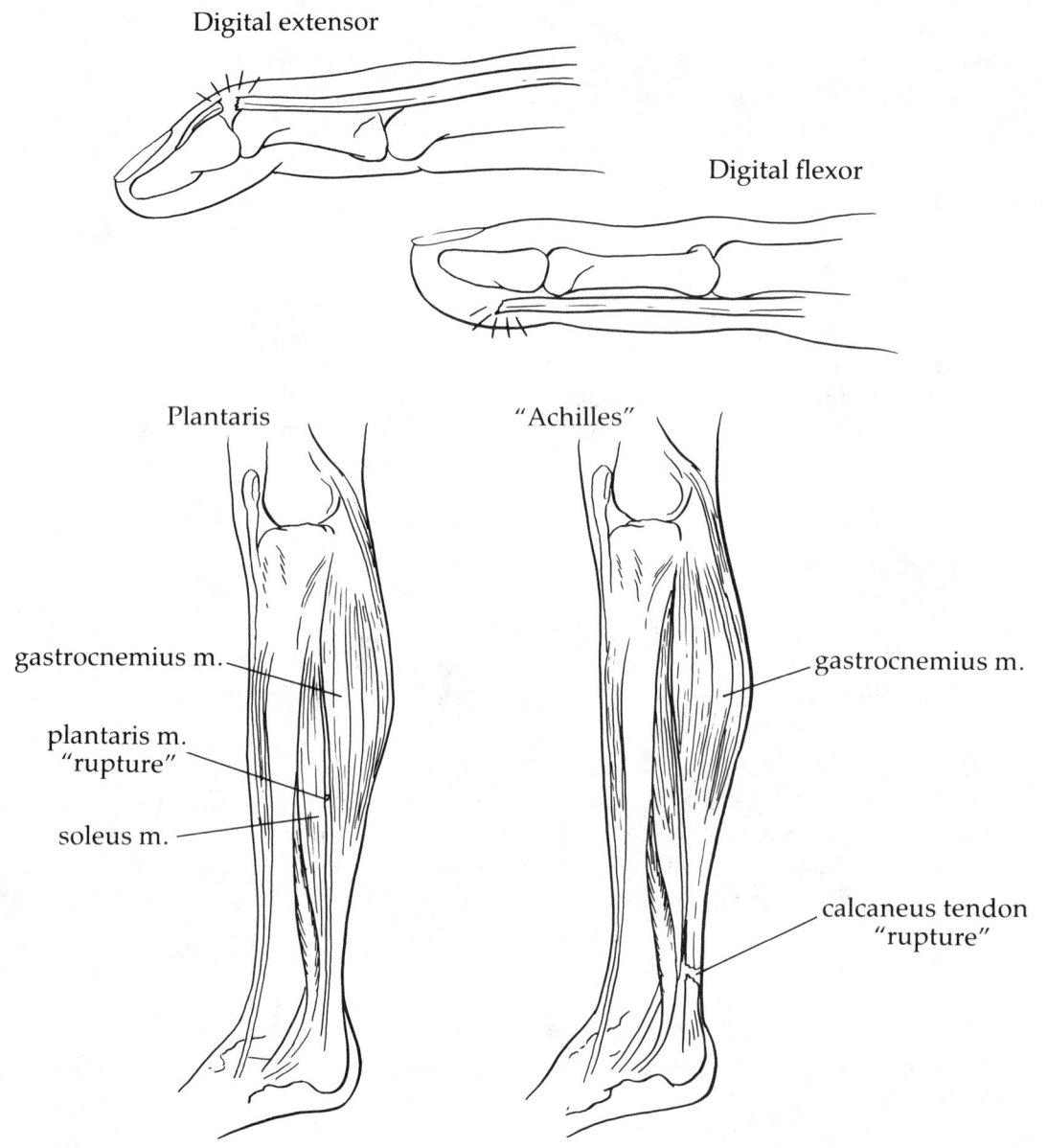

Figure 7-30. Sites of tendon rupture. Either the digital extensor or the digital flexor tendon may rupture, most commonly at its site of insertion into the distal phalanx. In the lower limb, the plantaris tendon may rupture and cause pain consistent with acute thrombophlebitis. Great force is required for the calcaneal tendon to rupture—it usually ruptures within its substance.

musculotendinous junction under circumstances similar to plantaris rupture.

(1) Signs
  (a) Laxity of Achilles tendon
  (b) Hollowing of lower one-third of muscle at the site of musculotendinous separation
  (c) Weak flexion of the foot against gravity. (A false impression of normal function can be gained if the test is done with leg dependent, as the foot will flex passively with relaxation of the anterior group.)

(2) Treatment. Treatment depends on the severity of the injury. Complete ruptures should probably have surgical repair. Although some functional return can be anticipated in extreme ankle flexion by casting, a specialist should be consulted. Incom-

plete ruptures can be treated by casting for 3 to 4 weeks with gradual lengthening of casted position. Another site of rupture is the "rotator cuff" of the shoulder.
2. Tendinitis. Closed trauma can cause inflammation of a tendon or its sheath. More commonly these symptoms are related to excessive repetitive movements. Any tendon can develop symptoms of inflammation, but inflammation occurs most commonly where tendons pass through a fascial or bony tunnel.
    a. Signs
        (1) Tenderness and swelling at site of tendinitis
        (2) Pain on passive stretch of the specific muscle
        (3) Limitation of movement or weakness with active use of the muscle
        (4) Popping or catching of tendon, producing a ratchet-like sudden movement termed *triggering*
    b. Sites. Some of the common sites of tendinitis are:
        (1) Bicipital tendon, at shoulder
        (2) Extensor of elbow, at lateral epicondyle (tennis elbow)
        (3) Abductor pollicis longus, at "snuff box" of thumb (de Quervain's tendinitis)
        (4) Flexor digitorum profundus and superficialis, at proximal flexor sheath (trigger finger)
    c. Treatment
        (1) Acute
            (a) Rest and immobilization (sling, cast) for 3–7 days
            (b) Antiinflammatory medications, such as aspirin, indomethacin (Indocin), and phenylbutazone (Butazolidin)
            (c) Heat
            (d) Careful reactivation of muscle
        (2) Chronic. Chronic, recurrent tendinitis, particularly if accompanied by popping or locking in a canal, may require either surgical release of the investing canal or systemic or injected cortisone. These are problems to be evaluated by the orthopedic, plastic, or hand surgeon and are not in the scope of emergency care.

VESSELS

Blunt trauma to major vessels of the extremities rarely results in complete disruption unless associated with severe avulsion injuries. More commonly associated with blunt injuries are spasm, which can be severe enough to cause vascular occlusion, or the development of early or late true or pseudoaneurysms.

1. Vasospasm. Occasionally severe spasm may follow relatively limited closed injuries, such as a direct blow over a relatively superficial vessel (e.g., the radial artery of the wrist).
    a. Diagnosis. The diagnosis of vasospasm is based on the history and location of injury and physical signs. The physical signs include:
        (1) Absent or diminished distal pulse
        (2) Color change, such as pallor or cyanosis
        (3) Pain in the parts distal to the site of injury
        (4) Doppler confirmation, aided by Doppler ultrasound examina-

tion, comparing the abnormal limb or area to its normal counterpart
        (5) Arteriography for definitive diagnosis
    b. Treatment
        (1) Intraarterial injection of a vasodilator such as dipyridamole (Persantine) to relax spastic vascular smooth muscle
        (2) Chemical stellate ganglion blocker to relieve sympathetic-mediated spasm
        (3) Operative resection of the damaged segment, with or without interpositioning vein grafting, if conservative measures fail
2. True or pseudoaneurysm. These pathologic conditions usually present as a pulsatile tender mass overlying the course of a major vessel. Referral to a vascular specialist is needed.
3. Thrombosis. Blunt trauma can cause intimal and endothelial damage leading to thrombosis. This is most common in the lower extremity but can also occur in the subclavian vein.

    The thrombosis is not apparent in the acute phase but develops from *vascular stasis* and progressive platelet clumping.

    Treatment for venous thrombosis may require anticoagulation, but consultation with consideration of other injuries is important.

NERVES

The three types of nerve injury, neurapraxia, axonotmesis, and neurotmesis have been defined. Acute injuries to nerves frequently follow blunt or closed trauma. The site of nerve damage is where the nerve is close to the surface, confined, or adjacent to a rigid area.

1. Median nerve (forearm and wrist). The median nerve can be compressed at the wrist (carpal) tunnel or in the forearm in the flexor compartment. *Carpal tunnel syndrome* is the most common neurologic sequela of blunt injury (followed closely by superficial peroneal nerve syndrome). The median nerve passes from the distal forearms into the hand through a rigid anatomic area, termed the *carpal tunnel*. The tunnel is composed of a bony floor and walls and is covered by a stiff fibrous ligament, the transverse flexor retinaculum. Any traumatic event that results in edema within this confined space can cause compression of the median nerve. The most frequent causes of injury are falls onto the heel of the hand and blows to the palm.
    a. Diagnosis
        (1) Numbness, pain, or paresthesias (tingling) in the median nerve distribution
        (2) Weakness of the median-innervated intrinsic muscles (i.e., those that permit abduction and rotation of the thumb away from the plane of the palm)
    b. Treatment
        (1) Treatment is initially conservative and involves:
            (a) Splinting the wrist in slight extension
            (b) Elevation
            (c) Corticosteroids to reduce edema. A common method of administration is:

(i) 30 mg of prednisone per day for 2 days
(ii) 20 mg of prednisone per day for 3 days
(iii) 15 mg of prednisone per day for 3 days
(iv) 10 mg of prednisone per day for 2 days
(v) 5 mg of prednisone per day for 1 day
   (2) If no improvement is seen in 5 to 7 days, referral to a surgeon for reevaluation, and possibly, surgical decompression is indicated.
2. Radial nerve (arm and wrist). Injury to the superficial sensory branch of the radial nerve at the wrist is very common and follows a direct blow to the nerve or compression of the nerve (e.g., handcuffs fastened too tightly about the wrist). Anesthesia in the distribution of the nerve, and pain, are common presentations.

   The radial nerve in the arm lies in the spiral groove against the humerus. Humeral fractures can injure the nerve at this site.
3. Ulnar nerve (elbow and wrist). The ulnar nerve can be compressed at two sites at which it passes through bony canals: the elbow medial epicondyle (funny bone) and the wrist ulnar tunnel of Guyon.
   a. Elbow. Direct trauma or compression can injure the ulnar nerve as it passes behind the medial epicondyle. The signs are:
      (1) Paresthesia of ulnar nerve (dorsal and volar)
      (2) Paresis of ulnar wrist flexor, ulnar superficialis, and intrinsics
   b. Wrist
      (1) Paresthesia of ulnar nerve (volar only)
      (2) Paresis of ulnar intrinsics
4. Peroneal nerve. Injury to the peroneal nerve is usually secondary to direct trauma about the fibular head. Hypesthesia of the dorsum of the foot and a foot drop are common clinical signs.

JOINTS AND LIGAMENTS

The management of injuries closed to joints is not within the scope of this volume. We can offer only general guidelines to diagnosis and treatment of partial ligament stretch injuries (sprains) and more serious complete ligamentous ruptures.

1. Diagnosis
   a. History of the mechanism of injury
   b. Physical examination to elicit points of maximum tenderness, joint instability, or ligamentous laxity to stress, hemarthrosis, or ecchymosis
   c. Pain elicited by stretch, rather than compression as in a fracture
   d. X-rays to look for subluxation (partial joint malalignment), dislocation (complete joint malalignment), fractures, or bony avulsions
2. Treatment. For simple injuries, treatment usually includes compression dressings, splinting, elevation, cold (initially), analgesics, and rest.

   Severe injuries and those associated with dislocation require consultation regarding emergency relocation and ligament repair.

BONES

The response of bone to closed blunt injury is typically a fracture. The management of fractures is not within the scope of this book.

8. POSTOPERATIVE CARE AND DRESSINGS

Often a patient with a perfectly repaired laceration returns to the surgeon's office with a dehiscence, excessive scar, or infection. Postoperative care, such as dressing, elevation, immobilization, and medication, can be even more essential to a favorable result than the surgical repair. This chapter presents a method of choosing, designing, and applying a dressing.

Equally important in postoperative care is the need to educate the patient and family. A cooperative patient who participates in his or her own care and understands the signs of infection and other complications can greatly facilitate a favorable outcome. No patient should be discharged from care after leaving the emergency room or even after sutures are removed. The physician's responsibility ends only when the preinjury state has been obtained, or the lack of this attainment prompts referral to a specialist.

Postoperative care and dressing application follow a specific sequence.

1. Patient assessment and education
2. Wound assessment
3. Determination of general goals and specific objectives
4. Design of a dressing
5. Choice of materials
6. Application technique
7. Reassessment

PATIENT ASSESSMENT AND EDUCATION

The involvement of the patient in postoperative wound care is essential to a successful outcome. An assessment must be made of the patient's social and intellectual capabilities and ability to contribute to postoperative care. The following section is a guide to instructions for the patient.

Anticipated Events and Course of Wound Healing

Common nonmedical terminology is used to describe the anticipated normal and potential abnormal healing events, including pain, swelling, infection, bleeding, scar quality, and function. Possible long-term outcomes that may affect appearance and function are described, but specific or implied guarantees are not given.

Activities and Elevation

The specific instructions depend on the nature and location of an injury. For most situations, a period of decreased activity and elevation is beneficial. Excessive activity increases cardiac output, which may cause bleeding and result in physical stress or trauma that could disrupt the wound. *No matter how minor the wound, the injured part should be elevated so that there is minimal edema and pain.* Specific instructions are given regarding return to work or school and limitations of activity.

Dressing Care

Patients should be instructed regarding changing their own dressings or leaving the dressing intact until the next appointment. In most situations, the patient should avoid exposure to sunlight to reduce the possibility of hyperpigmentation or hypertrophy of the scar; avoid prolonged contact in the water as in bathing or swimming because of the increased risk of infection and maceration of a wet wound; and avoid dusty environments or environmental chemicals.

Complications (Infection, Hematoma)

Patients should be told of the usual signs of local infection, including erythema, increased swelling, local heat, drainage, pain, and fever. Circulatory or neurologic dysfunction caused by compression from a hematoma or too tight a dressing also should be described. The patient should understand the normal anticipated amount of postoperative suture-line oozing and bleeding and what constitutes an abnormal amount.

Diet and Drugs

Most patients can have a normal diet, although patients with lacerations around the oral cavity should have a soft or liquid diet. Patients should be instructed regarding avoidance of drugs that could affect the healing process adversely. Cortisone and antimetabolites may retard healing; *anticoagulants, including aspirin,* may result in hematoma. The emergency physician must provide additional instruction regarding antibiotics or other medications.

Follow-up

The patient should be given a follow-up appointment after an interval appropriate to the type and magnitude of the injury. An emergency telephone number is also provided.

WOUND ASSESSMENT AND CLASSIFICATION

The wound conditions should be evaluated and described according to the classification system outlined in Chapter 1. The wound is either open or closed, tidy or untidy, clean or contaminated, vascular or avascular. From the description of the wound condition, an overall goal is arrived at; the dressing should be designed to maintain favorable conditions or improve unfavorable conditions.

ESTABLISHING OBJECTIVES

A dressing has many distinct benefits, but the overall objective can be characterized as either *maintenance*—preserving favorable conditions in the clean, tidy, closed, vascular wound, or *therapeutic*—improving unfavorable conditions in the open, avascular, contaminated, untidy wound. Specific objectives are then determined, including protection, support, antisepsis, debridement, granulation, and hemostasis.

Maintenance Dressing

The following objectives should be attained with a properly designed maintenance dressing. We also suggest some of the common methods and materials for achieving the objectives.

PROTECTION (PREVENTION OF TRAUMA)
A dressing can protect the wound from physical trauma, which can cause disruption or dehiscence. The protective element can be in all three layers of the dressing.

1. Avoidance of surface shearing—inner layer
2. A bulky padding to absorb direct impact—middle layer
3. Hard encasement (cast) to repel major impact—outer layer

POSITION (PREVENTION OF CONTRACTURE)
Proper positioning is most important for periarticular injuries that require prolonged immobilization. For example, if the fingers are not properly positioned, the collateral ligaments and tendons become foreshortened. Even if the wound heals well, the ultimate result may be joint contractures and compromised function.

Proper positioning is also important after nerve repair, tendon repair, fractures and dislocations, and skin grafts.

IMMOBILIZATION (PREVENTION OF WOUND SEPARATION)
Immobilization maintains the proper positioning of the injured tissues and allows progress of healing with lessened risk of disruption. Moreover, there is less wound pain. Immobilization is achieved with bulky dressings, splints, casts, or Kirschner wires.

SUPPORT (PREVENTION OF MALPOSITIONING OF BONE AND CARTILAGE)
Support is required to prevent collapse of unstable bone, cartilage, or soft tissue of the face into an air space such as nasal, oral, or sinus cavities. This is usually achieved with gauze packing, balloon catheters, or foam rubber.

CONTOUR (PREVENTION OF ABNORMAL SKIN POSITION)
Injuries with elevation of a skin flap or with a skin graft require that the graft or flap contour into the wound bed. This can be achieved by careful packing and light pressure wraps.

PRESSURE (PREVENTION OF EDEMA AND CAPILLARY OOZING)
Pressure dressings are important for minimizing edema and low-pressure capillary oozing. The physician must learn the subjective clinical feel of properly applied pressure dressings. Because the wound environment is constantly changing, the injured area may swell from inflammation, bleeding, edema, or transudation, or it may loosen and the pressure may be

reduced because of movement or elevation. Therefore, it is extremely critical and quite difficult to achieve and maintain ideal pressure. The pressure dressing is often used for preventing capillary oozing under skin flaps and skin grafts. It should not be used in larger arterial or venous bleeding sites.

ANTISEPSIS (PREVENTION OF WOUND AND SUTURE INFECTION)

A dressing can incorporate an antiseptic or antibiotic for the purpose of minimizing the growth of bacteria on the skin surface. Antiseptics can reduce bacterial growth, prevent suture abscess, and prevent suture marks. However, subsurface wound infection in dermis and subcutaneum is not prevented by antiseptic dressings. Wound infection is usually the result of bacterial contamination within the wound at the time of original injury or closure rather than contamination after application of the dressing. Commercially prepared antiseptic and antibiotic gauze, such as nitrofurazone (Furacin), Xeroform, and scarlet red, are poor antiseptic agents when used as a single application. However, direct application to the wound of antibiotic ointments or creams, such as nitrofurazone (Furacin), gentamicin, povidone-iodine (Betadine), Neosporin, sulfadiazine, and mafenide (Sulfamylon), is more effective.

Furthermore, antibiotics must be applied several times a day to maintain effective levels of the agent. A single application is of minimal benefit and may provide a moist culture medium after several days.

AESTHETIC CONSIDERATIONS

Although it is unlikely that a bloody or sloppily applied dressing may be particularly harmful, such a dressing does indicate inattention to detail. Furthermore, a neat-appearing dressing provides the patient with additional confidence in the capability of the physician and thus enhances the doctor-patient relationship.

COMFORT (INDUCING BETTER HEALING WITH HEAT AND COLD)

The healing and comfort of wounds can be affected by application of heat or cold. This requires the design of an occlusive reservoir or the direct application of heat or cold over the underlying dressing.

Because cold diminishes swelling and pain, it is used during the first 24 hours after injury. Application of cool water to a minor burn relieves pain and conducts heat out of the burn wound, thus minimizing the depth of the burn. Although cooling is most commonly done by immersing the injured part in water, the same effect can be achieved by application of a dressing with an incorporated catheter for application of water into the gauze. The use of dry cold with the application of a cold water bag on top of a dressing is more appropriate for sprains and nonthermal soft tissue injuries.

ELEVATION (PREVENTION OF EDEMA, PAIN, AND HEMATOMA)

Elevation is particularly important at night when the normal muscle pump mechanism is inactive. An edematous wound heals more slowly, is at greater risk of infection, and develops unnecessary postinjury scar and stiffness. An injured upper extremity should be elevated above the level of the heart; if a sling is used for the upper extremity it should maintain the elbow at an angle greater than 90° and the shoulder adducted somewhat across the chest. This can be achieved with a length of cloth or specifically designed commercial sling.

At night an injured part can be propped up on pillows. Likewise, following injuries to the head or neck, the head of the bed should be elevated on wooden blocks or books.

Therapeutic Dressing

In injuries with adverse conditions—open, contaminated, untidy, bleeding, or avascular wounds—a dressing should improve wound conditions. Adverse wounds undergo constant changes, which must be recognized so that appropriate alterations in the dressing can be made. The dressing should be constructed in such a way that maximum information can be obtained. For example, if there is concern about bleeding or purulence, a drain may be required. It would be unwise to surround the injured area with enormous amounts of absorptive gauze because the bleeding or infection may not become apparent until irreversible damage has occurred.

DESICCATION (DRYING OUT A WEEPING CONTAMINATED WOUND)

Wounds such as weeping dermatitis and contaminated abrasions require desiccation to reduce moist conditions, which favor bacterial growth.

Desiccation is best achieved by exposure to the air but can be achieved by application of chemical agents such as scarlet red or Xeroform.

EPITHELIALIZATION (MOISTURE AND OCCLUSION)

Abraded skin and skin graft donor sites heal by regeneration of the epithelial layer from hair follicles and other skin appendages. Reepithelialization can be more rapid in an environment that is moist from an occlusive dressing than with a dry, open method. Rapid reepithelialization is desirable on large surface areas to reduce metabolic and fluid loss, on deep abrasions, to prevent desiccation of epithelial elements, and on any wound to reduce the pain. An open, dry wound reepithelializes at a deeper plane within the dermis, whereas a moist, occluded wound reepithelializes on the wound surface. However, an occlusive dressing has a higher risk of inducing wound infection. The risk of infection can be reduced by frequent dressing changes and the use of antibiotic solutions in the moist environment. Occlusion and moisture can be achieved with the use of synthetic membranes (Opsite, N-terface, Biobrane) or with thick layers of antibiotic ointments, gauze, and plastic covers.

DEBRIDEMENT (REMOVAL OF NECROTIC TISSUE)

Debridement of untidy, ischemic, and necrotic tissue is most effectively achieved by surgical excision. However, various circumstances may preclude surgical debridement, and the dressing may serve the same therapeutic objective. Burn eschars, contaminated abrasions, and extensive untidy wounds are examples. Moreover, dressing debridement may be of benefit when conservation of tissue, anesthetic risk, or associated injuries make surgical debridement undesirable. Debridement of a wound with a dressing can be achieved by mechanical or enzymatic methods.

1. Mechanical debridement—the wet-to-dry dressing. Foreign material and necrotic debris can be mechanically removed. The gauze is applied to the wound surface and allowed to desiccate. The dry gauze and incorporated debris is then pulled off the wound surface. This can be painful and may require sedation or topical anesthetic. The process is repeated frequently until the wound is adequately debrided.
2. Enzymatic debridement. Another method of wound debridement makes use of proteolytic enzymes. The more commonly used enzymes are Travase, which is a nonspecific protease, and Subtilase, which is a bacterial collagenase. An occlusive dressing with the enzyme is applied to the wound. The dressing is removed, the wound cleansed, and a repeat application done 2 to 4 times daily. A more detailed description of topical enzymes is in this chapter. Enzymes are rarely used in initial emergency care except for circumferential full-thickness injuries with the potential for a compressive eschar.

GRANULATION (PROMOTION OF VASCULARIZATION)
If an open wound that cannot be closed is poorly vascularized (such as bone or tendon), healthy granulation should be stimulated before it is grafted. Granulation tissue is enhanced by a moist environment and the absence of infection. This is achieved by an occlusive antibiotic gauze dressing or a temporary skin graft (thin split autograft, allograft, or xenograft). Although skin grafts can be placed directly on granulation, they should not be placed on sites of heavy contamination or infection. Because excess granulation produces a poor bed for a graft, the excess should be removed.

HEMOSTASIS (PREVENTION OF HEMATOMA)
The site of bleeding and vessel type and size determine the need for a hemostatic dressing. Surface capillary ooze can be controlled with a firm pressure dressing similar to that used for controlling edema. Deep bleeding and bleeding from high-pressure large vessels usually should not be treated by pressure dressing alone; they may require a drain or suction.

1. Open packing and delayed closure. This method is often used when bleeding is associated with heavy bacterial contamination or an untidy or open wound. It is particularly useful for skin abrasions.

    Pressure dressings can be used for venous or arterial bleeding. However, a pressure dressing can be detrimental by creating ischemia and edema. A pressure of 25 to 60 mm stops venous capillary bleeding but doesn't cut off arterial flow. Pressure above 60 to 80 mm can cut off prearterial capillary flow. The use of pressure may be beneficial on a short-term basis for control of bleeding from superficial abrasions and for capillary bleeding under a skin graft. Pressure should be avoided for deep subcutaneous or intramuscular bleeding. This type of postoperative bleeding is better handled by drainage.
2. Rubber drains. Rubber drains are used when there is minimal bleeding from deep sites or a risk that delayed bleeding might occur. A rubber (Penrose) drain inserted in a corner of the wound does not usually provide adequate drainage of a hematoma. Nonetheless, it can be used as an indicator that bleeding is occurring and that more definitive mea-

sures must be taken. If staining of the dressing with blood occurs with a Penrose drain, the dressing should be removed and the wound inspected to determine if a large hematoma is developing.
3. Suction catheters. Primary wound closure and a suction catheter are particularly useful for deep wounds under flaps and on bone or muscle. If the wound is clean and has a slight ooze, a catheter can be used under skin flaps, undermined wounds, or deep lacerations into muscle. It is usually better to place the catheter through a separate stab wound. The catheter tubing should be flat, should not collapse with high suction pressures, and should have a lumen size large enough to evacuate the blood without plugging with clot. Suction can be created with a bulb or mechanical suction.

ABSORPTION (FOR DRAINAGE OF BLOOD OR PUS)

Drainage of sanguinous, serous, or purulent exudates from a wound requires an absorbent pad. Absorptive dressings must be changed frequently because the materials accumulating within the absorptive layer provide an excellent nutrient medium for the growth of bacteria and therefore perpetuate infection.

ANTISEPSIS (FOR TREATING OR PREVENTING WOUND INFECTION)

An untidy, ischemic wound, such as a burn, crush, abrasion, bite, or avulsion, is susceptible to secondary infection. Although systemic antibiotics may be indicated, a topical antiseptic is an important component of a dressing. The antiseptic or antibiotic agents must be in direct contact with the injury site, and the dressing requires frequent change or constant irrigation. The bacteriostatic effect of most agents persists for a few hours but gradually diminishes because of absorption or inactivation. The characteristics of some medicaments are described in the section on materials in Chapter 2. The three methods of applying medication are:

1. Direct application, followed by removal and reapplication
2. Gauze packing impregnated with antiseptic
3. Irrigation—closed continuous or intermittent

VASODILATION (FOR BETTER HEALING WITH LOCAL HEAT)

Heat increases local circulation and accelerates healing by local vasodilation and increase in metabolism. Inflammatory and infectious processes and soreness around muscles and joints are improved by the use of heat. Wet heat in an occlusive dressing is suggested for cellulitis, lymphangitis, and other nonpurulent infectious processes because of the greater capability of water to conduct heat from the environment into the tissues. In contrast, air is a poor conductor of heat, and a dry dressing is less effective.

DRESSING DESIGN—THE THREE-LAYER CONCEPT

Objectives

Our method of designing a dressing involves conceptualizing three layers: an inner contact layer, a middle layer, and an outer layer. Each layer can

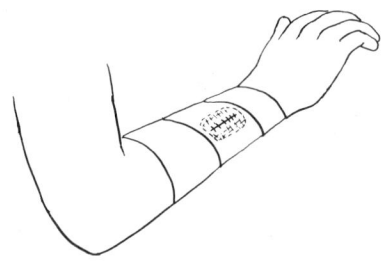

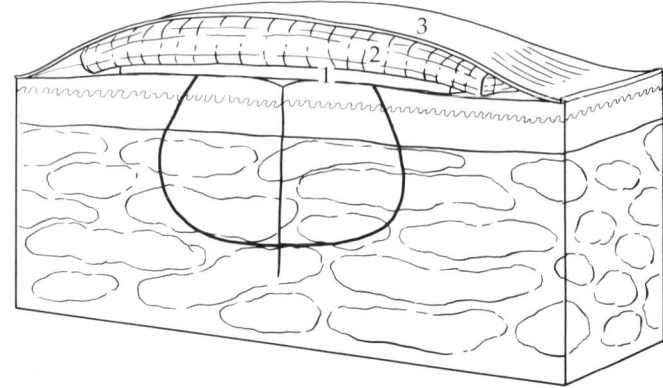

Layer	Objective	Method
1. inner	non-adherence, antisepsis	ointment or non-adherent gauze
2. middle	protection	4 × 4 gauze
3. outer	immobilization and pressure	tape or wrap

Figure 8-1. Components of a simple three-layer dressing for tidy lacerations.

achieve the specific objectives outlined for a maintenance or therapeutic dressing, although sometimes all three layers are not required. The choice of material and method is made on the basis of wound conditions, available materials, and personal preferences. Different methods or materials may achieve the same objectives.

The inner layer is called the contact layer because it is in direct physical approximation with the wound. Topical medicaments and gauzes are the most common contact materials. The middle layer is usually directed toward physical protection or absorption of wound fluids, and absorbent cotton gauze is commonly used. The outer layer is used for compressing, positioning, and immobilizing the inner and middle layers. This is usually achieved with elastic wraps, plaster splints, or tape.

A plastic bandage such as the Band-Aid is an example of a commercial product with an easily applied component three-layer dressing. The inner layer is Telfa, a nonadherent material, the middle layer is absorbent cotton, and the outer layer is adhesive tape.

Specific Wound Conditions

LACERATIONS AND SMALL FLAPS
1. Tidy, clean wound—maintenance dressing (Fig. 8-1). The primary objectives for a clean laceration are as follows:
   a. The inner layer prevents adherence of the sutures and transudate to the dressing. This can be achieved by application of a fine-mesh gauze impregnated with petrolatum-based ointment or synthetic membrane.

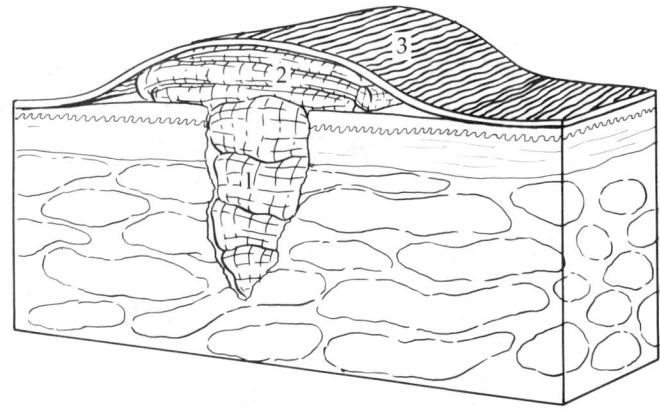

Figure 8-2. Components of a simple three-layer dressing for untidy, contaminated lacerations.

   b. The middle layer minimizes trauma, which could cause dehiscence or hematoma, and absorbs any blood or serum. A single layer of 4 × 4 cotton gauze serves this purpose.
   c. The outer layer immobilizes the underlying layers and provides pressure. Tape, gauze wraps, and elastic wraps can be used, depending on the anatomic site. Splints are used on the extremities when the wound is adjacent to a joint.
2. Untidy, contaminated, or ischemic laceration—therapeutic dressing (Fig. 8-2). An untidy laceration that cannot be converted to a tidy laceration by surgical debridement should have a delayed wound closure. For example, this may be used on a human bite on the hand. The objective of the dressing in this type of wound is to debride necrotic and infected tissue. The gauze is left in place for 4 to 12 hours. The gauze is removed dry, thus debriding the incorporated tissue of the contaminated wound. Packing and removal are repeated until a healthy wound is achieved. Usually the wound is secondarily closed in 3 to 7 days. Once debridement and a clean wound are achieved, a delayed closure is carried out. This is done by direct suturing, skin graft, or flap, or by allowing the wound to heal by contracture and reepithelialization.
   a. The inner layer provides debridement and antisepsis. A fine-mesh gauze impregnated with an antiseptic or antibiotic is packed into the crevices of the wound.
   b. The middle layer is made of cotton gauze pads to absorb drainage.
   c. The outer layer immobilizes the wound and provides slight pressure for hemostasis if there is a persistent capillary ooze. A gauze wrap is effective for this purpose.

BLEEDING (LACERATIONS AND FLAPS)

Bleeding usually subsides with pressure, time, and surgical hemostasis. However, a persistent ooze or intermittent, recurrent bleeding is likely to persist from muscle, large skin flaps, scar, and bone. When bleeding has not completely stopped before wound closure, there are four alternative surgical dressings that can be used:

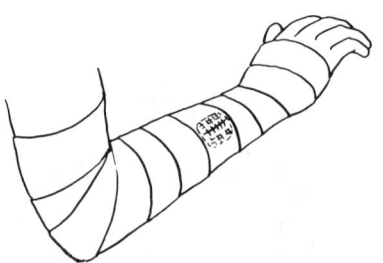
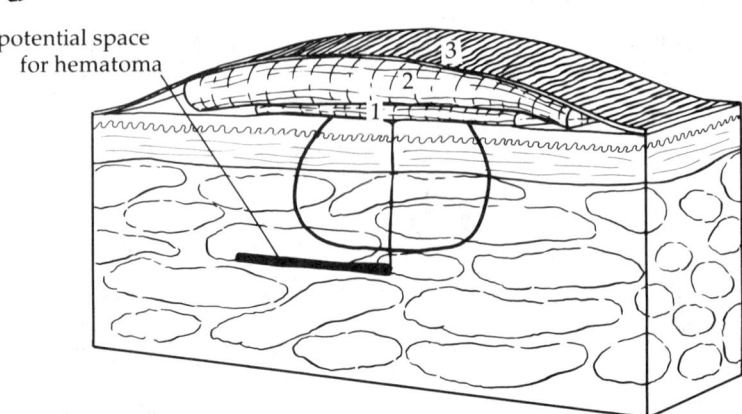

Layer	Objective	Method
1. inner	non-adherence	ointment gauze
2. middle	protection and contour	gauze pad
3. outer	immobilization and pressure	elastic wrap

Figure 8-3. Components of a simple three-layer dressing for tidy flaps or oozing lacerations.

Primary closure with pressure dressing
Primary closure with rubber drain
Primary closure with suction catheter
Delayed closure after packing

Immobilization and elevation are used for all bleeding wounds.

The appropriate method is chosen by evaluation of the clinical variables and the reliability and accessibility of the patient. Some of the wound factors to be considered are:

Severity of bleeding
Associated tissue ischemia
Anatomic site as it relates to applying pressure
Size of wound
Risk of associated infection
Type of tissue
Ability to immobilize and elevate the area

1. Primary closure with pressure dressing (Fig. 8-3). This technique is used for most simple wounds.
    a. Indications
        (1) Minimal capillary ooze
        (2) Tissues not likely to bleed postoperatively (fat, normal dermis)
        (3) Small wounds
        (4) Anatomic sites in which pressure and elevation can be achieved (extremities, scalp)
        (5) Tidy, uncontaminated wounds
        (6) Immobile areas

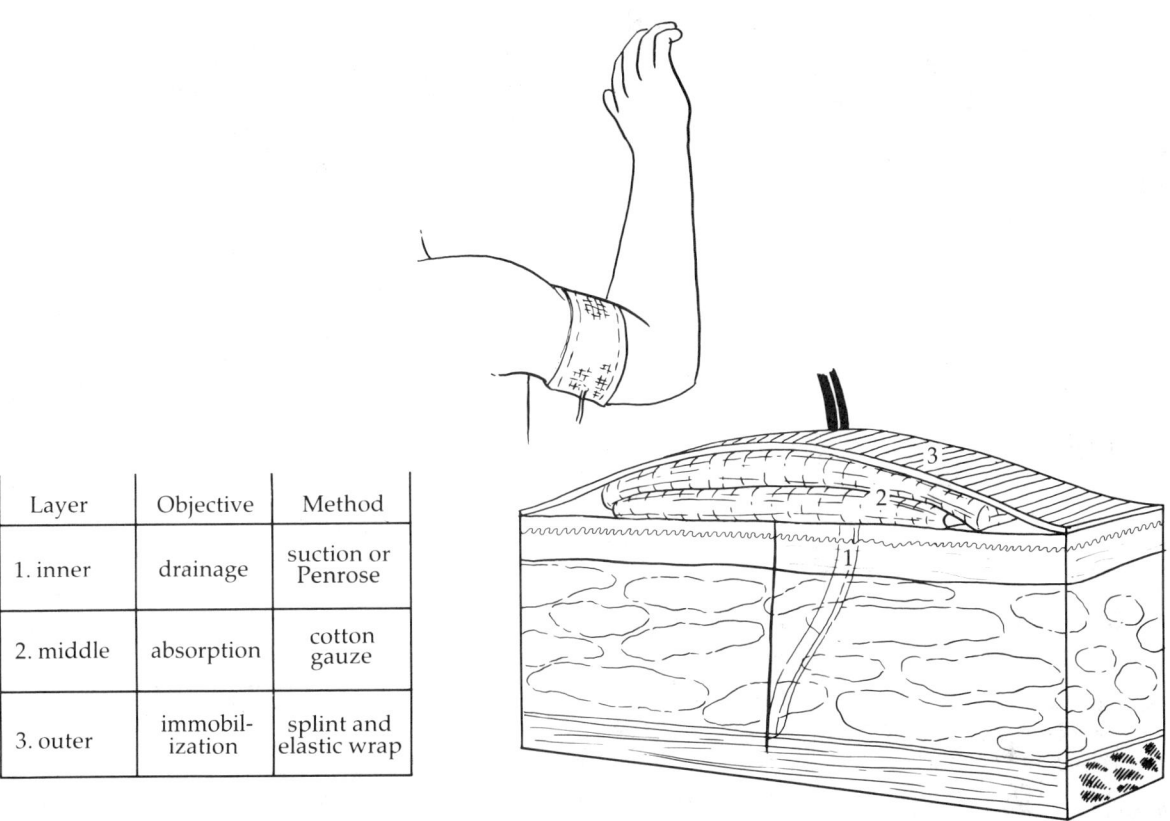

Figure 8-4. Components of a simple three-layer dressing for bleeding lacerations in which pressure cannot be applied.

Layer	Objective	Method
1. inner	drainage	suction or Penrose
2. middle	absorption	cotton gauze
3. outer	immobilization	splint and elastic wrap

b. Layers
  (1) The inner contact layer and middle layer are the same as for a clean laceration.
  (2) The outer layer is a pressure wrap. Under the skin flap, there is a *potential* space for hematoma. A firmly wrapped outer gauze layer contours the flap, obliterates the dead space, reduces the risk of capillary ooze, and minimizes edema. If there is uncontrolled bleeding under the skin flap or a very high risk of bleeding, the wound should be treated as one with deep bleeding and may require a drain or catheter instead of a pressure wrap.
2. Primary closure with rubber drain (Fig. 8-4). A drain is used in situations similar to those in which pressure dressings are used, but the wounds are larger, and there is a potential space for hematoma. Because a Penrose drain does not completely remove fresh blood, a hematoma may form in spite of the drain. However, the drain can serve as a *warning signal* of recurrent or persistent bleeding.
  a. Indications
    (1) Minimal oozing
    (2) Tissues that may bleed postoperatively but are inactive at the time of closure (muscle, around mobile joints)
    (3) Sites at which pressure or elevation is difficult or limited (neck, face, fingers, axilla, trunk)
    (4) Intermediate-sized wounds
    (5) Tidy, uncontaminated wounds

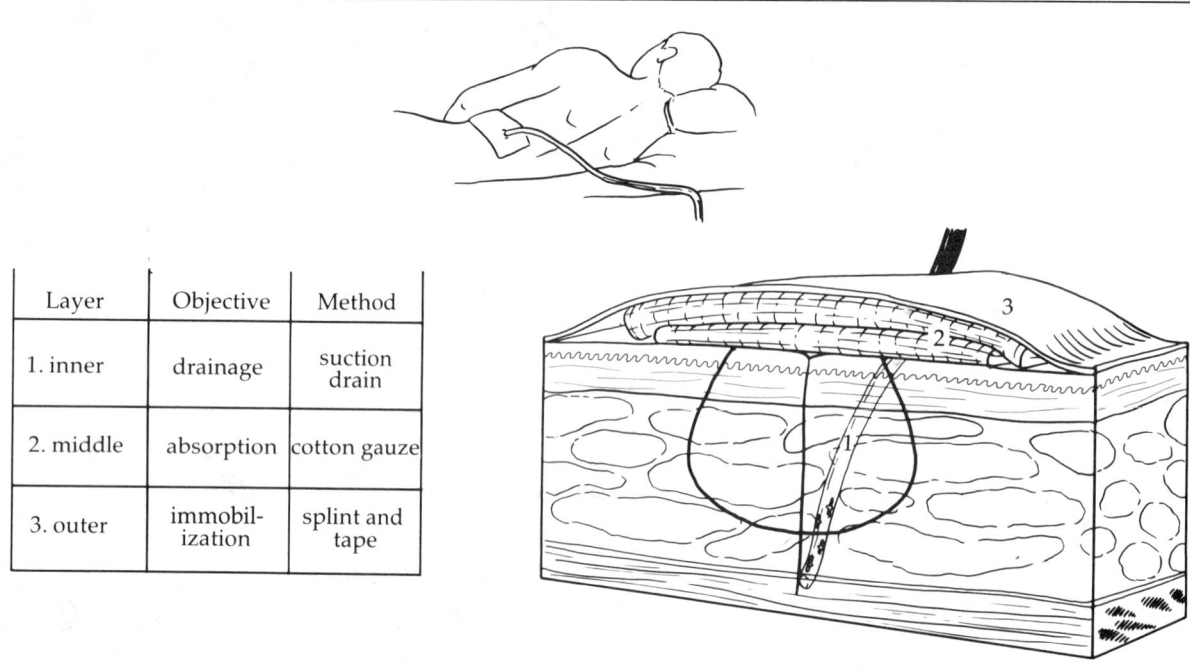

Figure 8-5. A minimally bleeding wound or a large flap that has the potential for accumulating a hematoma is dressed with a suction catheter. The catheter is usually a large, flattened silicone or plastic tube that will not collapse with negative pressure or become occluded with clot.

Layer	Objective	Method
1. inner	drainage	suction drain
2. middle	absorption	cotton gauze
3. outer	immobilization	splint and tape

    b. Layers
      (1) Inner contact layer. A rubber drain (1/8–1/2 inch wide) is inserted through the laceration or a separate stab incision. In addition, nonadherent gauze is applied over the suture line *except* for the drain site.
      (2) Middle layer. A small amount of gauze is used to contour the anatomic site. A flat 4 × 4 gauze pad is used on a convex or flat surface, and packed fluffed gauze is used in concave areas. Because the small volume of gauze limits the amount of bleeding that can occur, the bleeding is rapidly visible on the dressing. The use of "flats" or "fluffs" is related to the need for an outer pressure wrap and for the ideal configuration for smooth, even application of pressure.
      (3) Outer layer. A firm pressure wrap of an estimated 20 to 30 ml of water should be used. Ace bandage, Kling, bias-cut stockinette, or Elastoplast can be used, depending on the anatomic site. Splints also may be useful on the extremity.
  3. Primary closure with suction catheter (Fig. 8-5)
    a. Indications
      (1) Risk of bleeding is relatively high (hypertensive patients), but actual bleeding is minimal
      (2) Bleeding site is not amenable to pressure (abdomen, neck, chest)
      (3) Occurrence of a hematoma would be a serious complication (large skin flaps)
      (4) Injury to muscle, or scarred or irradiated tissue
      (5) Mobile areas
    b. Layers
      (1) The inner layer is a suction catheter, which comes in various sizes. The shape and material we prefer is flat, flexible, but non-

POSTOPERATIVE CARE AND DRESSINGS

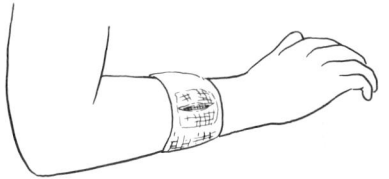

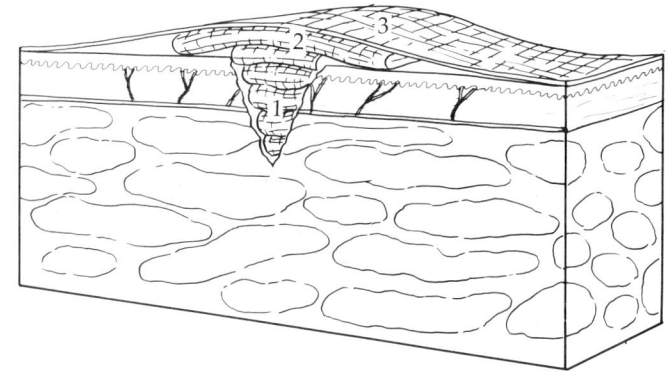

Layer	Objective	Method
1. inner	drainage and non-adherence	wide-mesh non-adherent gauze
2. middle	absorption	cotton gauze
3. outer	pressure hemostasis and immobilization	gauze wrap and splint

Figure 8-6. The actively bleeding wound is not closed, but a compressive dressing with gauze packs is used.

collapsible silicone of at least 7 mm in width. The catheter can be brought through one corner of the traumatic wound or through a separate stab wound, but the wound must be airtight. An ointment gauze over the suture line and around the catheter exit achieves a seal for suction.

(2) The middle layer is either an absorbent cotton gauze or, if a suction catheter is used, a protective layer of gauze.

(3) The outer layer is a splint or bulky dressing for immobilization. Immobilization prevents disruption of the newly formed clots and thus avoids the possibility of secondary bleeding from trauma or movement.

We should emphasize, however, that it is *often contraindicated to use a pressure dressing in combination with a suction catheter*. The reason is that some suction catheters (particularly round catheters) are quite firm. When pressure is applied with a tight wrap, the skin is compressed between the outer wrap and the catheter and therefore occludes the venous outflow, causing vascular congestion, wound ischemia, and finally, necrosis.

4. Packing and delayed closure (Fig. 8-6). In situations of persistent major bleeding or high risk because of extensive damage to muscle and bone, or if a hematoma would cause compromise of tissue viability, the wound can be packed and closed within a few days. Antiseptic gauze and systemic antibiotics are often used in these circumstances.
   a. Indications
      (1) Actively bleeding wound
      (2) Contaminated, untidy wound
      (3) When pressure cannot be applied to skin without increasing risk of ischemia
   b. Layers
      (1) The contact layer and middle layer are usually included as a combined unit. An antiseptic or antibiotic is incorporated into a

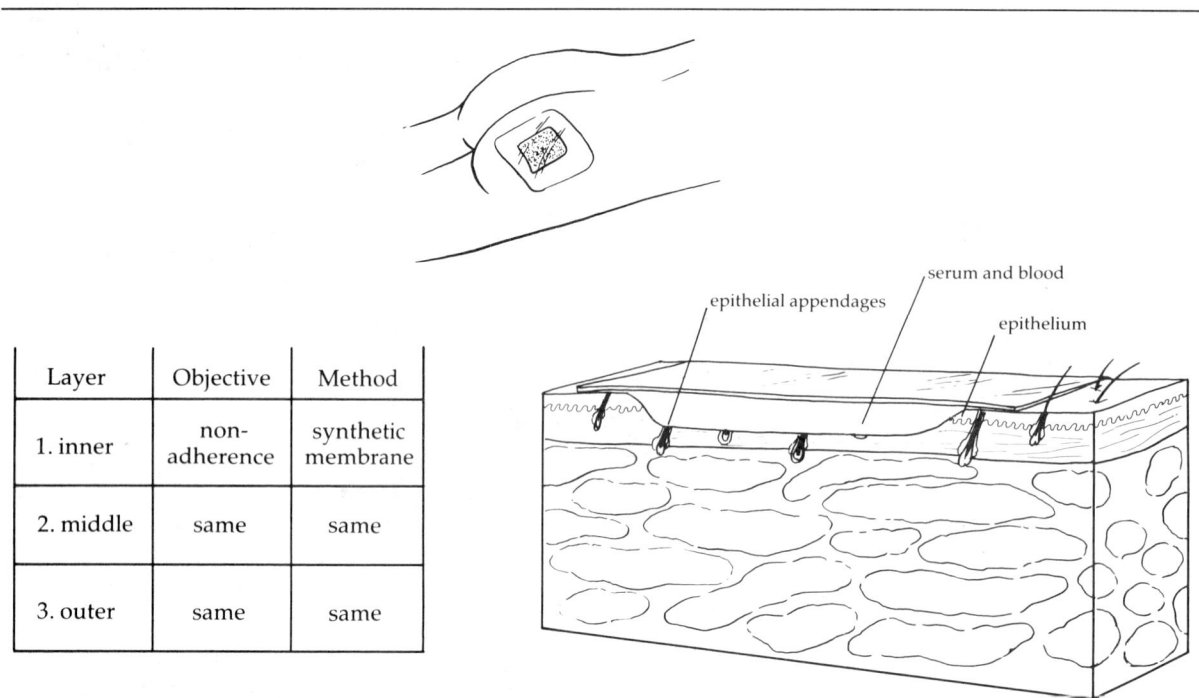

Figure 8-7. Clean abrasions and split-graft donor sites are dressed with synthetic membranes.

Layer	Objective	Method
1. inner	non-adherence	synthetic membrane
2. middle	same	same
3. outer	same	same

fine-mesh gauze, which is carefully and firmly packed into the contours of the wound. Alternatives are an iodophor ointment impregnated into gauze and an antibiotic ointment. Ointment is somewhat preferable to a cream-based product because it does not dry out as readily and prevents adherence of the gauze to the wound. If the gauze does adhere, it can reactivate bleeding when removed.

(2) The outer layer provides pressure and immobilization. On the extremities, a splint firmly wrapped with cotton gauze, elastic bandage, or bias-cut stockinette provides pressure against the wound. When wrapping to obtain hemostasis, it should be remembered that there is the danger of causing venous congestion. Wrapping should begin distally and progress proximally. The amount of pressure cannot be measured objectively but is learned by experience and by questioning of the patient. If the patient complains of pain, paresthesias, or numbness, or if the distal extremity appears congested or ischemic, the wrapping should be removed immediately, the wound checked, and the dressing reapplied.

Although the primary focus in this section is on the use of dressings for hemostasis, elevation and immobilization are also integral parts of the postoperative care of bleeding.

ABRASIONS (TRAUMATIC) AND SKIN GRAFT DONOR SITES

1. Clean, tidy abrasions (Fig. 8-7). A clean abrasion has no foreign matter embedded in the wound after debridement and sandpapering. A tidy abrasion is smooth without irregular fragments and gouges. A surgical split-graft donor site has anatomic features identical to a traumatic abra-

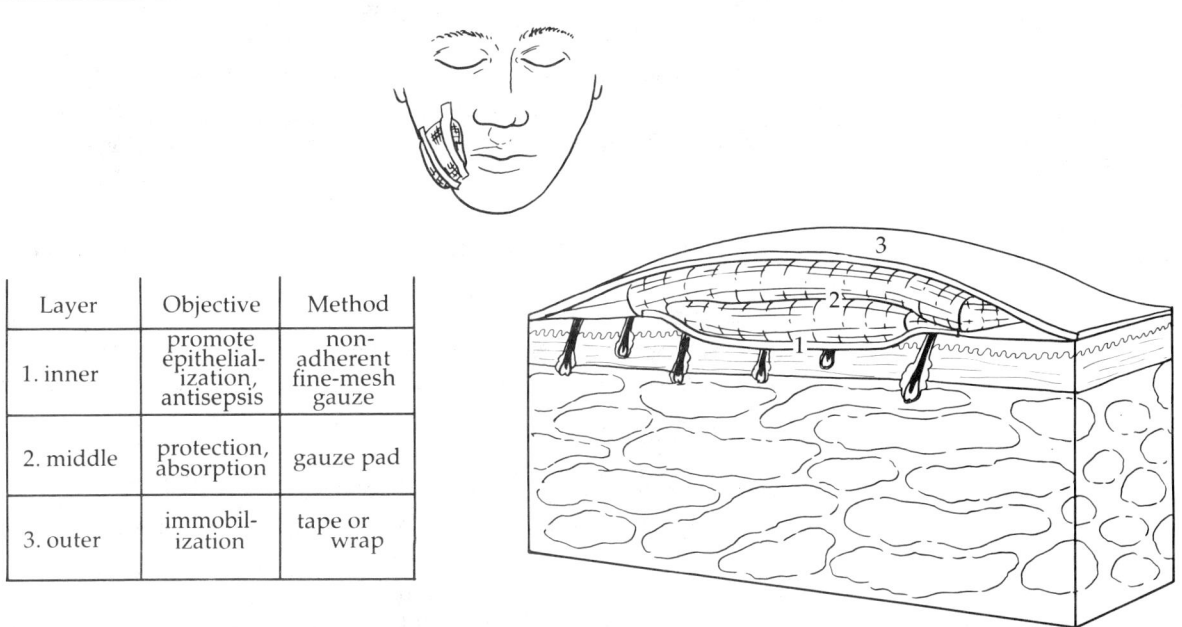

Figure 8-8. Noncontaminated traumatic abrasions. A nonadherent gauze impregnated with antibiotic is applied to the wound and covered with absorbent gauze. Frequent changes may be necessary.

sion: the epithelium has been removed along with a part of the dermis, but epithelial appendages are retained in the deep dermis.

  a. The inner layer promotes reepithelialization and hemostasis and prevents infection. This can be achieved with a nonadherent occlusive membrane or fine-mesh gauze.

    Our preference is for synthetic membranes such as Opsite, Biobrane, or N-terface (see Fig. 8-7). These are particularly suitable for skin graft donor sites but may not be suitable for traumatic abrasion because of the difficulty of application to the face and hands. In these areas, an occlusive mesh and wrap is used (Fig. 8-8). The inner contact layer may be the only layer of the dressing in areas such as the lips and eyelids.

    Alternative gauzes are scarlet red, nitrofurazone (Furacin), Xeroform, Xeroflo, and Aquaflo, "parachute silk," or cotton gauze that has been impregnated with antibiotic ointments.

  b. The middle layer protects against trauma and provides moisture retention and absorption. This is an inherent component of synthetic membranes.

  c. The outer layer immobilizes the underlying layers. A cotton gauze wrap or elastic bandage is suitable for either a synthetic membrane or a gauze dressing.

2. Untidy abrasions (traumatic). Untidy abrasions that have irregular surfaces with gouges, tissue fragments, and possible foreign body contamination *in spite of surgical attempts at sandpapering and scrubbing* should be treated differently from clean, tidy abrasions. The objectives are to obtain a smoother wound contour, avoid infection, and avoid tattooing of the abrasion with grease and dirt particles. There are two alternatives for this type of wound. One is to *use no dressing at all and allow the wound to heal as an open, desiccated wound.* If this is done, the contaminated, injured skin, which is irregular, ischemic, and filled with debris, will desiccate and therefore not be incorporated under the epithelium. Instead, the epithelium migrates deep to this ischemic and irregular tissue. If a dressing is to be used because of drainage, a variation of the method for tidy abrasions is acceptable.

  a. The inner layer should be a wide-mesh dry gauze. The gauze is incorporated into the crust, and epithelium grows underneath the gauze and crust. Because adherence to the wound is desirable, no ointment is used. If there is extensive irregularity and contamination, the gauze should be removed once or twice a day so that the necrotic tissue and debris are removed with the gauze and crust. This dry-gauze debridement technique is repeated until a clean smooth surface is obtained. This technique delays reepithelialization because epithelium is torn off when the gauze is removed. However, delay in epithelium reformation is an acceptable outcome in this circumstance.
  b. The middle layer should be no more than a fine thin gauze pad to absorb drainage.
  c. The outer layer can be a light cotton gauze wrap or tape around the periphery but not overlying the wound.

OPEN WOUNDS AND AMPUTATIONS

1. Clean, tidy wounds. Most clean open wounds should be covered immediately with an appropriate skin graft or skin flap. If this cannot be done immediately, however, the wound should be dressed to prevent infection while waiting for permanent surgical skin grafting.
   a. Inner, contact layer. A protective gauze is placed on the wound to maintain antisepsis. Any topical antibiotic or antiseptic can be laid on the wound.
   b. Middle layer. Cotton mesh gauze absorbs the drainage.
   c. Outer layer. Tape or gauze wrap is used to immobilize the underlying layers.
2. Hypovascular avulsion wounds. A hypovascular wound occurs if there has been desiccation of hypovascular tissues, such as tendon, cartilage, or cortical bone. Normal periosteum and perichondrium are excellent beds for a skin graft; delay is not required. An avulsion injury to a hypovascular surface is dressed to prevent desiccation and promote granulation in preparation for skin grafting. In most circumstances, however, it is more appropriate to cover an avascular area immediately with a graft or skin flap. The specific indications for a dressing followed by a delayed skin graft or for an immediate graft or flap are discussed in the section on tissue avulsion.
   a. The inner layer promotes granulation and avoids desiccation by maintaining an aseptic moist environment. The use of fine-mesh gauze impregnated with an antibiotic ointment is one alternative. The other is to use cotton gauze impregnated with a liquid antibiotic solution and frequently change it. Allogeneic cadaver skin or xenogeneic pigskin are the most effective temporary wound covers. They must be removed within 3 days to avoid an immunologic response that is detrimental to the donor site as well as destructive to the graft.
   b. The middle layer is primarily a reservoir for the antibiotic solution if

POSTOPERATIVE CARE AND DRESSINGS

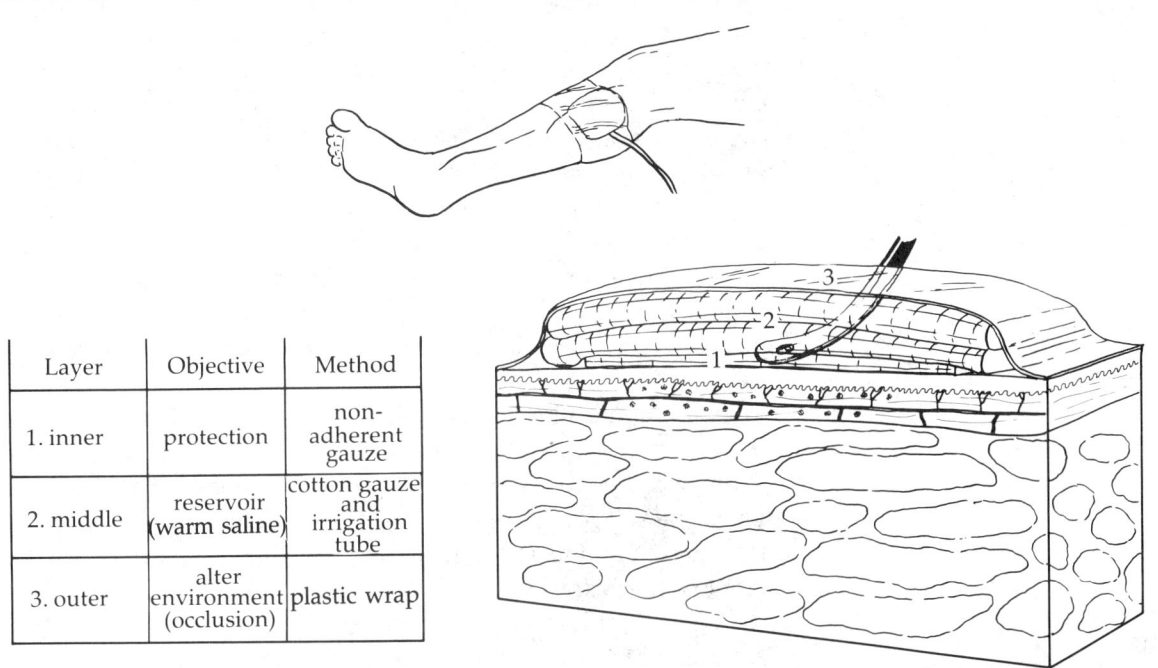

Figure 8-9. Closed cellulitis requires application of moist heat with irrigation either through a catheter as shown here or simply with a hot water bottle or pad.

Layer	Objective	Method
1. inner	protection	non-adherent gauze
2. middle	reservoir (warm saline)	cotton gauze and irrigation tube
3. outer	alter environment (occlusion)	plastic wrap

the wet dressing technique is used. If the fine-mesh gauze is used, the intermediate layer should also be kept moist to avoid desiccation. Most antibiotic-impregnated gauze is not adequate to prevent dehydration of the wound if used without additional occlusion.

  c. The outer layer can provide additional occlusion by the use of plastic films or multiple gauze layers covered with tape.

3. Untidy, contaminated open wound. The emergency objectives for this type of wound are the same as for the contaminated untidy laceration except that the wound is subsequently covered with a skin graft or skin flap rather than reapproximating the edges for delayed closure of the laceration. The technique of dressing is essentially the same as described for the untidy laceration except for a variation in the inner layer that should be considered.

  The inner layer can be covered with a gauze dressing as described for contaminated lacerations or with a temporary mesh skin graft. A very thin split graft (either an autograft, homograft, or xenograft) is removed within 3 or 4 days. The biologic skin graft technique is best used when there is contamination of exposed nerve, tendon, cartilage, or other important structures that do not tolerate desiccation.

INFECTION

1. Closed, nonpurulent wound (cellulitis, phlebitis) (Fig. 8-9). A nonpurulent soft tissue infection or inflammation such as cellulitis, lymphangitis, dermatitis, or phlebitis requires an environment that is conducive to resolution of the infection. This dressing technique is only an adjunct to the use of systemic antibiotics, elevation, and immobilization.

  The cellulitis may progress to an abscess, and this process, too, is accelerated by the use of the following dressing technique.

a. An inner layer is usually not required on an intact skin surface.
b. The middle layer is a reservoir for warm water or a heating pad. Bulky cotton gauze with a catheter as a conduit for continuous warm solution is designed.
c. The outer layer is an occlusive covering with plastic film wrap, cellophane, or other material that can contain the liquid. This technique is most appropriate for an extremity that is easily occluded. It can, however, be used on the trunk, but it is rarely used on the face.

   An alternative is a hot water bottle or dry heating pad. These self-contained units are somewhat less effective in heat conduction. Dry heat (100°–106°F) is applied with a hot water bottle over a cotton gauze.

2. Open, draining, purulent wound (drained abscess). If an abscess forms, the pus is first drained by appropriate incision. The dressing for an open infection promotes continued drainage from the infected area and does not allow the surface epithelium to close over the infection. The dressing is similar to that used for an actively bleeding wound (see Fig. 8-6). Frequent changes are required.
   a. The inner layer and middle layer are a single unit. It can be either a cotton gauze wick, such as plain or iodoform gauze, or any other type of drain or catheter. The packing regardless of type should be placed in such a way that the opening through the surface is nearly as large as the underlying subcutaneous abscess cavity. The gauze should not be packed in so tightly that it prevents drainage. The dressing should be bulky enough to absorb purulent drainage. This is achieved with cotton pads.
   b. The outer layer immobilizes the underlying inner and intermediate layers and immobilizes the infected area. A splint over the contralateral surface of that extremity plus a wrap is quite effective.

      This type of dressing must be changed frequently (2–5 times a day) to remove the necrotic material and accumulated purulence. At the dressing change, the wound is irrigated with an antibiotic solution or the injured part placed in a Hubbard tank or other form of agitated water solution. The dressing is then reapplied.

      Frequency of dressing change depends on the severity of infection and, therefore, the rate of accumulation of pus within the dressing.

3. Infection in joints, bursal spaces, and bone (Fig. 8-10). A continuous lavage with antibiotic solutions should be used for open joint infection. The choice of antibiotic solution depends on the origin of the infection and the probable infecting organism. Careful monitoring of dose, blood levels, and toxic effects is required.
   a. Inner contact layer. The antibiotic is instilled through a catheter and exits through a separate catheter or through the wound. The size and position of the catheter depend on the joint size. A separate catheter for intermittent suction is preferred because this allows alternation of antibiotic contact and removal.
   b. Middle layer. Large wads of absorbent cotton and/or a collection basin catch the lavage solution as it exits.
   c. Outer layer. The area should be immobilized with a cast or splint, with a window over the infected area.

Layer	Objective	Method
1. inner	irrigation	indwelling catheter–antibiotic solution
2. middle	absorption reservoir	gauze pads
3. outer	immobilization	casts, splints, or wrap

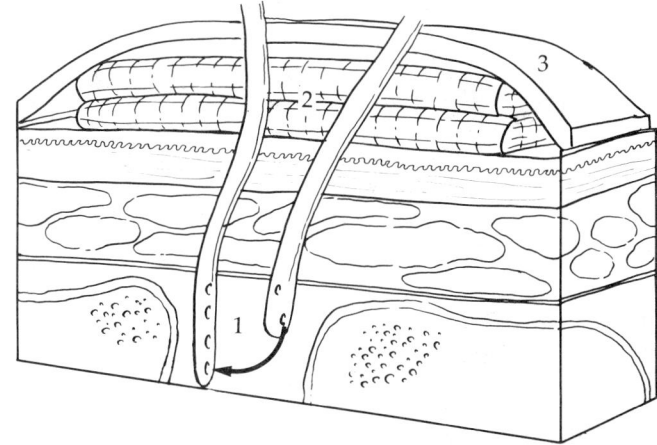

Figure 8-10. Bone and joint infections may require continuous antibiotic irrigation using inflow and outflow catheters.

SKIN GRAFTS

A detailed discussion of skin graft biology and techniques is included in Chapter 1. The basic principles of the graft dressing are as follows (Fig. 8-11):

1. The inner layer prevents adherence of overlying dressing to the skin graft. This requires a nonadherent ointment–impregnated gauze or a synthetic membrane. Our preference is for the N-terface gauze.
2. The middle layer is designed primarily to assist in contouring of the graft against the underlying bed. This is particularly important when the underlying wound has irregular surfaces. Our preference is for cotton wadding, which is applied dry or impregnated with glycerine or mineral oil. We avoid the use of wet cotton because it becomes extremely hard as it dries, and shearing can occur. Sponges or rubber Reston foam padding are also effective but do not absorb blood.
3. The outer layer puts pressure against the graft to minimize capillary bleeding and obliterate dead space. Immobilization and pressure can be obtained with either a tie-over dressing (Fig. 8-12) or a circumferential wrapping, depending on the anatomic area.

MATERIALS AND MEDICATIONS

Various commercial gauzes, antibiotics, enzymes, and other materials are available, and their characteristics must be understood so that appropriate materials and medications may be chosen to achieve the predetermined objectives.

Wound Contact—Inner Layer

The many commercially available gauzes vary in material, tightness of weave, thickness, added medications, and qualities of adherence, drainage, and antisepsis (Table 8-1).

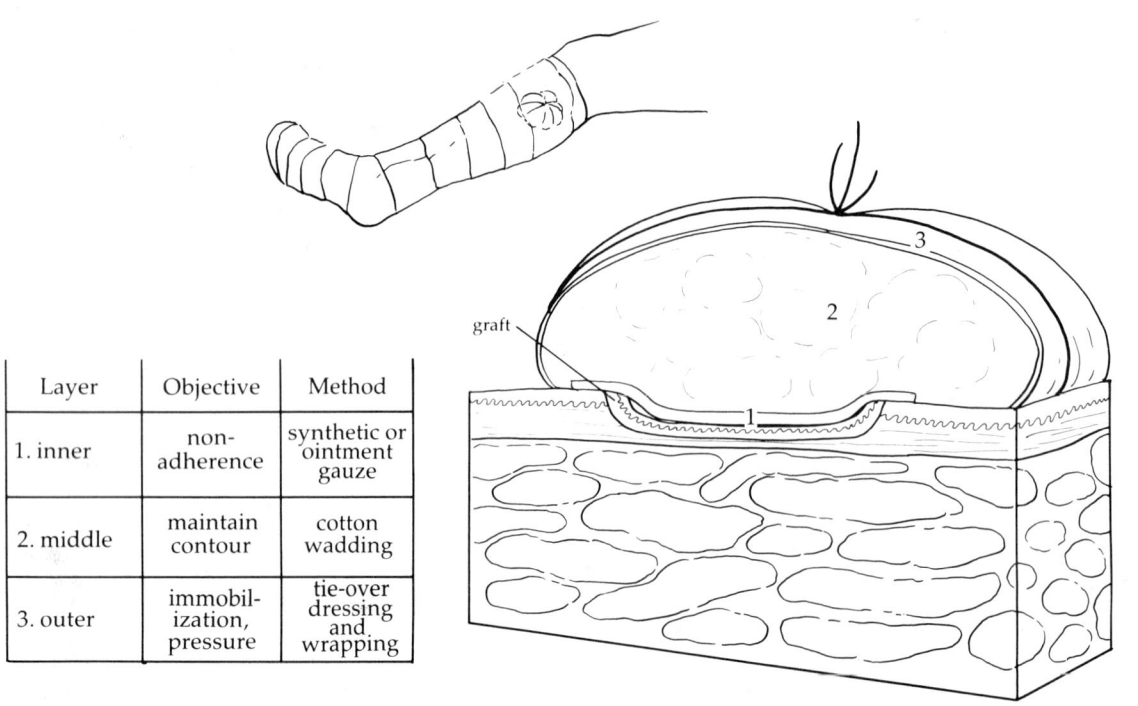

Layer	Objective	Method
1. inner	non-adherence	synthetic or ointment gauze
2. middle	maintain contour	cotton wadding
3. outer	immobilization, pressure	tie-over dressing and wrapping

Figure 8-11. Skin grafts are immobilized with a light pressure tie-over dressing.

Figure 8-12. Key points of the tie-over technique.
A. Careful smoothing of nonadherent gauze of large size.
B. Very bulky dry cotton packing that evenly distributes pressure.
C. Rolling the nonadherent gauze over the packing.
D. Grouping the sutures.
E. Tying over the gauze with moderate pressure.

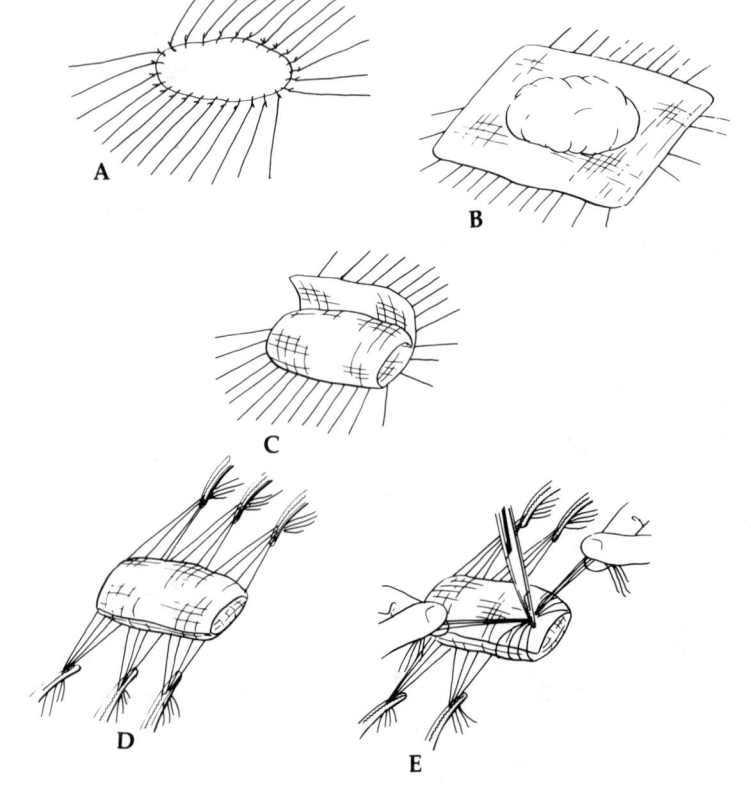

Table 8-1. Characteristics of commercial gauzes

Type	Antisepsis	Nonadherence	Occlusion	Desiccation
Adaptik	0	1	0	2
Aquaflo	0	2	2	2
Betadine	3+	2	2	2
Biobrane	0	0	3	0
Cotton gauze	0	3	2	3
Epigard	0	0	2	0
Furacin	3	2	2	2
N-terface	0	0	1	1
Opsite	0	0	3	0
Pigskin	1	2	3	0
Scarlet red	1	2	2	2
Silk gauze	0	1	2	1
Telfa	0	3	3	0
Vaseline gauze	0	2	2	1
Xeroflo	1	2	2	2
Xeroform	1	2	2	2

0 = none; 1 = minimal; 2 = moderate; 3 = extreme.

PLAIN GAUZE
1. Cotton gauze is by far the most commonly used material. It has a very loose weave that allows drainage and desiccation but is adherent, nonocclusive, and nonantiseptic. The gauze is usually referred to by size in inches (2 × 2 or 4 × 4).
2. Silk gauze ("parachute") is a much more tightly woven material with smaller interstices, which minimizes drainage and adherence. It is also more occlusive.
3. N-terface (Winfield) is a new synthetic composite material with excellent nonadherent qualities that nonetheless allows for drainage.

LAMINATED COMPOSITE MATERIALS
1. Epigard (Parke-Davis) is a polytetrafluoroethylene (polytef) sheet externally laminated to a polyurethane microporous foam. It allows absorption and debridement through the foam in contact with the wound, and protects against fluid loss and desiccation through the Teflon outer laminate.
2. Telfa (Kendall) is a combination of a thin polytef (Teflon) film on a cotton fiber pad. This is highly occlusive and nonadherent but does not allow for extensive drainage.

MEDICATED OR OINTMENT-COVERED MATERIALS
1. Adaptik (Johnson & Johnson)—petrolatum on a wide-mesh cotton gauze
2. Aquaflo (Chesebrough-Pond's)—oil emulsion on a fine-mesh cotton gauze
3. Betadine (Purdue Frederick)—povidone-iodone (iodophor)
4. Furacin (Eaton)—nitrofurazone, in a water-soluble base
5. Scarlet red (Chesebrough-Pond's)—scarlet red in a lanolin, petrolatum base

6. Vaseline (Chesebrough-Pond's)—petrolatum without antiseptic
7. Xeroflo (Chesebrough-Pond's)—oil emulsion with 3% tribromophenate; allows drainage and is mildly antiseptic
8. Xeroform (Chesebrough-Pond's)—petroleum base with 3% tribromophenate; more occlusive and mildly antiseptic
9. Unna boot (zinc oxide emulsion impregnated into cotton gauze)—(Edwards Lab). This material has been used in the treatment of chronic stasis ulcers. Its efficacy may be related to the zinc content, the compression application, or the occlusion. It has not been extensively used for acute ulcers.

MEMBRANES—OCCLUSIVE

Synthetic membranes are available with pore size permitting movement of gases but restricting large molecules, including liquids and bacteria. Several different brands are available, including Opsite and Biobrane.

Topical Medications

ANTIBIOTICS

Numerous antibiotic creams and ointments can be used directly on the wound or in gauzes. They all may be helpful for minimizing suture infection or to protect against infection on open wounds or burns. However, overgrowth with resistant bacteria is common, and hypersensitivity can develop. The spectrum of antibacterial activity for some topical agents is given in Chapter 2. Some common agents used in dressings are as follows:

1. Creams
   a. Silver sulfadiazine
   b. Mafenide (Sulfamylon)
   c. Gentamicin
   d. Neosporin-Polysporin
2. Ointments
   a. Neosporin
   b. Bacitracin
   c. Iodophor
      (1) Septisol (Vestal)
      (2) Povidone-iodine (Betadine) (Purdue Frederick)
      (3) Prepodyne (West Chemical Products)

VITAMINS AND HORMONES (Steroids)

Topical vitamins have no proven benefit, although some have an antiinflammatory effect and reduced scar has been attributed to vitamin E. We do not recommend their use in acute wound care. Cortisone is the only agent that is useful for topical application. This is generally used for allergic inflammatory reactions to other agents in the original dressing. However, its value in emergency wound care has not been proved except in instances of known contact to allergens such as poison oak or ivy.

ENZYMES AND DEBRIDING AGENTS

Travase (Flint), a protease, and Santyl (Knoll), a collagenase, can be used for burns, necrotic ulcers, and other wounds requiring debridement. They are of minimal value in acute outpatient care. These enzymes are partially inactivated by many topical antibiotics and are ineffective in acid environments (below pH 6.0). Allergic reactions and fever can be caused by their use, and thus they are not as effective in infected or inflamed wounds. In fact, infection rates and tissue destruction may be increased by enzymes. A possible use of enzymes in the emergency room is in clean circumferential burns with a constricting eschar that may cause vascular insufficiency of an extremity or for a chest burn that may prevent adequate chest expansion and pulmonary ventilation.

Debrisan (Pharmacia) is a dextran polymer formulated as small hydrophylic absorbent beads. It has been recommended for absorption of excessive drainage of chronic wounds. Its value in acute traumatic or infected wounds is questionable.

The comparative qualities of these contact materials are discussed and outlined in Table 8-1.

QUALITIES OF TOPICAL MEDICATIONS

1. Occlusion versus drainage. Cotton gauze impregnated with various agents is commercially available. Most of these gauzes are fine cotton mesh, which allows some drainage. The exception is Adaptik, which has a much looser weave and therefore allows drainage more freely. Also, the synthetic multilaminated gauze, N-terface, also allows for wound drainage, whereas Biobrane, Telfa, and Opsite are the most highly occlusive synthetics. Thus, if occlusion without drainage is desired, Opsite, Biobrane, and Telfa are most useful; if drainage without occlusion is required, Adaptik or N-terface can be used.
2. Adherence. Because in most circumstances (tidy, clean wounds) nonadherence of the contact gauze with the wound is required, N-terface, Telfa, and Adaptik are useful. When debridement is required, an adherent cotton gauze, plain or impregnated, is chosen.
3. Antisepsis. Minimal antisepsis is achieved by most commercial gauzes, particularly if used as a single application and not changed for several days. Povidone-iodine (Betadine) has the most antiseptic qualities, but it must be changed several times daily for maximum effect. If an antiseptic contact layer is desired, therefore, it is best to put an antibiotic cream directly on the wound and then apply the cotton gauze; this should be washed and changed 2 to 3 times daily.
4. Desiccation. Desiccation is generally not achieved by occlusive dressings and is best achieved by nonocclusive wide-mesh gauzes.

Padding and Absorbing Materials (Middle Layer)

ABSORBENTS
1. Cotton gauze
2. Cotton wadding
3. Dextranomer (Debrisan) beads

CONTOUR MATERIALS
1. Cotton gauze and fiber wads are used when absorbency and drainage are desired. They can be used dry or with water soaks or glycerin. We prefer to use them dry or with glycerin.
2. The Reston foam sponge (3M) is a foam pad with glue on one surface. The adherence allows stacking of several layers and/or direct application to the skin. It is a useful material for skin grafts or as a protective pad but does not allow absorption and is very occlusive.
3. Steel wool is occasionally used for hand dressing. It is stiff and difficult to contour but encourages drainage.

Wrapping Materials

The outer wrap materials are various combinations of cotton gauze, nylon, and elastics. Each component provides specific characteristics. The greater the amount of cotton the more absorbent, but less equal pressure can be achieved. Elastics allow more even pressure, but tend to be occlusive.

Many wraps are made in preformed tube shapes of different size. They encircle the part rather than being wrapped around. These tube gauzes are particularly suited to finger and some facial dressings.

COTTON GAUZE WRAPS
1. Kerlix (Kendall) is a very bulky, soft, wide-mesh gauze useful for protective cushioning against direct trauma or absorption but difficult to use when compression is required.
2. Kling (Johnson & Johnson) is a thin, less bulky wrap that is better for slight compression and immobilization but not as protective as Kerlix.
3. Stretch gauze (Parke-Davis) is similar to Kling in its application characteristics but stretches somewhat more, like Kerlix gauze.
4. Bias-cut stockinette is a very soft, stretch cotton fabric, often used under casts.

ELASTIC WRAPS
1. Ace bandage (Ace) or Tensor (Kendall)
2. Elastoplast (Beiersdorf) is a wrap similar to the Ace bandage but with an adhesive on one surface. It can be used as a tape or a wrap when unraveling or bunching occurs with the Ace bandage.
3. Coban (3M Corp.) is a nonadhesive self-adherent bandage because of its weave pattern. It has the advantage of relative stability without adhesive but has a more irregular surface.
4. Flexoplast (Edward Taylor) is similar to the Ace bandage.

TUBED GAUZES
Surgitube (Carlton Corp.), Diffuson (Dressinet), and Hyginet (Western Medical) are tubed meshed gauzes of various sizes (Fig. 8-13). The gauze is designed for fitting specific anatomic areas. These gauzes are easy to apply and in some instances can be used instead of tape to immobilize the underlying layers. The most useful is the finger tube.

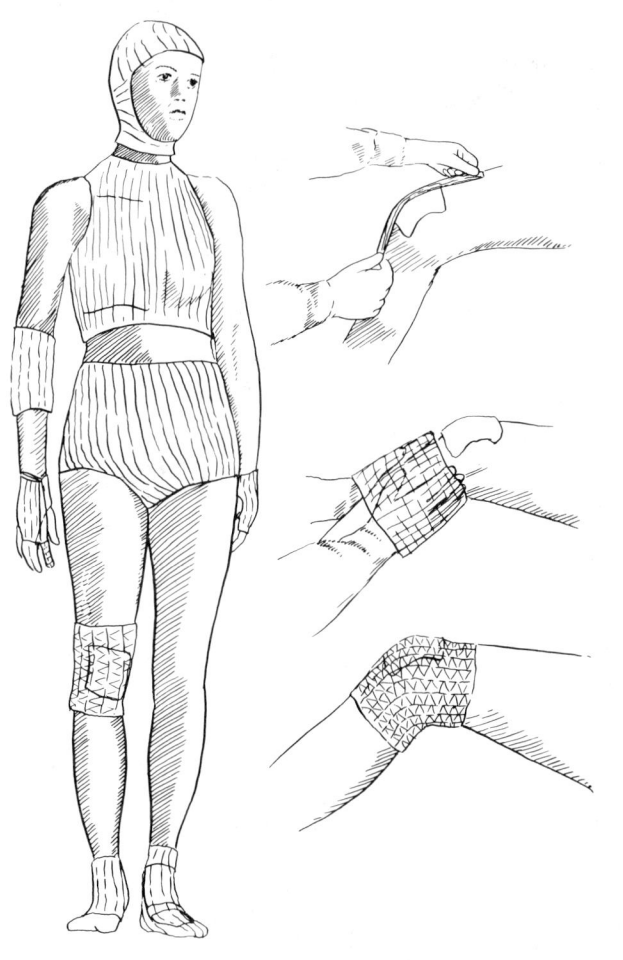

Figure 8-13. Net gauzes can be used for simple immobilization of large areas in which pressure is not required and frequent changes are necessary.

Tapes

Tapes vary in their material, adhesive, sterility, and other medicaments. Because many patients have allergies to tape, careful observation and history are important. The following is a list of some available tapes.

FABRIC ADHESIVE

These are the most commonly used tapes. The fabric has some elasticity and usually has perforations for aeration of underlying skin but may be treated. The fabric is usually cotton or silk. Characteristics are as follows:

1. Elastic
2. Pressure can be applied
3. Nonocclusive
4. Adapts to contours
5. Adapts to mobile area
6. Some are "hypoallergenic"

PAPER AND PLASTIC TAPE

These tapes are made of paper or synthetic materials. The papers have relatively little flexibility and can cause shearing and friction blisters if applied to a mobile area. The plastic and foam tapes are easy to conform, don't cause shearing, but are occlusive, similar to paper. Even porous synthetic tapes limit water/paper movement.

Some of the available tapes are:

1. Blenderm (3M)—hypoallergenic, plastic, occlusive
2. Micropore (3M)—hypoallergenic, paper, occlusive
3. Transpore (3M)—hypoallergenic, plastic, perforated
4. Microfoam—hypoallergenic, foam, nonocclusive, stretchable
5. Cordran (3M)—cortisone, paper, occlusive
6. Durapore

Splints and Casts

SPLINTS

Splints are strips of rigid material formed to immobilize a joint or mobile area. They can be made from plaster, plastics, metal, or wood. Four types of finger splints are shown in Fig. 8-14.

1. The aluminum trough is adequate for most wounds, but the finger must be kept extended. It is good for wounds that require soaks or frequent changes.
2. The wood tongue blade is most difficult to prepare and relatively uncomfortable but can be adequate when nothing else is available.
3. Plaster can fit any size or position, is very comfortable and adaptable, but is difficult to use with wet wounds. Because it allows water vapor transmission, it has less maceration.
4. Synthetic plastics are easily contoured and strong but do not allow evaporative water loss.

Techniques of Dressing Application

The dressing must be applied in a proper technical fashion with an understanding of important anatomic and functional factors.

Facial Dressing Techniques

EYE DRESSING

Dressings for a periorbital injury are designed to immobilize the lids (Fig. 8-15). Blinking and other lid movement may inhibit the healing process and cause discomfort. An eye dressing is *not* designed to apply pressure for hemostasis or reduce edema, because there is a danger of excessive pressure on the globe. *The lids must be closed!* It is essential that the eyelid be completely closed so that the eye is totally protected from desiccation or contact injury during the period it is hidden under the dressing.

EAR DRESSING

The ear dressing protects against trauma and provides pressure to the contours and convolutions of the ear to prevent hematoma formation (Fig. 8-16). Hemorrhage under the perichondrium can lead to a "cauliflower ear." This can be avoided by careful intraoperative hemostasis and postop-

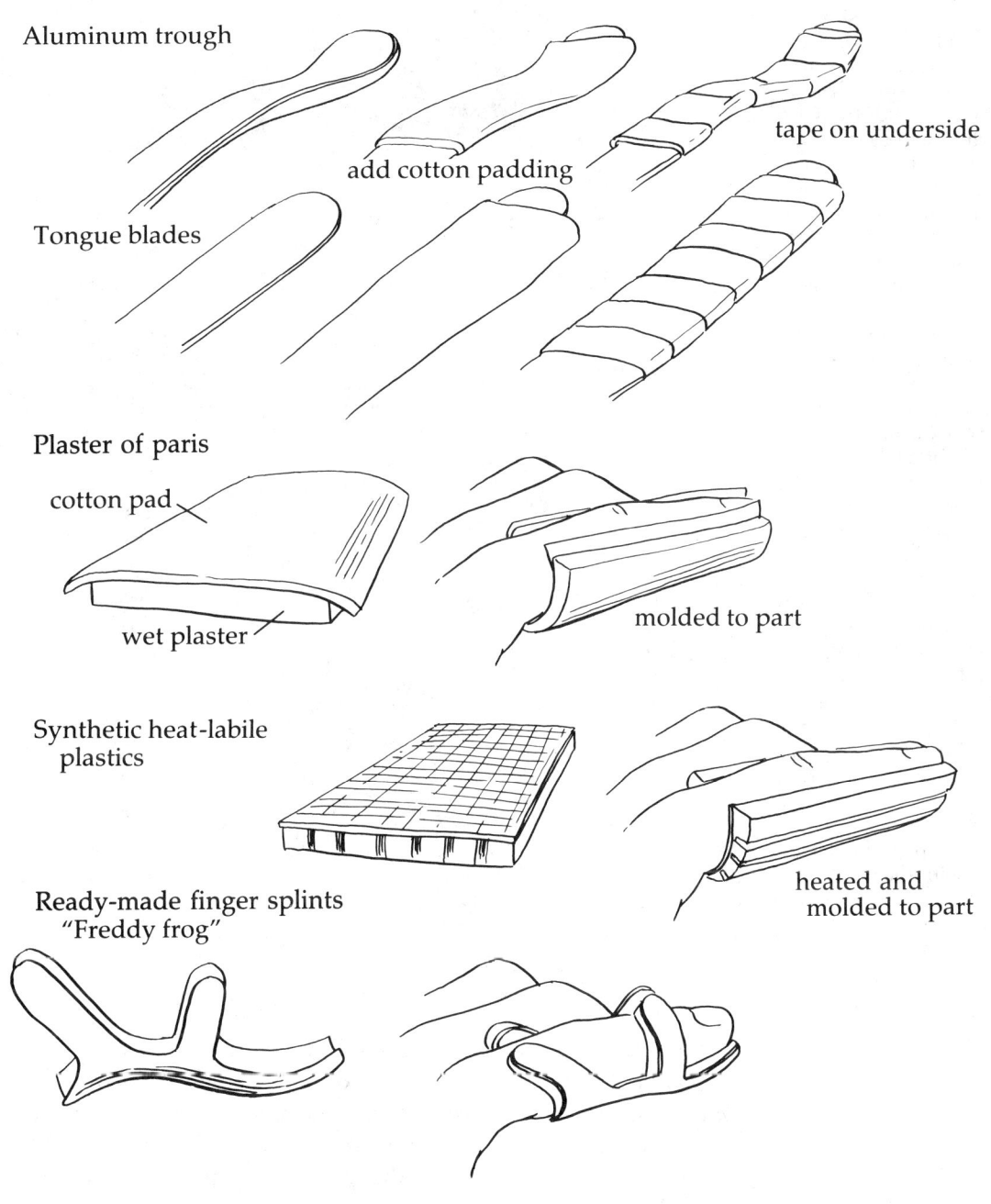

Figure 8-14. Examples of finger splints.

erative pressure and contouring. If a hematoma develops, it must be evacuated before the dressing is applied.

FACIAL DRESSING

This dressing is used for immobilization or light pressure on any facial or scalp laceration (Figs. 8-17 and 8-18). This includes the immobilization of dressings applied to the ear, eye, face, or scalp. It is generally not used for lip lacerations. The dressing is usually more secure if it is wrapped around the ears, under the chin, over the top of the cranium, and behind the occiput.

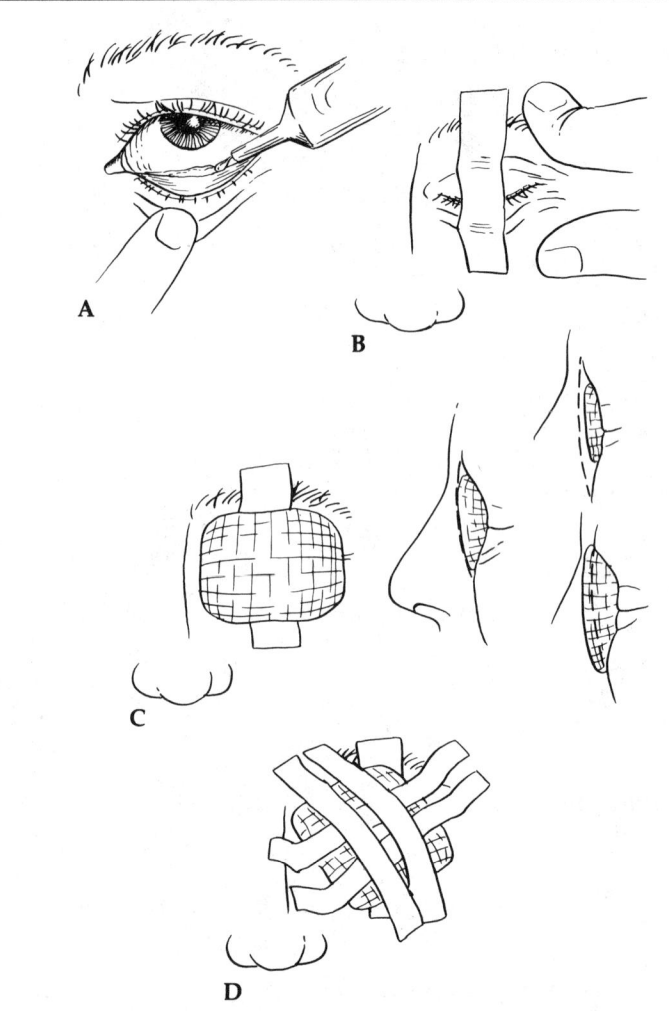

Figure 8-15. Eye dressing with ointment and eye pad.
A. Place boric acid or other ointment in the sulcus of the lower lid, from which it disperses onto the globe. The ointment protects against desiccation if there is accidental opening of the lid under the dressing and also causes the lids to adhere to each other.
B. Firmly close the lids by taping from the brow to the cheek (not lid-to-lid). Pull the brow down and the cheek upwards; then tape together.
C. Put one or two eye pads over the lids to protect against trauma. The pads are not to be used for pressure. Enough pads should be applied so that the dressing extends to the level of the orbital rims. If too many pads are applied and the dressing extends beyond the orbital rim margins, the globe may be more susceptible to injury than it is without any pads.
D. Lightly tape the pads in place with diagonal strips extending from the nasal glabella to the cheek and strips from the nasal bridge to the temple.

NOSE DRESSING

This dressing is used for through-and-through lacerations of the nasal tip or in association with nasal fractures (Fig. 8-19). An intranasal pack is used for unstable fractures, evacuated septal hematomas, or persistent bleeding.

A nonadherent antibiotic ointment–impregnated gauze (½-inch) is preferred. The antibiotic gauze reduces bacterial growth and the resultant odor.

Hand

POSITION

Sterling Bunnel stated: "Edema is the mother of scar." To avoid edema the injured part should be elevated above the level of the heart until there is no longer any throbbing when the hand is placed in a dependent position. Elevation is particularly important at night when the normal muscle pump mechanism is inactive. An edematous wound heals more slowly, is at greater risk of infection, and is subject to unnecessary postinjury stiffness and morbidity. If a sling is selected, it should maintain the elbow at greater than 90° and the shoulder adducted somewhat across the chest (Fig. 8-20).

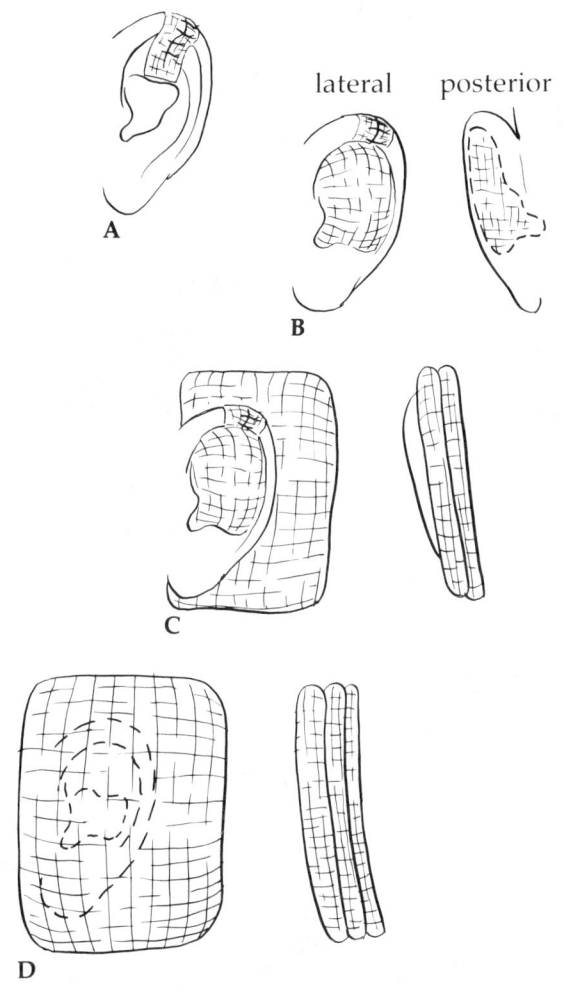

Figure 8-16. Ear dressing.
A. Cover the skin wound with a nonadherent gauze.
B. Fill the contour of the concha of the ear with dry cotton wadding.
C. Pad the retroauricular sulcus with cotton wadding, cotton gauze, or sponge. The ear is thus sandwiched between the retroauricular and conchal gauzes. Only the rim of the helix and the earlobe should be exposed.
D. Cover the ear with a 4 × 4 gauze pad or sponge. Wrap the ear with the circumferential figure-eight gauze head dressing or cover with net tube.

The function of a dressing is primarily determined by the local wound environment. The immobilized wound heals rapidly and with less edema and inflammation than a wound that is allowed movement. For the hand, however, more specialized and careful dressings must be designed because of functional and anatomic requirements.

1. Position of injured hand (Fig. 8-21). The injured hand usually falls into an abnormal, nonfunctional position because of comfort, gravitational effect on the wrist, and edema of the dorsal hand. The wrist is flexed, and metacarpophalangeal (MP) and interphalangeal (IP) joints are extended. Even though it is a natural occurrence, this position causes MP joint contracture and hand dysfunction. Therefore, hand repositioning with splints should be done.
2. Position of function for most injuries (Fig. 8-22). In most circumstances the hand and wrist are immobilized in the so-called position of function.

   The position of function is chosen because both intrinsic and extrinsic muscles are placed under a balanced tone. The supporting (collateral) ligaments of the MP joints are stretched with MP flexion preventing contracture during the period of immobilization. A wide first web space

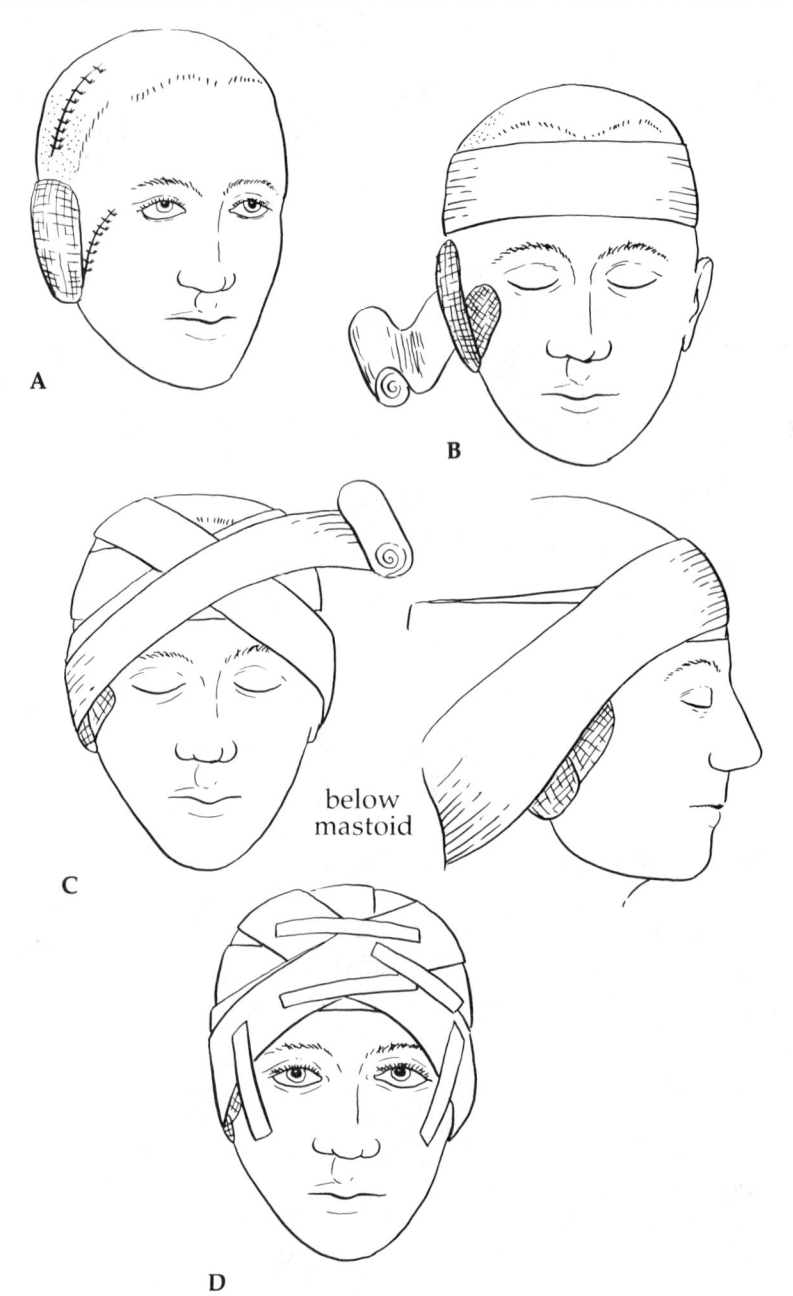

Figure 8-17. Facial dressing.
A. Padding should be placed behind the ears so that the cartilage of the ear is not bent back on itself in an uncomfortable position. The method of protecting the ear is essentially that described for the typical ear dressing, with gauze in both the ear contour and the retroauricular sulcus.
B. Begin the wrap around the forehead and behind the occiput.
C. Wrap obliquely in a figure-eight fashion, going across the ear and behind the mastoid process on one side, then reversing the figure-eight to include the opposite ear.
D. The dressing can be stopped at this point and held in place by tape extending circumferentially around the dressing and from the dressing onto the cheek.

is maintained by abducting the thumb in the palmar direction. The concept of a functional position is a key element in the care of hand wounds. Whenever possible, the hand is immobilized as follows:

a. 30° wrist extension
b. 70° to 80° MP joint flexion
c. 20° to 30° IP joint flexion
d. 20° radial and 35° palmar abduction of the thumb

This position is comfortable and establishes and maintains the integrity of the transverse and longitudinal arches. All hand injuries except the most severe burns or the most minor hand and distal digital soft tissue wounds should be splinted in the position of function.

POSTOPERATIVE CARE AND DRESSINGS

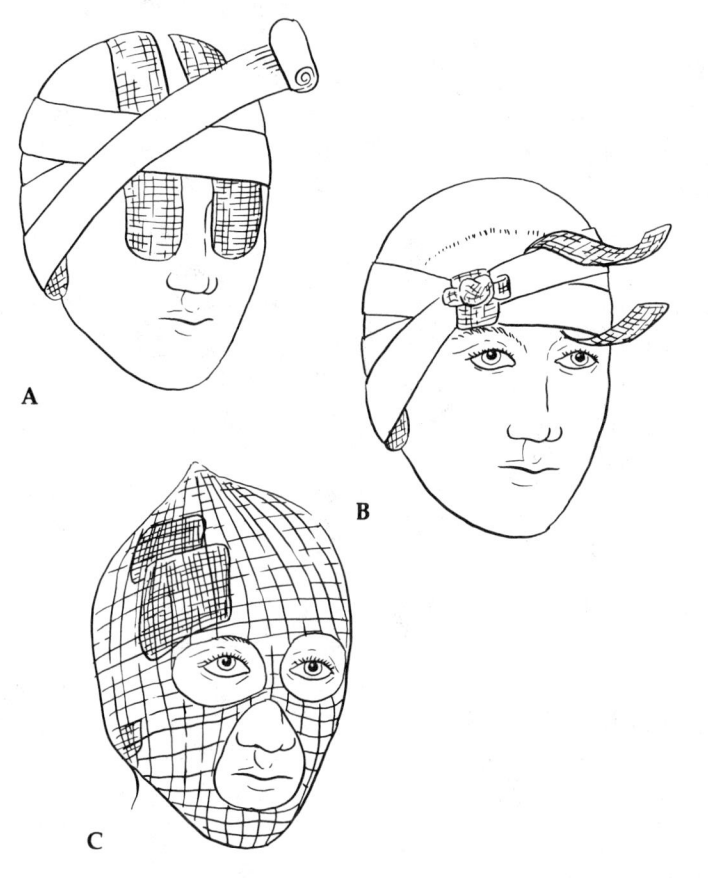

Figure 8-18. Alternative method of fixation of head dressing.
A. Before wrapping, drape 4 × 4's across the forehead.
B. Then tie the 4 × 4 to immobilize the roll and keep it from falling over the eyes.
C. Another alternative is to use a *gauze net* to hold the 4 × 4.

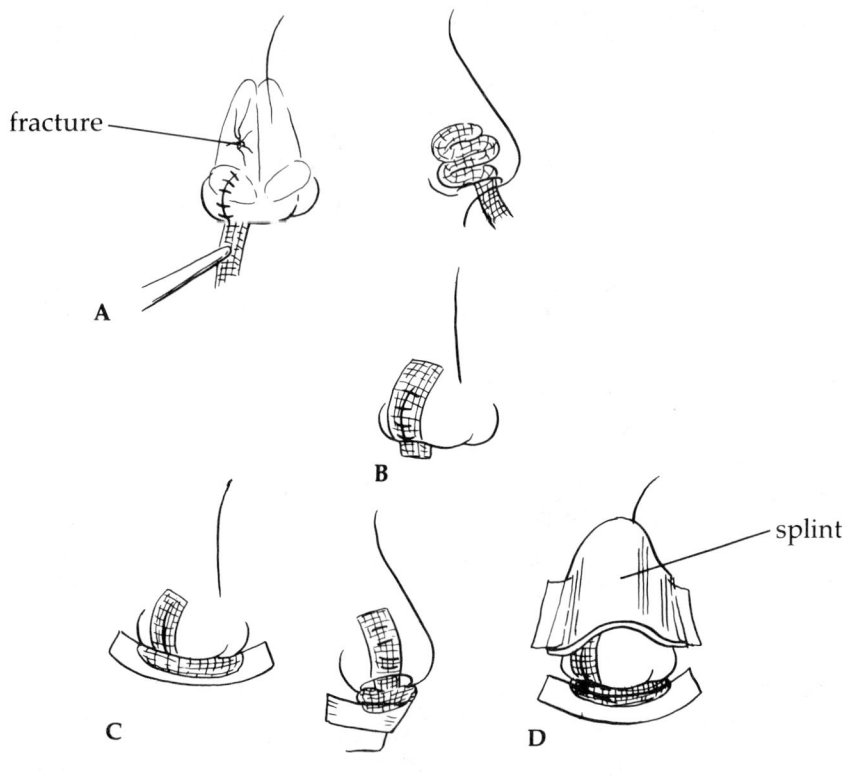

Figure 8-19. Nose dressing.
A. Begin packing on the nasal floor posteriorly and layer the gauze back and forth until the dome of the vestibule has been packed, causing a slight outward bulging of the nasal ala. Leave a small strip of gauze extending from the nasal vestibule.
B. Cover the external laceration with nonadherent gauze.
C. Place a 2 × 2 gauze pad underneath the nose to absorb any blood that may drip from the nasal cavity. Tape the drip pad in place with the tape extending from one cheek to the other. Also tape the nasal laceration.
D. Use nasal splints if there is a nasal fracture.

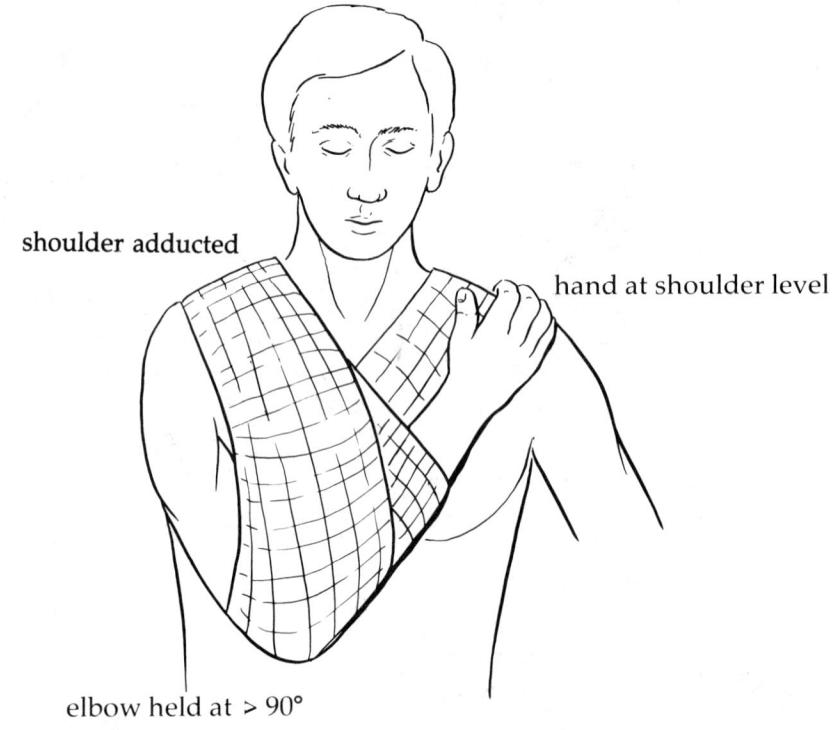

Figure 8-20. The hand position above the level of the heart.

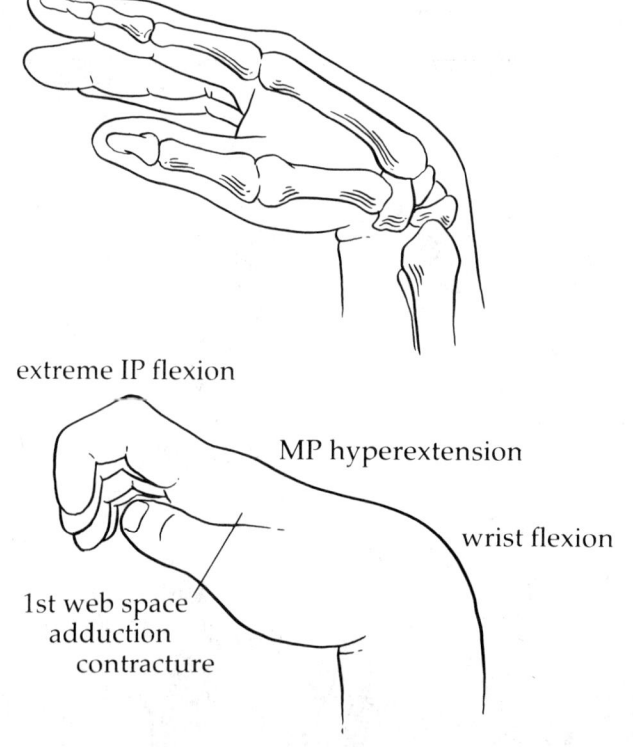

Figure 8-21. Position of the injured hand. Wrist flexion causes secondary MP extension, and thumb adduction. The resultant deformity from hand malposition can be the intrinsic minus (clawhand) position.

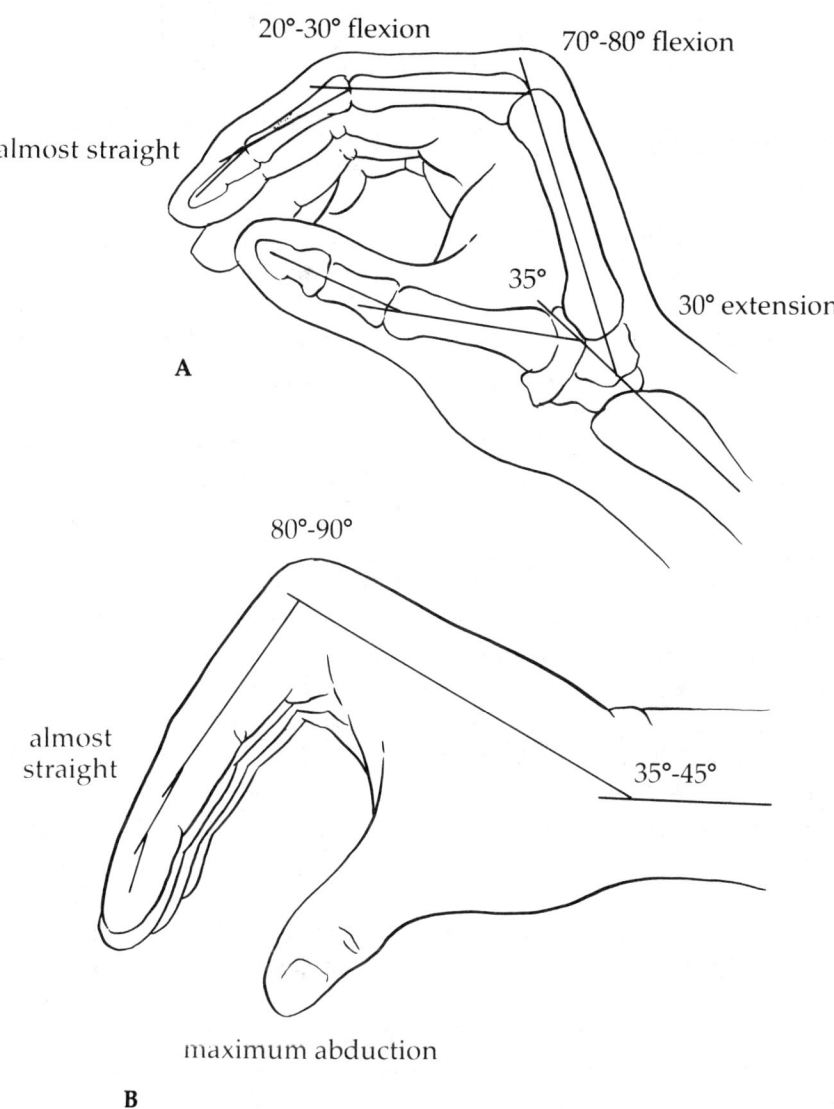

Figure 8-22. The position of function (A) and the intrinsic plus position (B) for hand splinting. The difference is in the degree of MP flexion, IP extension, and wrist extension. The intrinsic plus position is extreme and used primarily for hand burns or severe injuries that may lead to intrinsic minus, or clawhand, deformities.

3. Intrinsic plus (burned hand) (Fig. 8-22). The burned hand is immobilized in an even more extreme functional position because of high risk of joint exposure and damage, skin loss, and scarring. The burned hand tends to fall into the intrinsic minus (clawhand) position, which is extremely nonfunctional and must be avoided by immobilization in the intrinsic plus position. The intrinsic plus position of function is as follows:
   a. 35° to 45° wrist extension
   b. 80° to 90° MP joint flexion
   c. 10° to 15° IP joint flexion
   d. Thumb MP maximum palmar abduction

   Immobilization may require internal pinning or special splints. Simple soft dressings are not adequate.
4. Special positions—tendons and nerves. Tendon and nerve injuries may require special hand positions to relieve tension on the repair. For ex-

ample, injury to wrist and hand flexors or median and ulnar nerve requires slight wrist flexion. These positions must be highly individualized.

LENGTH OF TIME OF IMMOBILIZATION
The length of time of immobilization varies with the type of injury.

1. Soft tissue. Simple soft tissue injury or sprain may require a few days of immobilization until pain and swelling resolve.
2. Tendon and nerve. Tendon and nerve injuries require 3 to 4 weeks of immobilization to allow sufficient strength of repair for tendon movements. Prolonged immobilization can lead to adhesion of tendon to adjacent tissue.
3. Bone and joint. Fractures and severe sprains may require a month or more to allow for adequate strength of bone and ligament repair.

REMOBILIZATION
The patient should not be discharged from care when sutures are removed. The physician's responsibility ends only when the preinjury state has been obtained, or the lack of this attainment prompts referral to a specialist. *Inherent in immobilization of the hand is a responsibility to direct its remobilization.* For most minor injuries managed in the emergency department formal physical therapy is not necessary.

Easily followed exercises to recommend include mobilization of an injured hand in tepid water by squeezing a sponge, gripping smaller and smaller objects, kneading play-dough or "silly putty," and stretching rubber bands. The use of extreme heat is to be condemned, as is the advice to the patient simply to "use your hand" or "squeeze a hard rubber ball."

Remobilization following repair depends on the level of injury and associated injured structures. Remobilization may require 2 to 3 times the length of the immobilization (e.g., when there is persistent pain from a tender neuroma). Early identification of postinjury stiffness or problems and prompt referral to a specialist diminishes disability.

DESIGN AND APPLICATION
1. Finger dressing (Figs. 8-23 and 8-24)
    a. Soft tissue injuries—tubed gauze dressing (Fig. 8-23). Any digital injury (e.g., laceration, open crush, nail bed) heals better with some period of immobility. Soft dressings can immobilize IP joints adequately, and a firm wood or metal splint is unnecessary. When absolute immobilization is required, splints or internal wires should be used.
        (1) Advantages
            (a) Provides even compression
            (b) Splints joints
            (c) Neat, attractive dressing
        (2) Disadvantage. Circulation and wound cannot be assessed.
        (3) Other, similar tubed materials (e.g., Hyginet) can be used to hold 2 × 2 gauze sponges in place, but they do not provide compression. These materials are applied in a similar manner but with only one layer.

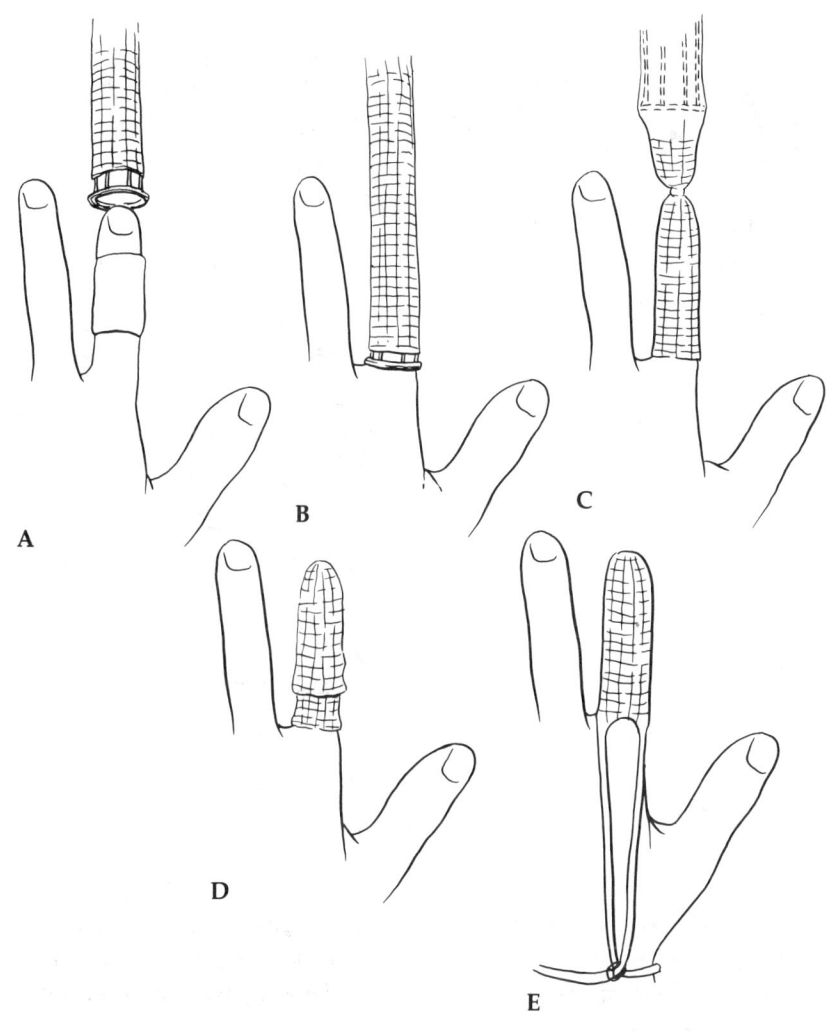

Figure 8-23. Finger dressing.
A. The inner layer is nonadherent gauze or whatever is required for soft tissue care. The middle layer is 2 × 2 gauze sponges wrapped circumferentially and held in place with a small strip of tape.
B. Begin #2 tube gauze at the base of the finger. It is useful to hold this end with one finger while the tube gauze applicator is pulled toward the fingertip. A twisting motion firms the wrap about the digit—generally about 90° is necessary. Excessive stretch or twisting can compromise circulation.
C. When the fingertip is reached, make a 360° twist.
D. Pass the applicator toward the finger base with an additional 90° twist. Repeat once more; thus three layers are in place.
E. Cut enough gauze to reach the base of the finger, and tape it there. As an alternative, pull the final layer beyond the tip, leaving it long enough to reach to and around the wrist (about three times the finger length). Split this gauze into two strands; bring them dorsally to the wrist; knot; and loosely wrap around the wrist.

   b. Distal injury, closed—simple splints (Figs. 8-14 and 8-24). Splints are required for closed injuries (undisplaced fractures, sprains, crush).
      (1) Advantages
         (a) Comfort
         (b) Sturdiness
         (c) Less expense
         (d) Easy to change
      (2) Disadvantages
         (a) Circumferential tape may constrict venous and lymphatic outflow.
         (b) Moisture may collect in the foam rubber or metal and macerate the skin.
      (3) Layers
         (a) Inner layer. None
         (b) Middle layer. None
         (c) Outer layer. Padded metal splints. These come in ½-inch sizes, ideal for finger splints. They should be molded to the exact joint position desired (e.g., in a mallet-finger deformity, minimal hypertension is desired).

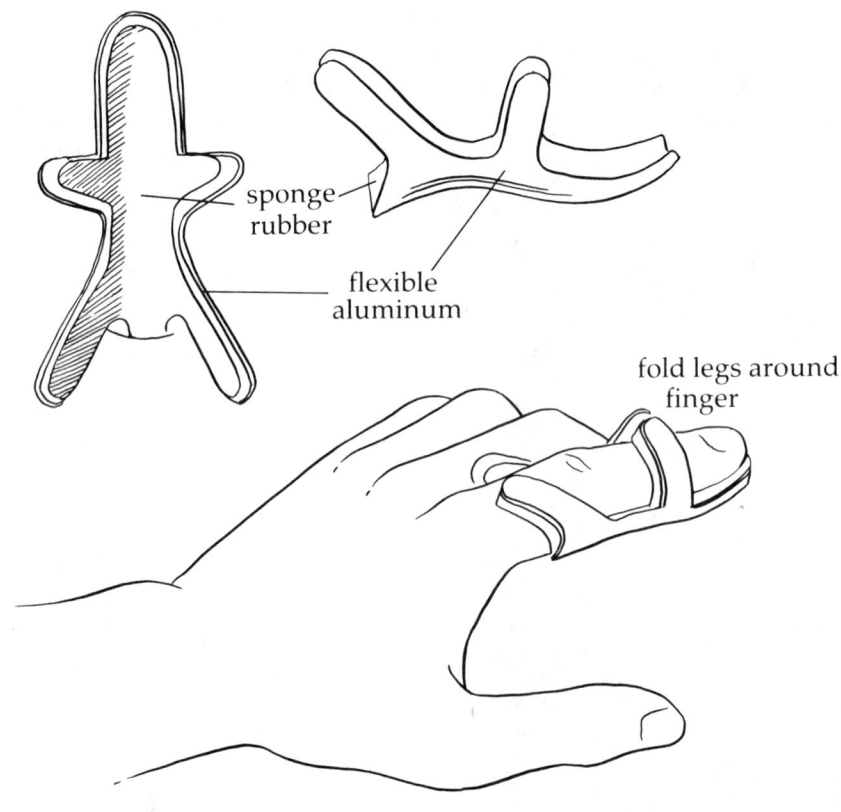

Figure 8-24. The frog-leg splint, which is useful for closed wounds, such as sprains, undisplaced fractures, and tendon tears. Choose an appropriate size and mold to the desired position.

    c. Proximal finger and metacarpal injury—gauntlet, splint, or cast (Fig. 8-25). *Proximal injuries cannot be adequately immobilized with a finger splint* because of the difficulty in immobilizing MP joints with such splints. A splint may be incorporated into a gauntlet-type cast to maintain immobilization, or a plaster gauntlet can be made. This type of splint can be windowed to allow observation and treatment of a soft tissue defect.

      (1) Inner layer. Whatever is appropriate for wound treatment

      (2) Middle layer. Reston foam, cast padding, or gauze protects the skin and any underlying bony prominence from pressure.

      (3) Outer layer. The necessary length and size of plaster cut from a strip and used as a splint or wrapped as a full cast. The plaster is dipped in water and held in place until firm.

2. Hand dressing

    a. Wrist—universal splint (Fig. 8-26). A number of so-called universal splints are marketed. These usually are designed to maintain the wrist in extension. Unfortunately, they fit no one perfectly, and, in fact, usually tend to extend the MP joints. Plaster of paris splints can be molded to fit the contour exactly and are best for maintaining the adaptable transverse arch so important for optimum hand function. Thus, universal splints are used for minor injuries, when hand position is unimportant, and when immobilization is of short duration and mainly for wrist comfort.

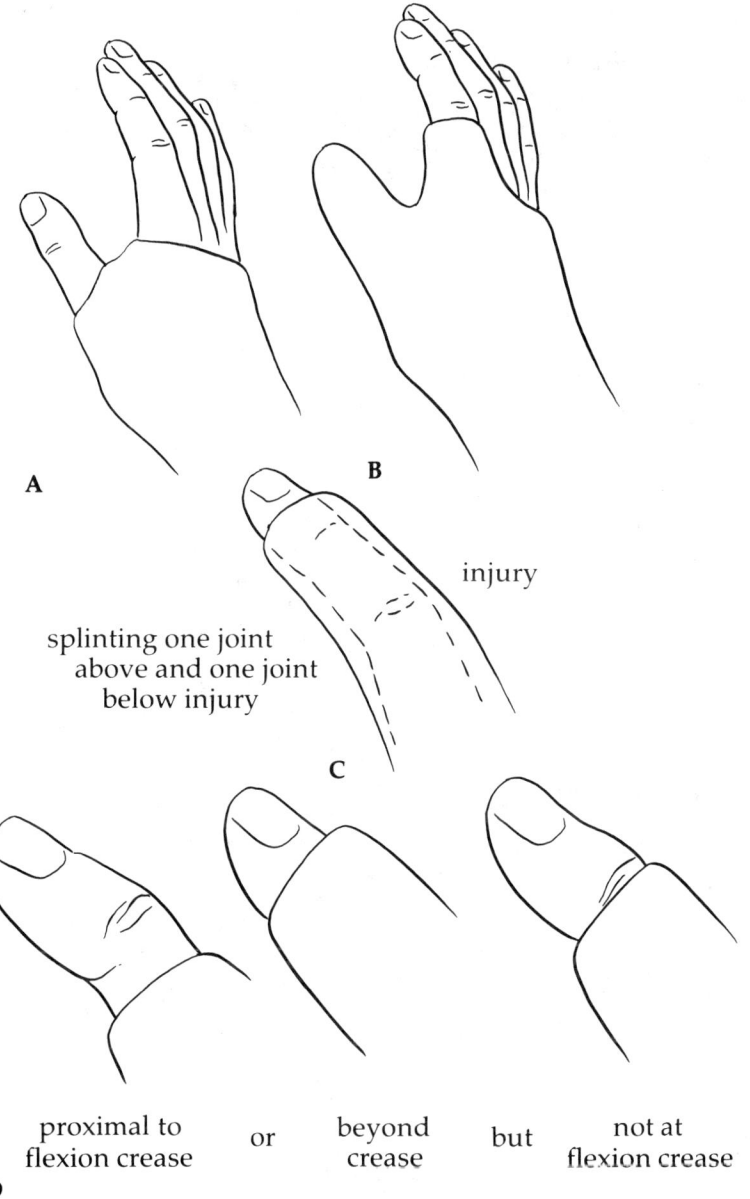

Figure 8-25. The gauntlet plaster splint, which is used for metacarpal injuries (A) and proximal digital injuries (B). The splint must include one joint beyond the site of injury (C) and should terminate distally on the digit, not on the joint crease (D).

  b. Soft tissue—"bulky" dressing (Figs. 8-27, 8-28). The so-called bulky hand dressing is both impractical and aesthetically unappealing. A large wad of material in the palm usually flattens the distal transverse arch and tends to extend the MP joints. The bulkiness prevents passing of the hand through coat or shirt sleeves, occasionally giving rise to a tailoring bill that surpasses the physician's bill. The soft tissue dressing is a maintenance dressing for minor wounds that do not require strict immobilization. A padded plaster splint can be placed over this dressing if greater immobilization is required.
    (1) Inner layer. Whatever is appropriate for wound treatment
    (2) Middle layer. Fully opened 4 × 4 gauzes
    (3) Outer layer. Elastic gauze (Kling)

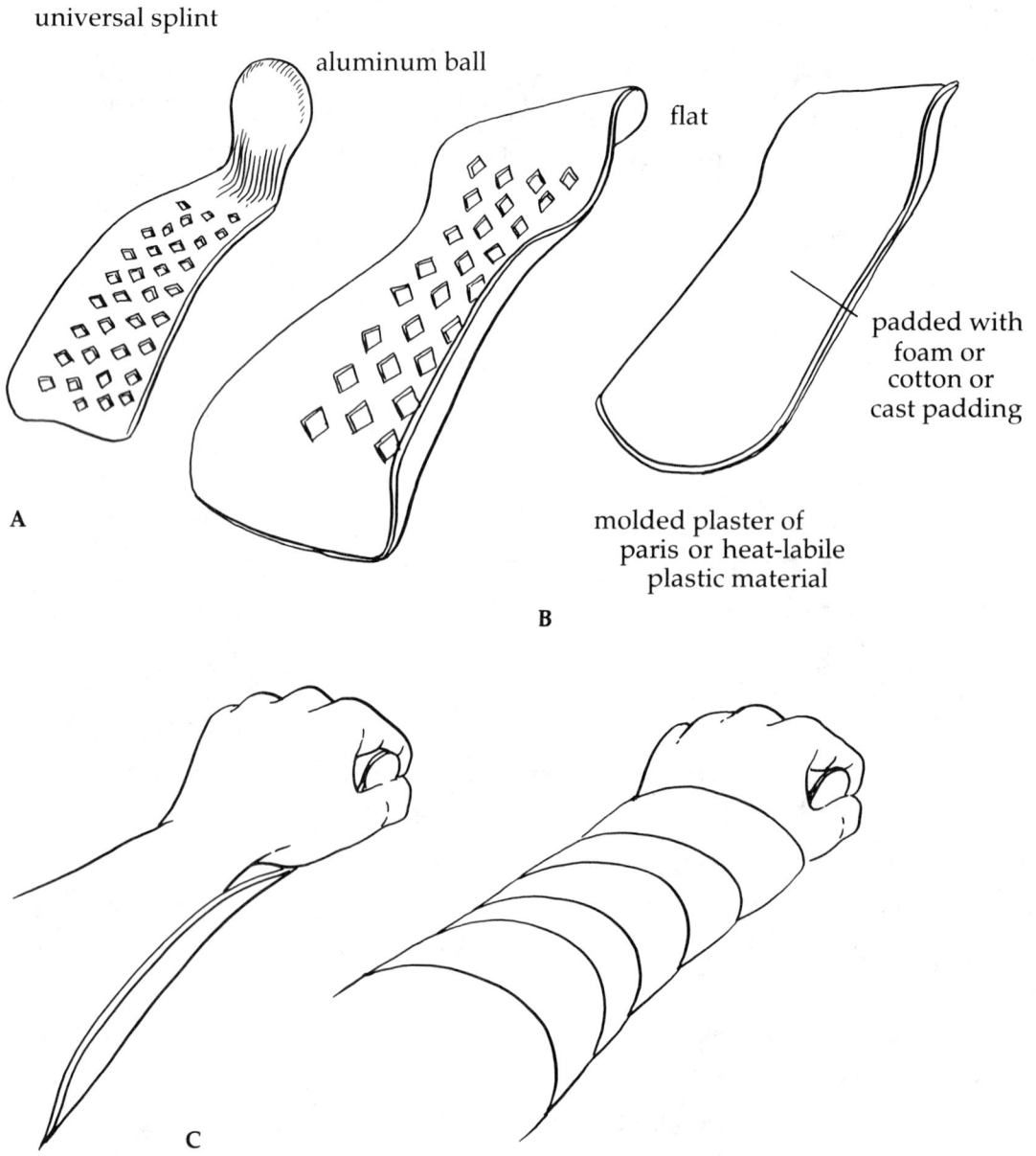

Figure 8-26. Universal splint for wrist.
A. Wrist splints are of different designs depending on desired wrist extension. Either an aluminum universal, plaster, or plastic splint is used.
B. The splint should be padded with cotton and/or foam.
C. It is lightly wrapped to maintain the position. The MP joints and fingers are free to move.

c. Forearm dressing (Fig. 8-29). Forearm injuries require a basic type of universal or plaster splint. If the digits do not require immobilization, the splint should extend from the midforearm to just proximal to the midpalmar crease, to avoid compromising MP joint motion. Usually a volar splint is more easily applied and molded to fit. It is made from eight to ten thicknesses of 3-inch or 4- × 15-inch splints premeasured to immobilize those joints necessary (i.e., always the wrist and any additional joints). Use cool water to wet the plaster, then mold the splint in the chosen position to maintain the proper longitudinal and transverse arches of the hand. Unless the digits require immobilization, the splint is stopped just proximal to the distal palmar crease. This is fixed with an additional Kling, 3-inch bias-cut stockinette, or Ace bandage.

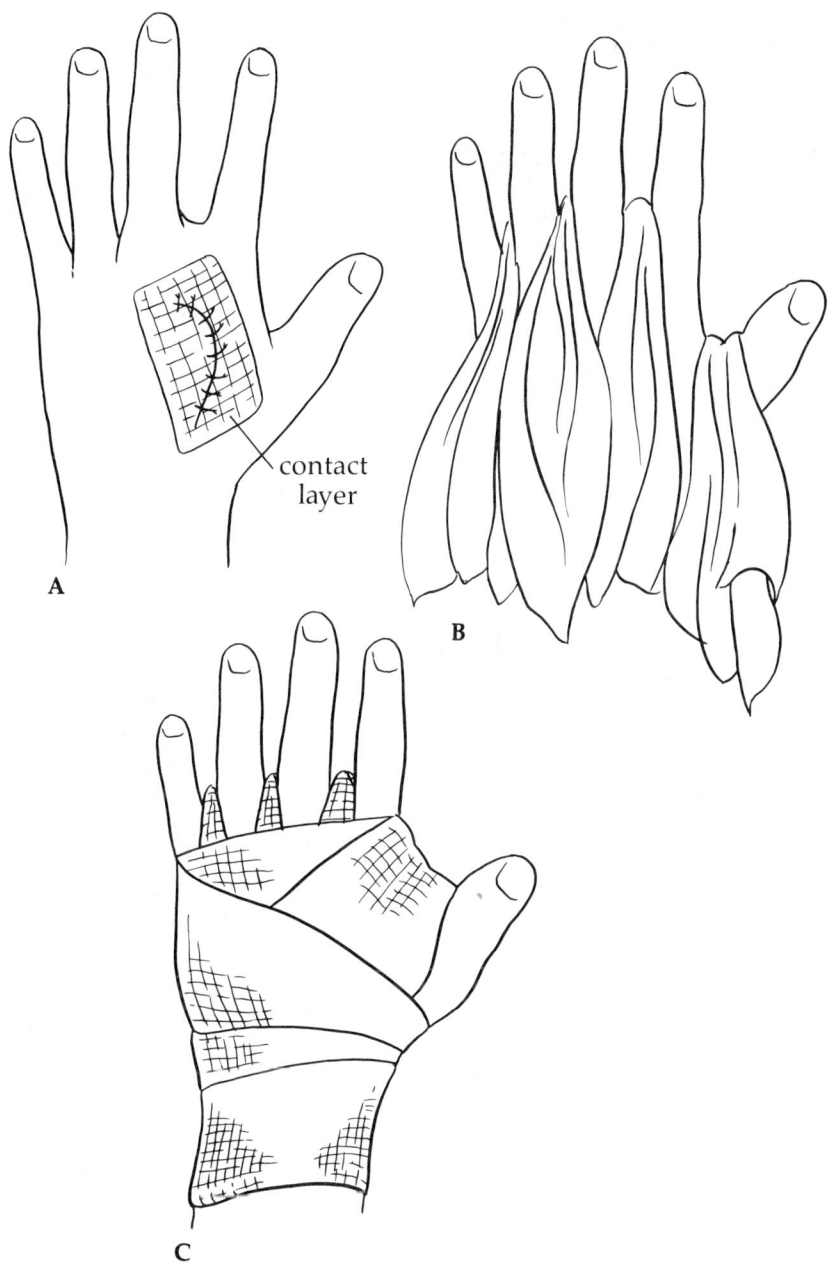

Figure 8-27. Compression dressing for hand.
A. Cover wound.
B. Loosely place a 4 × 4 gauze pad between each finger cleft with tips of gauze in opposite directions; do not force deeply into cleft. The purpose is to prevent maceration by maintaining separation of skin. Three or four gauze sponges maintain the first web space in abduction.
C. Wrap outer layer with gauze wrap (Kling, Kerlix, bias-cut stockinette).

(1) Inner layer. Whatever is appropriate for wound treatment
(2) Middle layer. Fully opened 4 × 4 gauze sponges (without paper filling) or "fluffs"
(3) Outer layer. Webril is applied (one layer only) over the Kling. Its function is only to prevent the plaster from sticking to the gauze.
   (a) 3-inch Kling or 3-inch bias-cut stockinette, wrapped as a figure-eight
   (b) Cast padding (Webril)
   (c) Cast. A circumferential plaster cast is not tightly applied but reinforces the hand dressing. When patient reliability is questionable, it may be greatly reinforced to keep out prying

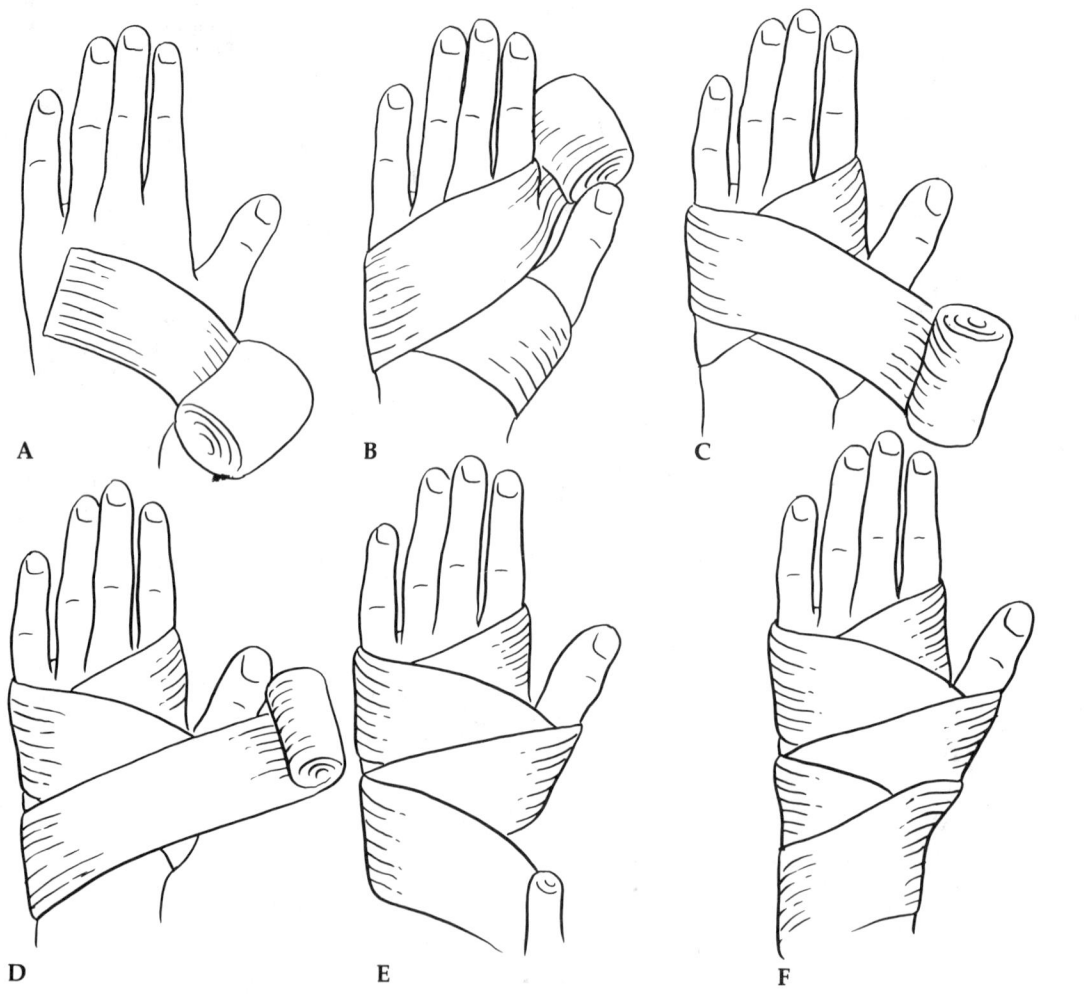

Figure 8-28. Compression wrap with Ace bandage or bias-cut stockinette.
- A. Fix in place with 3-inch gauze wrapped evenly about the hand and wrist.
- B. Pass through first web space but not between any other digits.
- C. The thenar eminence is left free in part unless the wound is located here. The wrap should be applied firmly but should not occlude venous outflow from the fingers.
- D, E, and F. A figure-eight pattern is less likely to bunch up than a parallel pattern.

fingers. It also cannot be removed easily without a cast saw, which sometimes ensures follow-up.

Two rolls of 3-inch plaster are wrapped circumferentially, leaving mobile the thenar eminence and distal palmar crease, if desirable.

Careful molding to anatomic contours is achieved with proper pressure while the plaster is setting. It is molded to fit the distal mobile transverse arch so it will be comfortable and worn without complaint. Avoid ending the plaster at a joint crease, because when the finger is flexed or extended, un-

POSTOPERATIVE CARE AND DRESSINGS

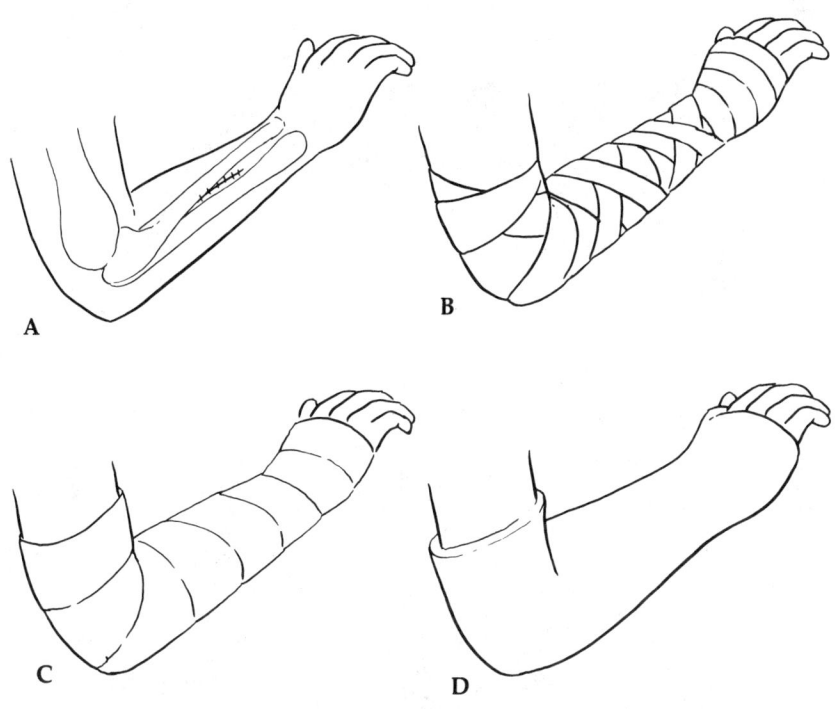

Figure 8-29. Forearm dressing.
A. Covered forearm injuries or undisplaced fractures with appropriate inner contact layer.
B. Wrap the forearm with cotton gauze from 3 to 4 inches above the elbow to the thenar crease.
C. Wrap a cotton pad or cast padding around the gauze.
D. Carefully mold circumferential plaster to contour. The plaster maintains forearm in slight pronation.

comfortable pressure occurs. Stop either before or beyond the crease.

d. Lower extremity dressing

(1) Position of immobilization. Most foot and ankle injuries require immobilization of the ankle at 90° of dorsiflexion with a volarly applied splint. This should be reinforced in an I-beam fashion.

Toes are immobilized by taping the affected toe to an adjacent one. Dry gauze between toes prevents maceration.

(2) Elastic bandages. The elastic bandage is frequently misused to the point of becoming a hazard to proper wound care. It is usually wrapped too tightly and in too many superimposed layers. When used properly (i.e., to maintain in place and splint) or wrapped carefully about an ankle, it is an excellent dressing.

The elastic bandage must be applied carefully as a figure-eight and wrapped without tension. No more than two layers should be applied. Holes cut in the bandage to allow approximation about digits may easily constrict circulation to such digits and are to be condemned. The figure-eight technique shown for the forearm in Fig. 8-28 is most effective. Wrapping should begin distally at the toes and proceed proximally to the knee.

DRESSING CHANGES AND REASSESSMENT

Wound and dressing conditions must be reassessed repeatedly and dressing changes made to coincide with changes in wound conditions.

Figure 8-30. Changing the dressing.

A. Soak the wound for 15 to 30 minutes so that the crust is thoroughly hydrated and the dressing can be gently teased away from the wound. Hydrogen peroxide can be used to remove some of the more adherent crusts.

B. Place a cotton-tipped applicator against the skin surface and gently push down on the skin while using a gloved hand or forceps to grab the inner layer of dressing and gently tease it away from the crust and sutures. It is important that the direction of pull when removing the dressing be parallel with the suture line rather than perpendicular to it. An alternative method is to use a water jet with a Water Pik or Jacuzzi-type agitator to assist separation of the dressing. Some minimal teasing of the dressing from the wound may still be required.

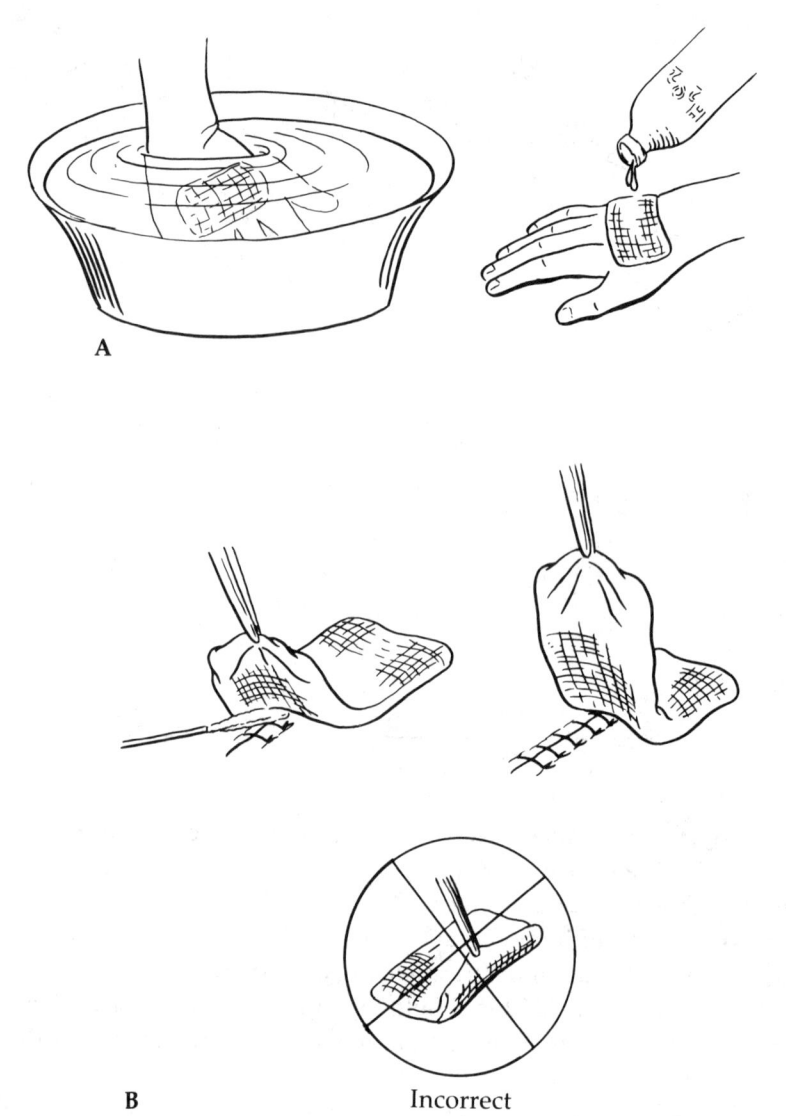

Timing

CLEAN, TIDY WOUNDS

The guidelines for determining when a dressing should be changed are based on the type of injury rather than type of dressing. Clean, tidy, lacerations, tidy flaps, and skin grafts usually do not need a dressing change for 3 days and sometimes not for 5 or 7 days unless there is a specific symptom or sign of bleeding or infection.

CONTAMINATED, UNTIDY, BLEEDING WOUNDS

Wounds with the potential for infection, hemorrhage, or necrosis may need frequent inspection and dressing changes. This may be as often as every hour when there is considerable hemorrhage or infection, or possibly, daily, for contaminated wounds. There is no absolute indication, but experience and good judgment are required.

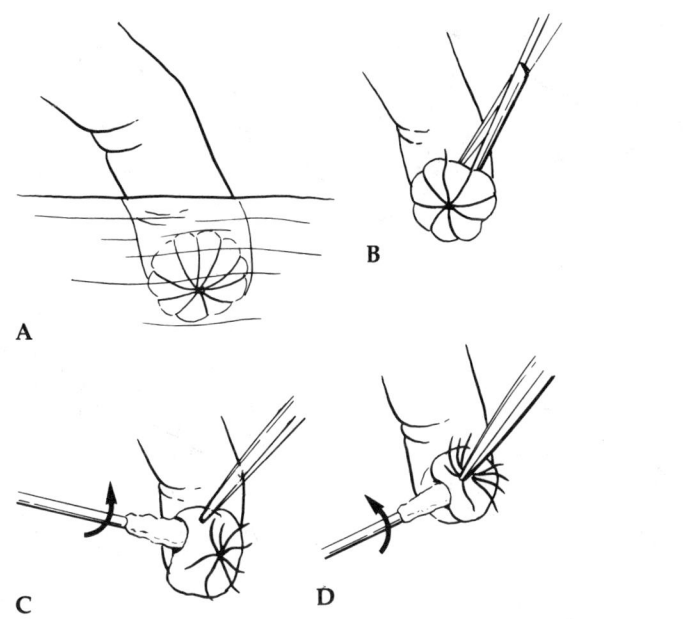

Figure 8-31. Removal of skin graft dressing.
A. *Thoroughly* soak the dressing.
B. If there is a tie-over stent, cut all sutures at the skin level.
C. Carefully separate the contact gauze layer from the suture line at one margin; using a cotton-tipped applicator or small blunt instrument (Freer elevator, dental probe), completely separate the "nonadherent" gauze from the sutures and suture line crusts by working around the margin of the graft.
D. After the suture lines are completely free, the cotton-tipped applicator can be slid under the dressing to hold the graft down against the bed and the applicator rolled between the graft and dressing. *Do not lift the dressing until it has been completely separated.* Even one area of attachment can cause disruption of the skin graft.

Technique

CLEAN, TIDY, OR BLEEDING WOUNDS

When removing a dressing from a tidy wound, it is important not to disrupt the healing epithelium, scar, blood vessels, or underlying anatomic structures (Fig. 8-30). There is a tendency for all dressings to desiccate and become incorporated into the wound crust, and there is a risk of removing the wound epithelial surface when the dressing is changed. Removal of the wound surface may be desirable if the wound is untidy, infected, or necrotic. This technique of wound debridement is referred to as the wet-to-dry method. Although it is effective in some cases, the method may be painful and may cause considerable bleeding. These disadvantages must be weighed against the advantage of additional debridement and the alternatives of surgical debridement or enzymes.

UNTIDY, NECROTIC WOUNDS

1. If adequate analgesia is obtainable or the patient can tolerate some discomfort, the dressing is *removed dry* to debride surface crust and necrotic infected tissue!
2. A similar dressing is reapplied to the wound and allowed to dry and incorporate into the crust. The procedure is repeated until the wound becomes debrided and is clean and tidy.

SKIN GRAFTS

The dressing on a skin graft must be removed with extreme care! A dressing on a clean wound is usually removed after 5 to 7 days. The graft is weakly adherent to the underlying soft tissue bed and can be easily separated, or a hematoma can form under the graft. A graft in a hypovascular site may not be adherent for 3 to 4 weeks.

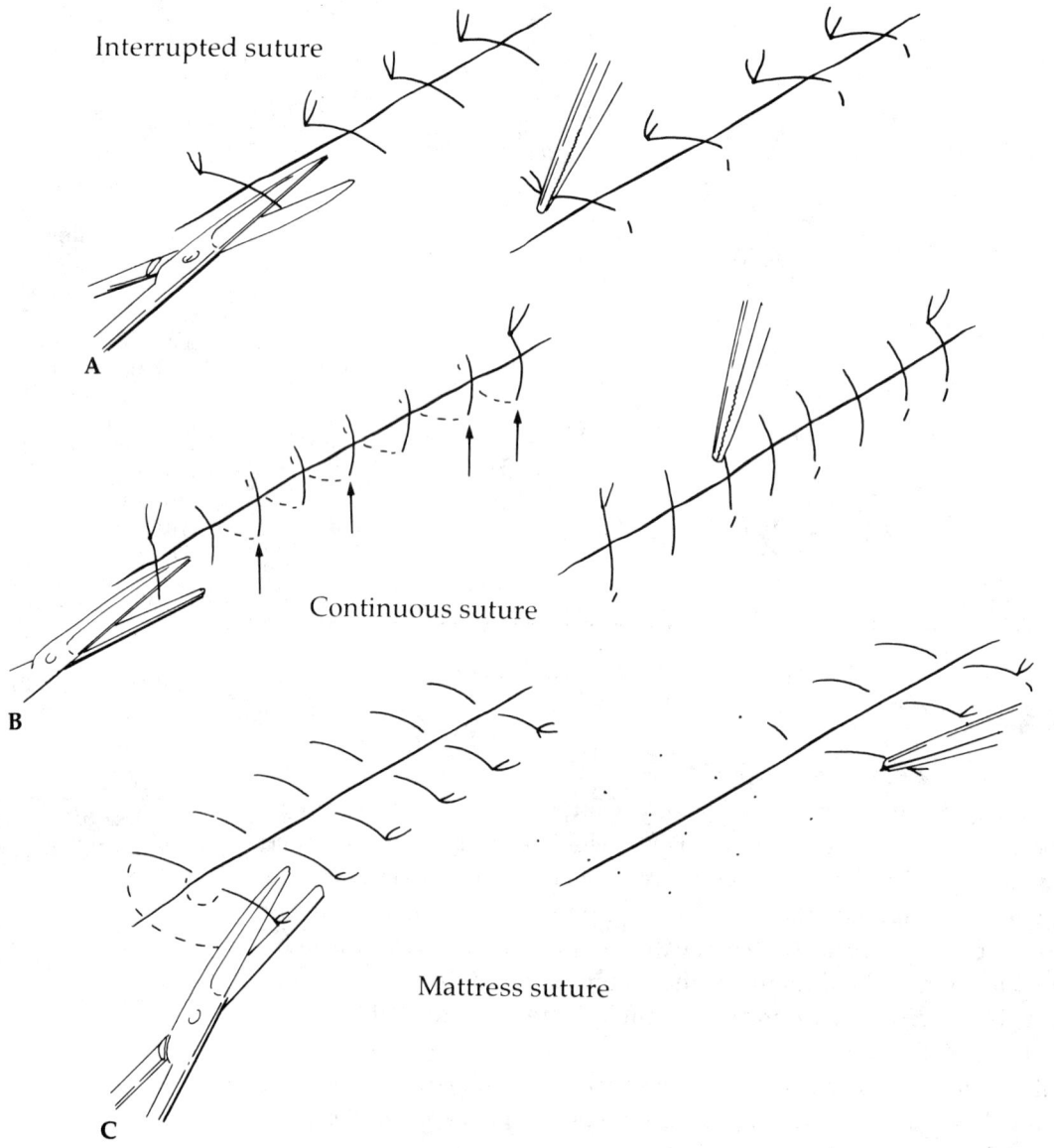

Figure 8-32. Suture removal.
A. Remove interrupted sutures by cutting each suture separately. Slide the sharp pointed scissor under the unknotted end and cut. It is not necessary to grasp the suture while cutting; in fact, grasping the suture causes pain. Cut all sutures that need to be removed before removal. Then grasp the sutures at the knot and pull perpendicular to the surface.
B. Cut continuous sutures in the same manner. Cut the end sutures and alternating loops. Grasp and remove the end sutures and uncut loops.
C. Remove mattress sutures by cutting the suture between knot and skin. If the suture does not slide out easily when pulled by the knot, the subcutaneous portion must be freed first by pulling on the exposed portion opposite the knot.

The method of removal is essentially the same as described for the tidy, clean wound (Fig. 8-31).

Changing Wound Conditions

Each dressing change requires a reassessment of wound conditions. Clean wounds can become infected, and contaminated wounds can become clean. A new objective and new dressing materials and methods may be indicated.

Suture Removal

The timing for suture removal depends on the nature and location of injury (Fig. 8-32). In general, the sooner the sutures are removed the less chance there is of developing a secondary infection and the less possibility of developing pinpoint suture marks. Suture marks begin to form after 5 days because the deposition of collagen around sutures leaves a scar at each site. If there is concern about separation of the wound edges, tape can maintain skin position. If subcutaneous and subdermal sutures have been used, there is considerable safety in removing sutures early. Wounds of the lower extremity heal slowly, and sutures there may be left in for a longer time.

Guidelines for suture removal of simple lacerations are as follows:

Eyelids	3 days
Face	5 days
Scalp	7 to 10 days
Trunk	7 to 10 days
Upper extremities	7 to 14 days
Lower extremities	14 to 21 days

These intervals reflect the differences in the rate of healing and tension encountered in the various areas. The techniques for suture removal are indicated in Fig. 8-32.

INDEX

Abdominal injuries, 188–189
Abrasions, 193–195, 306–308
Ace bandage, 316
Achilles tendon rupture, 287–288
Acupuncture, in pain control, 73
Airway obstruction, diagnosis and treatment of, 1, 2, 3–4
Alcohol antiseptics, 34–35
Allen's test, 212, 214
Allografts, 136
Aluminum, in antisepsis, 33
Amputations
 causes of, 8
 complete, 126–127
 definition of, 9
 dressings for, 308–309
 of ear, 162–163, 165
 of eyelid, 166–169
 of finger and fingertip. See Finger and fingertip amputations
 of forearm, 182
 of forehead, 164, 166
 of hand, 180–182
 of lip, 163–164, 166
 of nail, 182–184
 of nose, 160–162
 partial, 123–126
 and preservation of amputated part, 126–127
 principles of, 123
 of scalp, 164, 166
 and skin grafts. See Skin grafts
 and stump, management of, 132–134
 and transportation of amputated part, 126
 and use of amputated part
  discarding, 127
  replantation, 129–132
  salvaging, 127–129
Analgesics, dose schedules for, 27
Anesthetics
 local. See Local anesthesia
 regional intravenous, 72–73
 topical, 55, 99–100
Antibiotics
 choice of, 23
 dosages of, 24
 and dressings, 14
 guidelines for using, 22–23
 and infections, common, 25
 in penetrating injuries, 188
Antimony, in antisepsis, 33
Antisepsis, 31, 299
Antiseptics
 classes of, 32–35
 definition of, 31–32
Arm injuries. See Hand injuries; Upper extremity injuries
Arteriograms, 6
Autografts, 135–136
Avascularity, and delay in healing, 16–17

Axillary nerve block, 69–71
Axonotmesis, 240, 242, 251, 290

Bald spot, avoidance of, 104
Bias-cut stockinette, 316
Biguanides, in antisepsis, 35
Biscuit deformity, 107, 109, 112–114
Bismuth, in antisepsis, 33
Blanching-flushing, and tissue viability, 93
Bleeding
 dressings for, 301–306
 massive, 2, 4–5
 in penetrating injuries, 185–187
 of viable tissue, 94
Bleeding disorders, 18–20
Bleeding time test, 20
Blenderm, 318
Blisters, 252–253, 279
Blunt injuries. See also specific site of injury
 causes of, 249
 characteristics of, 249
 cutaneous, 251–256
 and tissue damage, 250–251
Bone grafts, 126, 129
Bowstring scars, 104, 106
Bruise, diagnosis and treatment, 253
Bullet wounds, 189–190

Capillary ingrowth, in graft healing, 153
Cardiopulmonary resuscitation, 3, 52
Carpal tunnel syndrome, 290–291
Cartilage grafts, 129
Cartilage injuries, 277–278
Casts, 318
CAT scan, 6, 188
Cervical spine, examination of, 2–3
Chest injuries, 188–189
Chlorine, in antisepsis, 33
Circumferential wraps, 155
Coagulation
 and collagen formation, 13–14
 disorders of, 56–57
 and wound healing, 18
Coban, 316
Collagen, formation of, 13–14
Complex lacerations
 abrasion-laceration, 99–100
 configuration of
  C-flaps, 114–116
  U-shaped flaps, 107, 109, 112–114
  unequal lengths, 116–121
 location of
  anatomic borders, 102–103
  on concave surfaces, 104, 111
  on convex surfaces, 104, 111
  on hair-bearing skin, 104
 multiple adjacent lacerations, 100–101
 tension, in repair of, 96–98
 untidy, 93–96

339

Composite grafts, 129–131, 135
Compression injuries, 249
Computerized axial tomography, 6, 188
Conjunctiva, trauma to, 257, 259
Contact lenses, in eye injuries, 259
  removal of, 259, 260
Contamination of wound, assessment of, 53–54
Contraction, of wound, 14, 132–134, 137
Contusion, diagnosis and treatment of, 253
Cordran, 318
CPR, 3, 52

Dacryocystograms, 263–264
Debridement. *See also* Undermining
  and dressings, 297–298
  enzymatic, 298
  mechanical, 298
  need for, 95
  of nerve ends, 243–244
  technique of, 96
Debrisan, 315
Degeneration, after repair of peripheral nerve, 245
Dental nerve block, 62
Dentoalveolar fracture, 276–277
Dermatomes, choice of, 144–146
Desiccation, of wounds, 297
Diffuson, 316
Digital nerve block, 67–69
Discarding, of amputated parts, 127
Disinfectants, 32
Dog-ears, 116–118
  treatment of, 118–121
Doppler flowmeter, 6, 212
Drapes
  extremity, 36–37
  head, 36
  purpose of, 35
Dressings
  absorptive, 299
  care of, 294
  and casts, 318–319
  change of
    need for, 333
    technique for, 335–337
    timing for, 334
  and debridements, 297–298
  design of
    for abrasions, 306–308
    for amputations, 308–309
    for bleeding, 301–306
    for infection, 309–311
    for lacerations, 300–301
    for open wounds, 308–309
    for skin grafts, 311–312
    for small flaps, 300–301
    three-layer concept, 299–300
  ear, 318, 320
  eye, 318, 320
  facial, 319, 322
  finger, 326–328
  forearm, 330–333
  hand
    design of, 328–333
    immobilization, time of, 326
    position of, 320–322, 324–326
    remobilization, 326
  lower extremity, 333
  materials for
    choosing of, 311
    elastic, 316
    laminated composite materials, 313
    medicated or ointment-covered materials, 313–314
    membranes, synthetic, 314
    plain gauze, 313, 316
    tubed gauze, 316
  nose, 320, 323
  padding materials
    absorbents, 315
    contour materials, 316
  for skin grafts
    donor site, 148–150, 306–308
    recipient site, 153–156, 311–312, 335, 337
  and splints, 318–319
  and tapes, 317–318
  techniques of, 318–323
  therapeutic, 297–299
  and topical medication
    antibiotics, 314
    debriding agents, 315
    enzymes, 315
    hormones, 314
    qualities of, 315
    vitamin E, 314
  wrist, 328–329
Durapore, 318
Dye passage test, 262

Ear injuries and amputations, 162–163, 165
  dressings in, 318, 320
Ecchymosis, 253
Edema, in cutaneous injury, 252
Elastoplast, 316
Elevation, of injured part, 293–294, 296–297
Emergency care
  ABCs of, 1
  and cardiopulmonary resuscitation, 3
  of head injuries, 2–5
  of neck injuries, 2–5
Epinephrine, 47–50
  advantages of, 47
  concentration of, 50
  disadvantages of, 48
  precautions for, 49–50
  reactions to, 48–49
Epithelialization, 14–15, 297
Erythema, in cutaneous injury, 252
Extremity injuries
  joints, 291
  ligaments, 291
  muscle and muscle compartments, 283–287
  nail, 282–283

INDEX

nerves, 290–291
and regional blocks. *See* Regional block, hand and upper extremity
skin, 279–280
subcutaneous tissue, 280–282
tendons, 287–289
vessels, 289–290
Eye injuries. *See* Facial injuries, ocular and periorbital injuries
Eyebrow lacerations, 104–105
Eyelid injuries and amputations, 103, 166–169

Facial injuries
and cartilage injury, 277–278
dressings in, 319, 322
fractures, 264
dentoalveolar, 276–277
diagnostic examination for, 264
mandibular, 271–273
maxillary, 270–271
nasal, 268–270
periorbital, 264–268
temporomandibular joint, 273–276
and muscle injury, 209
and neck injury, 199–202
and nerve injury, 199–202
ocular and periorbital, 257
conjunctiva, 257–259
and contact lens removal, 259
dressings in, 318, 320
extraocular muscles, 259–261
nasolacrimal apparatus, 262–264
orbit and globe injuries, 209
pain control in, 257
pupils in, 261–262
upper lid levator muscle, 259
visual acuity testing, 257–258
regional block in. *See* Regional block, facial
Fainting, 51
Fibrin split products, 20
Field block, 59
Finger and fingertip injuries
amputations
closure, 172
composite replants, 171–172
partial, 170–171
postoperative care, 184
skin and pulp deficit, 174–180
skin deficit only, 173–174
dressings, 326–328
hematomas, 279–280
Fishing hook injuries, 197
Flap surgery, 134
Flexoplast, 316
Flexor digitorum profundus, injury to, 287
Fluorescein dye test
and amputated parts, 125
and eye lacerations, 263
and nonviable tissue, 94
and skin death, 255–256
and vascular injuries, 213
Forearm injuries. *See also* Upper extremity injuries
amputations, 182
dressings, 330–333
Forehead amputations, 164, 166
Fractures, facial. *See* Facial injuries, fractures
Full-thickness skin grafts. *See also* Skin grafts
fat in, 135
sites for, 141–142
taking of, 142–144

Germicides, 32
Granulation, 298

Halogens, in antisepsis, 33–34
Hand injuries. *See also* Finger and fingertip injuries; Upper extremity injuries
amputations, 180–182
dressings for. *See* Dressings, hand
and palmar skin injury, 279–280
regional block of. *See* Regional block, hand and upper extremity
vascular injuries in, 212–215
Head injuries
and drapes, 36
examination for, 2–5
and radiology, diagnostic, 188
Heavy metals, in antisepsis, 32–33
Hematomas
diagnosis of, 253–254
fingertip, 279–280
palmar, 279–280
in postoperative care, 294
prefibrotic, 280–281
and revascularization, 157–158
treatment of, 254–257
and vascular injury, 6
Hemostasis, 73
causes for failure of, 55–57
and coagulation disorders, 56–57
and dressings, 298–299
in penetrating injuries, 186–187
process of, 12–13
Heterografts, 136
Hexachlorophene, 34
Homografts, 136
Hyginet, 316
Hypertrophic scars, 16, 17–18
Hypnosis, in pain control, 73
Hypovascular recipient bed, in skin graft failure, 156

Impact injuries, 249
Impaled objects, 197–198
Infection
antibiotics for, 26
and dressings, 309–311
and penetrating injuries, 185
in postoperative care, 294
prevention of, 22–25
and skin grafts, 149–150, 159
and sutures, 44–45
Inflammatory response, 13
Infraorbital nerve block, 61

Injury. *See also* Wound; *specific type or site of injury*
  assessment of, 5
  blunt. *See* Blunt injuries
  diagnosis of, 6–8
  history of, 5
  impact, 249
  penetrating. *See* Penetrating injuries
Inosculation, 153
Instruments, surgical
  basic, 37–38
  special, 38–39
Intermetacarpal nerve block, 67–69
Iodine, in antisepsis, 33
Iodoform, in antisepsis, 34
Iodophors, 33–34
Irrigation, of wounds, 57, 100
Ischemia, in compression and crush injuries, 249, 251
Isografts, 136

Joint injuries, 7, 291

Keloids, 17–18
Kerlix, 316
Kling, 316
Knives, choice of, 144
Knot slippage, 42
Knot tying, 81
Kutler flap, 175–176

Lacerations
  abrasion-dermal, 99–100
  causes of, 8
  clusters of, 100–101
  complex. *See* Complex lacerations
  definition of, 9
  dressings for, 300–301
  eyebrow, 104–105
  eyelid, 103
  facial muscles, 209
  multiple adjacent, 100–101
  and nail amputations, 183–184
  simple. *See* Simple lacerations
Lacrimal probes, malleable, 263
Laryngotracheal injuries, 209–210
Levator muscle injuries, 209, 259
Lifesaving, priorities for, 1
Ligament injuries, 8, 291
Lip amputations, 163–164, 166
Local anesthesia
  anesthetics in
    action of, 47
    allergy to, 50–51
    avoidance of reactions to, 52
    central nervous system toxicity and, 51–52
    characteristics of, 48
    composition of, 47
  methods of
    field block, 59
    infiltration, 58–59
    regional block. *See* Regional block
    regional intravenous, 72–73
  and vasoconstrictors, 47–50

Malleable lacrimal probes, 263
Mandibular fracture, 271–273
Maxillary fracture, 270–271
Median nerve block, 62–64
Median nerve injury, 290
Mental nerve block, 61–62
Mercurials, in antisepsis, 32
Mesh grafts, 137
Microfoam, 318
Micropore, 318
Microvascular anastomosis, 131
Multiple scars, 100
Muscle and muscle compartment injuries, 215–216, 283–287

Nail grafts, 128–129
Nails
  amputation of, 182–184
  injuries to, 282–283
Nasal trauma, 268–270
Nasolacrimal duct injuries, 206–210
Neck injuries
  examination for, 2–5
  and radiology, diagnostic, 188
Necrosis, in blunt trauma, 251
Needles, types of, 46
Neovascularization, and skin grafts, 153
Nerve grafts, 129
Nerve injuries, 239–242, 290–291. *See also specific nerve*
  anatomy in, 234
  diagnosis of, 7–8, 237–239
  repair of, 242–247
  and sensation, 234–237
  testing of nerves in, 234
Neurapraxia, 240, 242, 251, 290
Neurotmesis, 242, 251, 290
Nose injuries
  amputations, 160–162
  dressings for, 320, 323

Ocular and periorbital injuries. *See* Facial injuries, ocular and periorbital
Operative field preparation
  drapes, 35–37
  hair trimming, 30–31
  packing, 31
  skin preparation and, 31–35
Oxidizing agents, in antisepsis, 35

Packing, 31
Paint gun injuries, 191–192
Palmar skin injuries, 279–280
Parotid duct injuries, 202–206
Partial thromboplastin time, 19
Patient
  comfort of, 26–27
  postoperative education of, 293–294
  preoperative preparation of, 26–28
  stabilization of, 1
Penetrating injuries. *See also specific injuries and sites of injuries*
  and antibiotics, 188
  bleeding in, 185–187

from bullet wounds, 189–190
classification of, 189
definition of, 8, 9
diagnostic radiology in, 188
from fishing hooks, 197
from glass fragments, 197
from paint guns, 191–192
and prevention of additional damage, 187–188
and road dirt abrasions, 193–195
from shotgun injuries, 190–191
from splinters, 195–196, 197
from stabs, 193
Periorbital fractures, 264–268
Peroneal nerve injury, 291
Pharyngoesophageal injury, 209
Phenol, in antisepsis, 34
Phenolic compounds, in antisepsis, 34–35
Pinch grafts, 136–137
Plantaris tendon injury, 287
Plasmatic imbibition, 153
Platelet count and smear, 19
Plethysmography, 212
Postoperative care, 293–294
PTT, 19
Pupils, injuries affecting, 261–262

Quaternary ammonium compounds, in antisepsis, 35
Quick test, 19

Rabies vaccination, 24–25
Radial nerve block, 66–67
Radial nerve injury, 291
Radiology, diagnostic, 188–189
Reendothelialization, 153
Reepithelialization, 132–134
Regeneration, in wound healing, 11, 245–246
Regional block
  facial
    dental nerve, 62
    infraorbital nerve, 61
    mental nerve, 61–62
    supraorbital-supratrochlear, 60–61
  hand and upper extremity
    axillary nerve, 69–71
    digital nerve, 67–69
    intermetacarpal nerve, 67–69
    median nerve, 62–64
    radial nerve, 66–67
    ulnar nerve, 64–66
  principles of, 60
Reinnervation, in wound healing, 246–247
Replantation
  added flap blood supply, 131–132
  in complete amputations, 129–130
  composite graft, 129–131
  microvascular, 131, 170
  in partial amputations, 123–125
Revascularization
  and characteristics of graft, 138
  and healing of graft, 152–153
  and hematomas, 157–158

Road dirt abrasions, 193–195
Rongeur, 175
Running sutures. *See* Sutures and suturing, continuous

Salvaging, of amputated part, 127–129
Santyl, 315
Scalp amputation, 164, 166
Scars
  bowstring, 104, 106
  hypertrophic, 17–18
  multiple, 100
Scoring, in laceration repair, 76–77
Sedation, and reactions to local anesthetics, 52
S-excision, 114
Sheet grafts, 136–137
Shock, 4–5
Shotgun injuries, 190–191
Silver ion, in antisepsis, 32
Silver nitrate, in antisepsis, 32
Silver sulfadiazine, in antisepsis, 32–33
Simple lacerations
  assessment of, 53–54
  definition of, 53
  irrigation of, 57
  preparation of, 54–57
  suturing of. *See* Suturing
Skin flaps, 133–134
Skin grafts. *See also* Amputations
  adherence of, 153
  in amputations, 128
  application of, 150–151
  and care of skin, 131
  characteristics of, 137–138
  classification of, 135–137
  definition of, 134–135
  donor sites
    common, 138–139
    dressings for, 148–150, 306–308
    for full-thickness skin grafts, 141–142
    for split-thickness skin grafts, 139–141
  dressings for
    closed antibiotic, 148–149
    closed occlusive, 149–150
    donor site, 148–150, 306–308
    open technique, 148
    recipient site, 153–156, 311–312, 335, 337
  of extremity, 142
  of eyelid, 166–169
  facial, 166–168
  failure of
    hematomas, 157–158
    hypovascular recipient bed, 156
    infection, 159
    technical errors, 158–159
  and open wounds, 133
  and preservation of skin, 126
  principles of, 123
  recipient site for
    defect in, 150–151
    dressings for, 153–156, 311–312, 335, 337

Skin grafts—*Continued*
　revascularization of, 152–153
　techniques
　　differences in, 142
　　for full-thickness graft, 142–144
　　for split-thickness graft, 144–148
Skin taping, 90, 92
Splinters
　single, superficial, 195–196
　subungual, 197
Splints
　definition of, 318
　finger, 319
　frog-leg, 328
　hand, 325
　plaster, 329
　wrist, 328, 330
Split-thickness skin grafts (STSG). *See also* Skin grafts
　description of, 135
　sites for, 139–141
　taking of, 144–148
Stab wounds, 193
Stabograms, 6
Staples, for wound closure, 92
Step deformity, 102–103
Sterilization, defined, 32
Steroids, in topical wound care, 314
Stretch gauze, 316
Supraorbital-supratrochlear nerve block, 60–61
Surgeon, preoperative preparation of, 37–39, 46
Surgical instruments. *See* Instruments, surgical
Surgitube, 316
Sutures and suturing
　continuous
　　half-buried mattress, 88
　　horizontal mattress, 88–89
　　intradermal "pull-out," 90–91
　　vertical mattress, 88–89
　definition of, 39
　and infection, 44–45
　and knot slippage, 42
　and knot tying, 81
　and layered subdermal closure, 78–80
　　methods of, 81
　materials for, 43, 45–46
　needles for, 46
　placement of, 73–74
　reactivity of, 44
　removal of, 336–337
　simple
　　depth of, 81–84
　　position of, 81, 85–87
　skin, 76
　and skin taping, 90, 92
　and staple use, 92
　strength of, 40–43
　technique of
　　and knot slippage, 42
　　and knot tying, 81
　　and layered closure, 81
　　and skin surface approximation, 81, 83, 87–88, 90, 92
　tissue handling in, 73–74
　types of, 39–40
　and wound approximation, 73–77

Tapes, types of, 317–318
Temporomandibular joint injury, 273–276
Tendinitis, 289
Tendon injuries. *See also specific tendon*
　diagnosis of, 8, 219–226
　healing of, 218–219
　and operation, 232–233
　penetrating, in upper limb, 216–233
　and tendinitis, 289
　and tendon transections, 226–232
Tensor, 316
Tetanus immunization, 23–24
T-excision, 115, 118, 119
Thrombosis, venous, in closed and blunt injuries, 290
Tie-over stents, 155
Topical anesthesia pack, 55
Torque, as cause of injury, 249
Tourniquets
　arm, 28–29
　finger, 29–30
　leg, 28–29
　purpose of, 28
　in regional intravenous anesthesia, 72–73
　use of, 29
Transpore, 318
Trap door configurations, of lacerations, 107, 109, 112–114
Travase, 315
Triiodomethane, in antisepsis, 34
Turgor, and tissue viability, 94

U-shaped flaps, 107–114
Ulnar nerve block, 64–66
Ulnar nerve injury, 291
Undermining
　guidelines for, 96–97
　levels for, 97–98
　problems with, 97
Upper extremity injuries, 211. *See also* Hand injuries; Forearm injuries
　to muscle and fascia, 212–215
　to nerves, 234–247
　and regional block. *See* Regional block, hand and upper extremity
　to tendons, 216–233
　　extensor tendons, 223–226
　　flexor tendons, 219–223, 232–233
　　transections, 226–232

Vascular injuries, 6, 185, 209, 212–215, 289–290
Vasoconstrictors. *See* Epinephrine
Vasodilation, in wound healing, 299
Vasospasm, in closed and blunt injuries, 289–290
Vasovagal reactions, 51
Venous thrombosis, in closed and blunt injuries, 290
Vessels, blunt trauma to, 289–290

Vitamins, in wound healing, 314
Volar advancement, 176–177

Wounds. *See also* Injury; *specific wounds*
  assessment of, in postoperative care, 294
  closed, 8
  condition of, 10–11
    abrasion-dermal laceration, 99–100
    clean versus contaminated, 10
    multiple adjacent, 100–101
    noncomplex versus complex, 10–11
    simple versus compound, 11
    tension and, 96–98
    tidy versus untidy, 10
    untidy, 93–96
  configuration of
    C-flaps, 114–116
    determining, 95–96
    unequal lengths, 116–121
    U-shaped flaps, 107, 109, 112–114
  and elevation of injured part, 293–294, 296–297
  healing of
    abnormal, 16–20
    and age, 15–16
    and drugs, 18
    and location, anatomic, 16
    normal, 12–15
    postoperative, 293–294
    and race, 16
    regeneration, 11
    and sex, 16
    surgical, 12
    and systemic diseases, 17–20
  high-energy, 9–10
  irrigation of, 57
  location of, 102–103
    on concave surfaces, 104, 106–108, 111
    on convex surfaces, 104, 106–108, 111
    on hair-bearing skin, 104
  low-energy, 9–10
  management of. *See* Wound management
  mechanism of, 9–10
  noncomplex, 10
  open, 8
    dressings for, 308–309
  preparation of, preliminary, 54–57
  simple, 11
  and skin creases, natural, 95–96
  tidy, 10
    dressing change for, 334–337
  types of, 8–9
  untidy, 10, 93–95
    dressing change for, 334–337
Wound management
  and classification of wounds, 8–11
  and healing of wound, 11–15
    abnormal, 16–17
    factors affecting, 15–20
  priorities in, 1–2, 8
Wrist, dressings for, 328–329. *See also* Hand injuries; Upper extremity injuries

Xenografts, 136
Xylocaine, 55, 100

Zinc, in antisepsis, 33
Z-plasty, 106–107
  correct method of suturing, 109
  treatment of dogear by ½ Z-plasty, 118, 120–121